ISSN 2332-3841

HIV/AIDS

Barbara Wexler

INFORMATION PLUS® REFERENCE SERIES
Formerly Published by Information Plus, Wylie, Texas

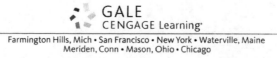

GALE
CENGAGE Learning·

Farmington Hills, Mich · San Francisco · New York · Waterville, Maine
Meriden, Conn · Mason, Ohio · Chicago

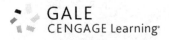

HIV/AIDS

Barbara Wexler

Kepos Media, Inc.: Steven Long and Janice Jorgensen, Series Editors

Project Editors: Kimberley A. McGrath, Kathleen J. Edgar, Elizabeth Manar

Rights Acquisition and Management: Sheila R. Spencer, Lynn Vagg

Composition: Evi Abou-El-Seoud, Mary Beth Trimper

Manufacturing: Rita Wimberley

For product information and technology assistance, contact us at
Gale Customer Support, 1-800-877-4253.
For permission to use material from this text or product,
submit all requests online at **www.cengage.com/permissions.**
Further permissions questions can be e-mailed to
permissionrequest@cengage.com

Cover photograph: © Susan Walsh/AP Photo.

Gale
27500 Drake Rd.
Farmington Hills, MI 48331-3535

ISBN-13: 978-0-7876-5103-9 (set)
ISBN-13: 978-1-56995-795-0

ISSN 2332-3841

This title is also available as an e-book.
ISBN-13: 978-1-56995-839-1 (set)
Contact your Gale sales representative for ordering information.

Printed in the United States of America
2 3 4 5 6   19 18 17 16 15

TABLE OF CONTENTS

projections, the effect of AIDS on birth and death rates, and patterns of infection. The status of the HIV/AIDS epidemics in Africa, Europe, Asia, Central and South America, the Caribbean, and the Middle East are also discussed.

CHAPTER 10

Surveys and polls reported on in this chapter illustrate how Americans feel about HIV/AIDS. Topics covered include concerns about HIV/AIDS, knowledge and tolerance, and persistence of misinformation about HIV/AIDS. Efforts to heighten public awareness, such as the AIDS Memorial Quilt, AIDS activist organizations, and celebrity activists, are also highlighted.

PREFACE

HIV/AIDS is part of the *Information Plus Reference Series*. The purpose of each volume of the series is to present the latest facts on a topic of pressing concern in modern American life. These topics include the most controversial and studied social issues of the 21st century: abortion, capital punishment, care of senior citizens, crime, the environment, health care, immigration, national security, social welfare, sports, women, youth, and many more. Although this series is written especially for high school and undergraduate students, it is an excellent resource for anyone in need of factual information on current affairs.

By presenting the facts, it is the intention of Gale, Cengage Learning to provide its readers with everything they need to reach an informed opinion on current issues. To that end, there is a particular emphasis in this series on the presentation of scientific studies, surveys, and statistics. These data are generally presented in the form of tables, charts, and other graphics placed within the text of each book. Every graphic is directly referred to and carefully explained in the text. The source of each graphic is presented within the graphic itself. The data used in these graphics are drawn from the most reputable and reliable sources, such as the various branches of the U.S. government and private organizations and associations. Every effort has been made to secure the most recent information available. Readers should bear in mind that many major studies take years to conduct and that additional years often pass before the data from these studies are made available to the public. Therefore, in many cases the most recent information available in 2014 is dated from 2010 or 2011. Older statistics are sometimes presented as well if they are landmark studies or of particular interest and no more-recent information exists.

Although statistics are a major focus of the *Information Plus Reference Series*, they are by no means its only content. Each book also presents the widely held positions and important ideas that shape how the book's subject is discussed in the United States. These positions are explained in detail and, where possible, in the words of their proponents. Some of the other material to be found in these books includes historical background, descriptions of major events related to the subject, relevant laws and court cases, and examples of how these issues play out in American life. Some books also feature primary documents or have pro and con debate sections that provide the words and opinions of prominent Americans on both sides of a controversial topic. All material is presented in an evenhanded and unbiased manner; readers will never be encouraged to accept one view of an issue over another.

HOW TO USE THIS BOOK

The spread of acquired immunodeficiency syndrome (AIDS) has become a global epidemic. As of 2011, an estimated 34.2 million people worldwide were living with human immunodeficiency virus (HIV), according to the Joint United Nations Programme on HIV/AIDS. That same year there were 2.5 million new HIV cases diagnosed and 1.8 million HIV-related deaths. This book includes information on the nature of HIV/AIDS and the HIV/AIDS epidemic; symptoms and transmittal; patterns and trends in surveillance; populations at risk; children, adolescents, costs, and treatment; people living with HIV/AIDS; testing, prevention, and education; HIV/AIDS worldwide; and knowledge, awareness, behavior, and opinion of those affected by HIV/AIDS.

HIV/AIDS consists of 10 chapters and three appendixes. Each chapter is devoted to a particular aspect of HIV/AIDS. For a summary of the information that is covered in each chapter, please see the synopses that are provided in the Table of Contents. Chapters generally begin with an overview of the basic facts and background information on the chapter's topic, then proceed to examine subtopics of particular interest. For example, Chapter 3: Patterns and Trends in HIV/AIDS Surveillance, begins with a description of how the Centers for Disease Control and Prevention keeps track of the number of people in the United States who are infected with HIV. The chapter then goes on to provide estimates of HIV infection and AIDS cases, which are important because they directly influence public health and medical resource allocation as well as political and economic decisions. The chapter also studies the nature of the epidemic and describes the people affected. It details the epidemiology of HIV in terms of specific populations by examining differences based on age, race, geography, sex, and transmission category. Readers can find their way through a chapter by looking for the section and subsection headings, which are clearly set off from the text. They can also refer to the book's extensive Index if they already know what they are looking for.

Statistical Information

The tables and figures featured throughout *HIV/AIDS* will be of particular use to readers in learning about this issue. These tables and figures represent an extensive collection of the most recent and important statistics on HIV/AIDS and related issues—for example, graphics cover clinical categories of AIDS infection, adult and adolescent HIV infection and AIDS cases, pediatric AIDS cases, AIDS-defining conditions, an HIV replication cycle, and the percentage of high school students tested for HIV. Gale, Cengage Learning believes that making this information available to readers is the most important way to fulfill the goal of this book: to help readers understand the issues and controversies surrounding HIV/AIDS in the United States and to reach their own conclusions.

Each table or figure has a unique identifier appearing above it, for ease of identification and reference. Titles for the tables and figures explain their purpose. At the end of each table or figure, the original source of the data is provided.

To help readers understand these often complicated statistics, all tables and figures are explained in the text. References in the text direct readers to the relevant statistics. Furthermore, the contents of all tables and figures are fully indexed. Please see the opening section of the Index at the back of this volume for a description of how to find tables and figures within it.

Appendixes

Besides the main body text and images, *HIV/AIDS* has three appendixes. The first is the Important Names and Addresses directory. Here, readers will find contact information for a number of government and private organizations that can provide further information on HIV/AIDS. The second appendix is the Resources section, which can also assist readers in conducting their own research. In this section, the author and editors of *HIV/AIDS* describe some of the sources that were most useful during the compilation of this book. The final appendix is the detailed Index. It has been greatly expanded from previous editions and should make it even easier to find specific topics in this book.

COMMENTS AND SUGGESTIONS

The editors of the *Information Plus Reference Series* welcome your feedback on *HIV/AIDS*. Please direct all correspondence to:

Editors
Information Plus Reference Series
27500 Drake Rd.
Farmington Hills, MI 48331-3535

CHAPTER 1
THE NATURE OF HIV/AIDS

The acquired immunodeficiency syndrome (AIDS) is the late stage of an infection caused by the human immunodeficiency virus (HIV). HIV is a retrovirus that destroys certain white blood cells. The targeted destruction weakens the body's immune system and makes the infected person susceptible to infections and diseases that ordinarily would not be life threatening. AIDS is a bloodborne, sexually transmitted disease because HIV is spread through contact with blood, semen, or vaginal fluids from an infected person.

Before 1981 AIDS was virtually unknown in the United States. That year, testing of blood and other samples for HIV began, and disease reporting became mandatory. In 1983 a research team at the Pasteur Institute in Paris, France, led by Luc Montagnier (1932–), Françoise Barré-Sinoussi (1947–), and Harald zur Hausen (1936–) first isolated HIV. Montagnier, Barré-Sinoussi, and zur Hausen were awarded the Nobel Prize in Physiology or Medicine for this discovery in 2008.

Over time, awareness grew as the annual number of diagnosed cases and deaths steadily increased. In "First 500,000 AIDS Cases—United States, 1995" (*Morbidity and Mortality Weekly Report*, vol. 44, no. 46, November 24, 1995), the Centers for Disease Control and Prevention (CDC) stated that the number of U.S. AIDS cases reported since 1981 reached the half-million mark in 1995. It also indicated that HIV infection was the leading cause of death among Americans aged 25 to 44 years.

By 1998, however, HIV/AIDS deaths among this age group had fallen dramatically, and HIV infection was the fifth most-common cause of death among people in the United States between 25 and 44 years old. It had dropped to eighth place by 2011, with the disease claiming 2,262 people aged 25 to 44 years. (See Table 1.1.)

By 2011 AIDS was no longer among the 15 leading causes of death among people of all ages in the United States. Donna L. Hoyert and Jiaquan Xu of the CDC observe in "Deaths: Preliminary Data for 2011" (*National Vital Statistics Reports*, vol. 61, no. 6, October 10, 2012) that although the age-adjusted death rate for AIDS decreased 7.7% from 2010 to 2011, it remained a public health concern for people aged 15 to 64 years, and among people aged 45 to 64 years it was the 13th leading cause of death in 2011.

Overall, HIV mortality (death) rates plateaued in 1995 and began to decline in 1996, even before the widespread use of effective drug treatments such as protease inhibitors. In 1997 HIV infection was the 14th leading cause of death overall in the United States. By 1999 HIV infection no longer ranked among the 15 leading causes of death in the United States. Figure 1.1 shows the sharp decline in deaths from HIV disease since the mid-1990s and the subsequent stabilization in the number of deaths attributable to AIDS between 1985 and 2010.

Although the overall decline in HIV/AIDS deaths between 1995 and 2000 was a positive trend for people infected with HIV and those suffering from AIDS, the reality is that the actual number of people living with HIV/AIDS increased during this period. In other words, even though not as many people were dying from HIV/AIDS, more people were living with the disease due to successful therapies.

The observed decline in HIV/AIDS deaths is no reassurance to the estimated 50,000 people who are diagnosed with an HIV infection each year in the United States. The CDC indicates in *HIV Surveillance Report: Diagnoses of HIV Infection in the United States and Dependent Areas, 2011* (February 2013, http://www.cdc.gov/hiv/pdf/statistics_2011 _HIV_Surveillance_Report_vol_23.pdf) that in 2011 there were 49,273 new cases of HIV infection in adults, adolescents, and children. In "Basic Statistics" (October 7, 2013, http://www.cdc.gov/hiv/basics/statistics.html), the CDC reports that an estimated 1.1 million people were living

TABLE 1.1

Deaths and death rates for the 10 leading causes of death by age groups, preliminary 2011

[Data are based on a continuous file of records received from the states. Rates are per 100,000 population in specified group.]

Rank	Cause of death (based on the International Classification of Diseases (ICD), 10th rev., 2008 ed., 2009) and age	Number	Rate
15–24 years			
...	All causes	29,605	67.6
1	Accidents (unintentional injuries)	12,032	27.5
...	Motor vehicle accidents	6,984	15.9
...	All other accidents	5,048	11.5
2	Intentional self-harm (suicide)	4,688	10.7
3	Assault (homicide)	4,508	10.3
4	Malignant neoplasms	1,609	3.7
5	Diseases of heart	948	2.2
6	Congenital malformations, deformations and chromosomal abnormalities	429	1.0
7	Influenza and pneumonia	213	0.5
8	Cerebrovascular diseases	186	0.4
9	Pregnancy, childbirth and the puerperium	166	0.4
10	Chronic lower respiratory diseases	160	0.4
...	All other causes	4,666	10.7
25–44 years			
...	All causes	113,341	137.5
1	Accidents (unintentional injuries)	29,424	35.7
...	Motor vehicle accidents	10,181	12.4
...	All other accidents	19,243	23.3
2	Malignant neoplasms	15,210	18.5
3	Diseases of heart	13,479	16.4
4	Intentional self-harm (suicide)	12,269	14.9
5	Assault (homicide)	6,639	8.1
6	Chronic liver disease and cirrhosis	2,919	3.5
7	Diabetes mellitus	2,474	3.0
8	Human immunodeficiency virus (HIV) disease	2,262	2.7
9	Cerebrovascular diseases	2,245	2.7
10	Influenza and pneumonia	1,341	1.6
...	All other causes	25,079	30.4
45–64 years			
...	All causes	505,730	610.9
1	Malignant neoplasms	161,072	194.6
2	Diseases of heart	105,013	126.9
3	Accidents (unintentional injuries)	34,621	41.8
...	Motor vehicle accidents	9,701	11.7
...	All other accidents	24,920	30.1
4	Chronic lower respiratory diseases	19,646	23.7
5	Chronic liver disease and cirrhosis	19,551	23.6
6	Diabetes mellitus	18,548	22.4
7	Cerebrovascular diseases	16,848	20.4
8	Intentional self-harm (suicide)	14,852	17.9
9	Septicemia	7,365	8.9
10	Nephritis, nephrotic syndrome and nephrosis	6,758	8.2
...	All other causes	101,456	122.6

...Category not applicable.
Notes: Rank based on number of deaths. Figures for 2011 are based on weighted data rounded to the nearest individual, so categories may not add to totals or subtotals.

SOURCE: Adapted from Donna L. Hoyert and Jiaquan Xu, "Table 7. Deaths and Death Rates for the 10 Leading Causes of Death in Specified Age Groups: United States, Preliminary 2011," in "Deaths: Preliminary Data for 2011," *National Vital Statistics Reports*, vol. 61, no. 6, October 10, 2012, http://www.cdc.gov/nchs/data/nvsr/nvsr61/nvsr61_06.pdf (accessed July 5, 2013)

with HIV infection in 2013. About 18% of these were unaware of their infection.

The American Foundation for AIDS Research notes in "Thirty Years of HIV/AIDS: Snapshots of an Epidemic" (2013, http://www.amfar.org/thirty-years-of-hiv/aids-snap shots-of-an-epidemic/) that between 1996 and 1997 the number of AIDS deaths declined 42%. This dramatic decrease was due to the introduction and use of effective antiretroviral drugs that slow the progression of HIV infection. This decline continued but slowed to 21% between 1997 and 1998, and to 5% between 1998 and 1999. This may be due to a combination of several factors, including complicated drug treatment regimens that were difficult for patients to maintain and a lack of access to prompt testing or treatment. In *HIV Surveillance Report*, the CDC indicates that an estimated 872,990 people in the United States were living with diagnosed HIV infection. Furthermore, in "Basic Statistics," the CDC notes that through the end of 2011, 635,000 people had died from AIDS.

The AIDS epidemic is not a U.S. phenomenon. According to the CDC, in 2011 there were approximately 2.5 million new cases of HIV worldwide and an estimated 34.2 million people were living with HIV/AIDS. In 2010 about 1.8 million people worldwide died of AIDS and a total of nearly 30 million deaths were attributable to the epidemic. Although the countries of sub-Saharan Africa continue to have the world's highest annual rates of HIV infection and death, the epidemic has also taken a toll on Southeast Asia, Central Asia, eastern Europe, and Latin America.

THE HUMAN IMMUNODEFICIENCY VIRUS

A virus is a tiny infectious agent composed of genes that are surrounded by a protective coating. Until a virus contacts a host cell, it is essentially an inert bag of genetic material. Viruses are parasites. They must invade other cells and commandeer the host cell's replication machinery to reproduce. A frequent outcome of viral infection is the destruction of the host cell, as the newly made virus particles burst out of the cell. The host cell destruction can harm the host (in the case of HIV, a human).

HIV belongs to a group of viruses called retroviruses. The name arises from the presence of a special enzyme— reverse transcriptase—that reverses the usual pattern of translating the genetic message. (See Figure 1.2.) In animals, genes consist of deoxyribonucleic acid (DNA). DNA is the blueprint from which another type of genetic material called ribonucleic acid (RNA) is made, in a process called transcription. In turn, the RNA serves as the blueprint for the proteins that are the structural building blocks of the virus. In contrast to animals, retroviruses store their genes in RNA. After HIV infects a human cell, the viral reverse transcriptase transcribes HIV RNA into DNA. The viral DNA then becomes part of the host DNA—a process called integration—and is replicated along with the host DNA to produce new HIV particles.

Before 1980 retroviruses had been found in some animals. As far back as 1911 Francis Peyton Rous (1879–1970)

FIGURE 1.1

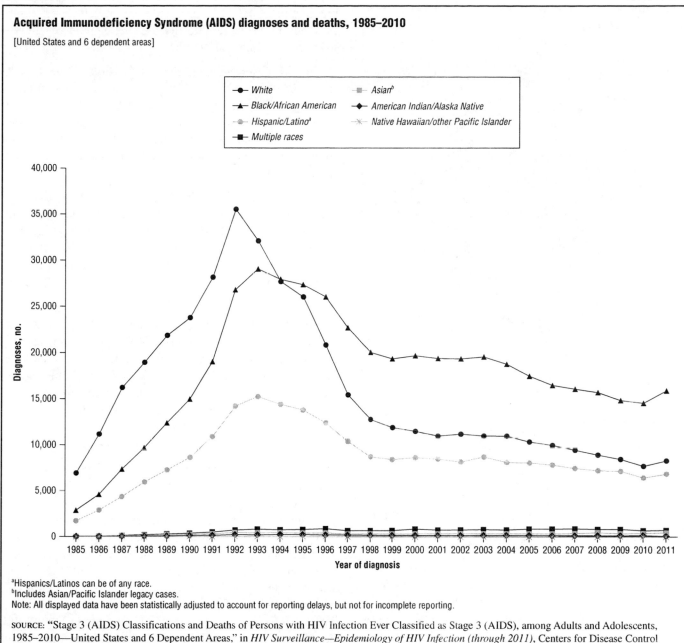

Acquired Immunodeficiency Syndrome (AIDS) diagnoses and deaths, 1985–2010

[United States and 6 dependent areas]

- ● White
- ▲ Black/African American
- ● Hispanic/Latino[a]
- ■ Multiple races
- ▧ Asian[b]
- ◆ American Indian/Alaska Native
- ✕ Native Hawaiian/other Pacific Islander

[a]Hispanics/Latinos can be of any race.
[b]Includes Asian/Pacific Islander legacy cases.
Note: All displayed data have been statistically adjusted to account for reporting delays, but not for incomplete reporting.

SOURCE: "Stage 3 (AIDS) Classifications and Deaths of Persons with HIV Infection Ever Classified as Stage 3 (AIDS), among Adults and Adolescents, 1985–2010—United States and 6 Dependent Areas," in *HIV Surveillance—Epidemiology of HIV Infection (through 2011)*, Centers for Disease Control and Prevention, June 11, 2013, http://www.cdc.gov/hiv/pdf/statistics_surveillance_Epi-HIV-infection.pdf (accessed July 5, 2013)

isolated an infectious and debilitating virus from a chicken. The Rous sarcoma virus was later shown to be a cancer-causing virus and the first known retrovirus. The first known human retroviruses, human T cell leukemia virus (HTLV-I) and the closely related human T cell lymphotropic virus (HTLV-II), were discovered in 1980 by Robert C. Gallo (1937–) and his colleagues at the National Cancer Institute (NCI). This breakthrough provided the groundwork for discovery of the virus that would eventually be known as HIV.

Identifying the Virus

In September 1983 Montagnier and his colleagues at the Pasteur Institute took a sample from a lymph node biopsy of a patient and identified a retrovirus they named lymphadenopathy-associated virus (LAV). Eight months later Gallo's group at the NCI isolated the same virus in AIDS patients, which they called HTLV-III. LAV and HTLV-III were found to be identical and are now referred to as HIV. A conflict arose about which researcher should be credited with the discovery. In 1991, in an intense, politically charged atmosphere, Gallo dropped his claim to the discovery of HIV.

The original HIV is now known as HIV-1. This is due to the 1986 discovery by scientists at the Pasteur Institute of another AIDS-causing virus in West Africans, which was labeled HIV-2. Although the two forms of

FIGURE 1.2

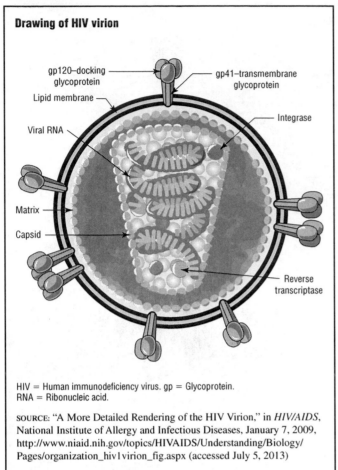

Drawing of HIV virion

gp120–docking glycoprotein

gp41–transmembrane glycoprotein

Lipid membrane

Viral RNA

Integrase

Matrix

Capsid

Reverse transcriptase

HIV = Human immunodeficiency virus. gp = Glycoprotein. RNA = Ribonucleic acid.

SOURCE: "A More Detailed Rendering of the HIV Virion," in *HIV/AIDS*, National Institute of Allergy and Infectious Diseases, January 7, 2009, http://www.niaid.nih.gov/topics/HIVAIDS/Understanding/Biology/Pages/organization_hiv1virion_fig.aspx (accessed July 5, 2013)

HIV have similar modes of transmission, the symptoms of HIV-2 were found to be milder than those of HIV-1. Furthermore, HIV-2 was shown to differ in molecular structure from HIV-1 in a way that ties it more closely to a virus that causes AIDS in macaque monkeys. Antoine Benard et al. indicate in "Immunovirological Response to Triple Nucleotide Reverse-Transcriptase Inhibitors and Ritonavir-Boosted Protease Inhibitors in Treatment-Naive HIV-2–Infected Patients: The ACHIEV2E Collaboration Study Group" (*Clinical Infectious Diseases*, vol. 52, no. 10, May 2011) that HIV-2 is generally diagnosed in western Africa, and small numbers of cases are diagnosed in Europe and North America each year. (Unless otherwise specified, the term *HIV* in the remainder of this edition refers to HIV-1.)

The Origins of the Virus

Montagnier and Gallo, along with other investigators, believed that HIV had been present in Central Africa and other regions for some time, and at some point the virus crossed the species barrier from primates to humans. The rural nature of these societies and limited access to the outside world by those infected with the virus may have confined the spread of HIV for decades. However, once the migration of tribal Central Africans to urban areas began, the more liberated sexual practices there promoted the spread of HIV. Within a comparatively short time, the once rare and remote disease was spread by globe-trotting HIV-infected people.

It was long speculated that HIV evolved from simian immunodeficiency virus (SIV), a retrovirus that infects monkeys. The theory was that HIV evolved from a human infection with a mutated form of SIV that was infectious to humans. Consistent with this theory was the finding that HIV is a part of the lentivirus family, which includes SIV.

In 1982 Isao Miyoshi (1932–) of Kochi University identified an HTLV-related virus in Japanese macaque monkeys. Genetically similar to HTLV, it was designated as the simian T-lymphotropic virus (STLV). Further studies identified STLV in both Asian and African monkeys and apes, with an infection rate ranging from 1% to 40%.

In 1988 Max Essex (1939–) and Phyllis Jean Kanki (1956–) of the Harvard School of Public Health discovered that the simian virus found in African chimpanzees and African green monkeys was more homologous (related in primitive origin) to the human virus than to the simian virus in Asian macaques. This discovery provided strong support for an evolved version of African STLV as being the origin of human HTLV.

In 1999 an international team of researchers at the University of Alabama announced that the genetic sequence of a simian virus isolated from a tissue sample obtained from a chimpanzee was virtually identical to the HIV discovered by Montagnier. Interestingly, chimpanzees are only rarely infected with SIV. This implies that chimpanzee may be temporary carriers of the virus, which normally resides in some other, as yet unidentified, primate species. A common chimpanzee subspecies, *Pan troglodytes troglodytes*, which along with the bonobo is the closest living species to humans, naturally harbors HIV-1, and there have been documented occurrences of cross-species transmission from them to humans. Because these chimpanzees are still poached for bushmeat, humans may be at risk for continued exposure. A complete understanding of the mechanisms of cross-species transmission and the ability of these chimpanzees to resist infection may help researchers develop strategies to protect humans from HIV as well as from other viruses such as H1N1, SARS coronavirus, hantaviruses, and the Ebola and Marburg viruses that originate in animals.

ATTACKING THE IMMUNE SYSTEM

As with other infections, HIV must evade the immune system, which functions to detect and destroy invaders. To learn how HIV first attacks healthy cells

FIGURE 1.3

How HIV attaches to an immune cell and reproduces

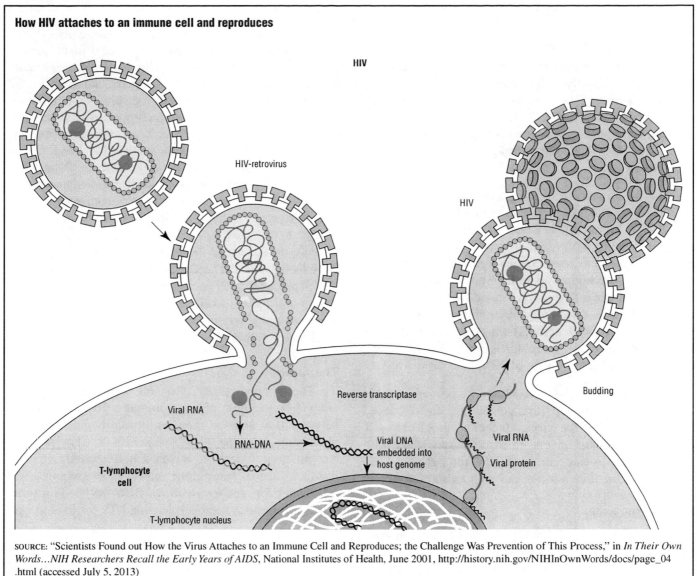

SOURCE: "Scientists Found out How the Virus Attaches to an Immune Cell and Reproduces; the Challenge Was Prevention of This Process," in *In Their Own Words...NIH Researchers Recall the Early Years of AIDS*, National Institutes of Health, June 2001, http://history.nih.gov/NIHInOwnWords/docs/page_04 .html (accessed July 5, 2013)

while evading attack by the immune system, it is important to understand the complex structure of HIV and how normal white blood cells work.

Healthy White Blood Cells at Work

White blood cells are major components of the coordinated system of organs and cells that make up the human immune system. These organs and cells work to prevent invasion by foreign substances. There are five types of white blood cells: macrophages (scavenger cells of the immune system), T4 or helper T cells, T8 or killer T cells, plasma B cells, and memory B cells. T and B white blood cells are also called lymphocytes. Lymphocytes bear the major responsibility for carrying out immune system activities.

Each type of white blood cell has a specific function. The macrophage, which begins as a smaller monocyte (single cell), readies the T4 cells to respond to particular invaders such as viruses. During a viral attack, the macrophage, which is sometimes referred to as the vacuum cleaner of the immune system, swallows the virus, but leaves a portion displayed so that the T4 cell can make contact. The macrophage also stimulates the production of thousands of T4 cells, which are programmed to battle the invader. Figure 1.3 shows how the virus attaches to an immune cell and reproduces.

When T4 lymphocytes attack an invading virus, they also send out chemical messages that cause the multiplication of B cells and T8 killer cells. These cells, along with the help of some T4 cells, destroy the infected cell. Other T4 cells, which are not actively involved in destroying the infected cells, send chemical messages to B cells, causing them to reproduce and divide into groups of either plasma cells or memory cells. Plasma cells make antibodies that cripple the invading virus, whereas memory cells increase the immune response if the invader ever attacks again.

HIV's Molecular Structure

HIV has nine genes. Three of these—designated env, gag, and pol code—form the structural components of the virus that surround the genetic material and the outer surface of the virus particle. The remaining genes—tat, nef, rev, vpr, vpu, and vif—are involved in regulating the genetic activities that are necessary to create copies of the infecting virus.

HIV's complement of nine genes is minuscule compared with the 30,000 genes in human DNA. Nevertheless, HIV is more complex than most other retroviruses, which have only three or four genes. Scientists believe these genes direct the production of proteins that make up parts of the virus and regulate its reproduction. The HIV core contains genes that are protected by a protein shell, and the virus is surrounded and protected by a fatty membrane dotted with glycoproteins (proteins with sugar units attached). (See Figure 1.2.) Figure 1.4 shows the steps in the replication cycle of HIV.

Once HIV enters the human body, its primary target is a subset of immune cells that contain a molecule called CD4. In particular, the virus attaches itself to CD4+ T cells and, to a lesser extent, to macrophages. Figure 1.5 shows the cell-to-cell spread of HIV through the CD4-mediated fusion of an infected cell with an uninfected cell.

Another Discovery

In November 1995 Ute-Christiane Meier et al. proposed in "Cytotoxic T Lymphocyte Lysis Inhibited by Viable HIV Mutants" (*Science*, vol. 270, no. 5240) that HIV defuses the killer cells that are supposed to destroy virus-stricken cells. The researchers isolated HIV from AIDS patients and demonstrated that the virus had undergone a mutation, or change, in its genetic structure. When killer T cells approached cells infected with the mutated virus, the T cells failed to kill the stricken cells, perhaps because they no longer recognized them. In fact, the T cells were unable to kill even cells infected with the original, unmutated virus. The mutations not only allowed the altered strains to multiply but also allowed unaltered strains to flourish.

AN ALTERNATE THEORY: "FRIENDLY FIRE." Not all researchers agree that the alteration of killer T cells is the underlying basis for the establishment of an HIV infection. Some believe that other cells in the immune system attack and kill CD4-containing cells. The CD4-containing cells that have not been invaded by the virus, but that display fragments of it, become targets for other cells—besides the killer cells—which see the infected cells as a camouflaged virus and kill them. In addition, HIV-infected cells may send out protein signals that weaken or destroy other healthy cells in the immune system.

It is, however, agreed that HIV subsequently exhibits various behaviors, depending on the kind of cell it has invaded and how the cell behaves. The virus can remain dormant in T cells for two to 20 years, hidden from the immune system. When the cells are stimulated, however, the viral genes that have been incorporated into the DNA of the T4 cells can be replicated and the gene products assembled into new virus particles that then break free of the T4 cells and attack other cells. Once a T4 cell has been infected, it cannot respond adequately and may reproduce to form as few as 10 cells. An uninfected T4 cell usually reproduces 1,000 or more times to form the army needed to fight the HIV invader. When these crippled T4 cells do encounter the invader, the virus inside them reproduces and the cells are destroyed. Worse still, HIV reproduces itself at a rate far greater than any other known virus. The T4 cells become factories for the invading enemy soldiers, ultimately producing them in overwhelming numbers.

The Attack

The immune system is unable to produce sufficient antibodies to fight off the complex HIV. The battle between HIV and the immune system begins when the virus slips into the bloodstream via a CD4 receptor enzyme on a T4 cell, to which it preferentially attaches itself. A CD4 receptor alone, however, is not enough to cause infection, and for years scientists searched for some other protein on the cell surface that HIV exploits to gain entry.

This protein was discovered in May 1996 by a team of scientists at the National Institute of Allergy and Infectious Diseases (NIAID). The scientists named the protein fusin because it helps the virus fuse with a healthy cell membrane and inject genetic material into the cell. The CD4-containing cell signals to killer T cells that it is infected by displaying fragments of HIV proteins on its surface. This triggers the killer cells to spring into action by multiplying and seeking out the infected CD4-containing cells to pierce them open and destroy them.

CONFIRMING A HIDING PLACE

Typically, an HIV infection begins with a sudden, flulike illness. Shortly after this first episode, the virus virtually disappears and symptoms may not materialize for as long as 20 years. Over time, the immune system eventually collapses and the virus appears in ever-increasing amounts of CD4-containing cells floating free in the patient's blood. Although previous studies focused on the presence of the virus in the blood, two independently conducted studies in 1993—Janet Embretson et al.'s "Massive Covert Infection of Helper T Lymphocytes and

FIGURE 1.4

HIV replication cycle

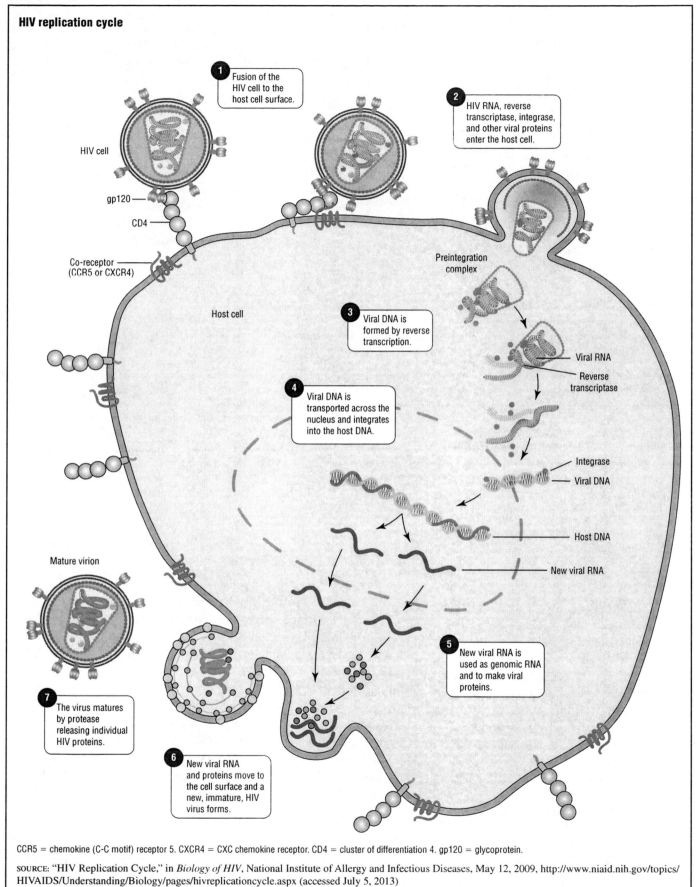

CCR5 = chemokine (C-C motif) receptor 5. CXCR4 = CXC chemokine receptor. CD4 = cluster of differentiation 4. gp120 = glycoprotein.

SOURCE: "HIV Replication Cycle," in *Biology of HIV*, National Institute of Allergy and Infectious Diseases, May 12, 2009, http://www.niaid.nih.gov/topics/HIVAIDS/Understanding/Biology/pages/hivreplicationcycle.aspx (accessed July 5, 2013)

FIGURE 1.5

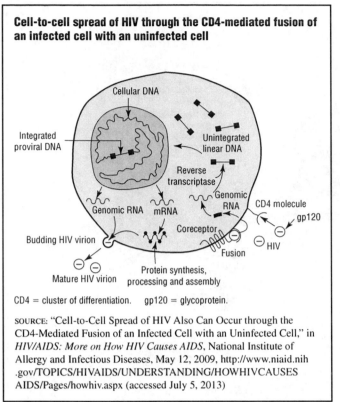

Cell-to-cell spread of HIV through the CD4-mediated fusion of an infected cell with an uninfected cell

CD4 = cluster of differentiation.   gp120 = glycoprotein.

SOURCE: "Cell-to-Cell Spread of HIV Also Can Occur through the CD4-Mediated Fusion of an Infected Cell with an Uninfected Cell," in *HIV/AIDS: More on How HIV Causes AIDS*, National Institute of Allergy and Infectious Diseases, May 12, 2009, http://www.niaid.nih.gov/TOPICS/HIVAIDS/UNDERSTANDING/HOWHIVCAUSESAIDS/Pages/howhiv.aspx (accessed July 5, 2013)

Macrophages by HIV during the Incubation Period of AIDS" (*Nature*, vol. 362, no. 6418, March 25, 1993) and Anthony S. Fauci et al.'s "Multifactorial Nature of Human Immunodeficiency Virus Disease: Implications for Therapy" (*Science*, vol. 262, no. 5136, November 12, 1993)—confirmed that HIV hides in a patient's lymph nodes and similar tissue during the first or early stage of infection.

Searching for an Active Virus

Research by Fauci et al. focused on the search for the virus in the blood and lymphoid tissue (the lymph nodes, spleen, tonsils, and adenoids) of 12 HIV-infected patients whose infections had progressed to varying severities. Initially, the virus is concentrated almost entirely in the lymphoid tissues. Fauci et al. believe the virus infiltrates the lymph nodes within weeks of the initial infection. Particles of the virus coated with antibodies adhere to the follicular dendritic cells, a group of filtering cells that trap foreign material. Nearby CD4-containing cells "see" the trapped material and are stimulated to attack the invaders. The stronger virus counterattacks and reproduces itself on some of these CD4-containing cells.

After this infiltration, performance of the immune system declines. This decline, which ultimately is dramatically debilitating, occurs over an extended period—up to 20 years in some people. During this decline the follicular dendritic cells also begin to deteriorate, and the quantity of HIV in the CD4-containing cells floating free

in the blood increases significantly. In the final stage of the disease, there is an almost complete dissolution of the follicular dendritic cell network. At this point the amount of HIV in the blood and in the CD4-containing cells has grown to equal the amount in the lymph nodes.

NOT JUST THE IMMUNE SYSTEM

For some time scientists believed HIV attacked and affected only the immune system. Many early AIDS cases that provided evidence of the involvement of other regions of the body were not counted due to the narrower definitions of AIDS that existed before 1993. However, after 1993 clear evidence showed that the free virus (not attached to any other cells) could appear in the fluid surrounding the brain and spinal cord and in the bloodstream. HIV can be found not only in T4 lymphocytes but also in other immune system cells, as well as in cells in the nervous system, intestine, and bone marrow.

CDC researchers proposed another reason HIV infections are so difficult to eliminate and why the immune system is so susceptible to them. HIV can infect and grow in immature bone marrow cells, offering no clues about what the mature HIV-infected cells will become. The virus reproduces without revealing itself to the immune system, which under normal circumstances would destroy it. By developing in immature bone marrow cells, a great quantity of the virus can be produced before the body ever attempts to resist it.

As they mature, the cells change, becoming infected monocytes and macrophages that may not only fail to fight infections but may also spread the virus to other immune system cells. Infected marrow cells can seed the virus into other parts of the body, including the brain.

SEARCHING FOR ANSWERS

Researchers have long been puzzled by the fact that AIDS is virtually always fatal, even though relatively small amounts of the virus are found in patients, compared with other lethal viral infections. How the virus kills cells has been hotly debated. Certainly, it is inconsistent with other retroviruses, which do not kill all the infected host cells. Although HIV is considered to be a slow virus (one that exerts its effect over a long period), some AIDS activity occurs quickly and may be associated with the coincidental presence of infectious mycoplasma (bacteria that lack a cell wall).

Restoring Immune Response

In December 1993 the NCI reported that the immune function had been restored to HIV-infected cells grown in a laboratory through the addition of interleukin-12 (IL-12). IL-12 is a member of a group of natural blood proteins called cytokines that were discovered in 1991 by scientists at the Wistar Institute and Hoffmann-La Roche Inc. Despite this promising result, the U.S. Food and Drug Administration (FDA) halted human testing of IL-12 in June 1995, after two patients died. After testing the protein on animals, researchers concluded that the problem was not in IL-12 itself, but in the timing of the doses. Consequently, human testing resumed in November 1995.

In December 1995 a new class of drugs called protease inhibitors received FDA approval. These drugs block the ability of HIV to mature and to infect new cells by suppressing the protein-degrading activity of a viral enzyme. Enzymes with this activity are classified as proteases, hence the designation of the enzyme blocker as a protease inhibitor. If protease inhibitors block the spread of HIV in the immune system, then AIDS will not develop. Although patients may be HIV positive the rest of their life, they may never die from HIV infection.

Theories of HIV/AIDS Progression

Even after three decades of research, there is no consensus among HIV experts about the origination and development of AIDS. There is, however, agreement that the latent period between the establishment of an HIV infection and the appearance of the symptoms of AIDS averages from two to 11 years, although some people remain symptom free for as long as 20 years. Furthermore, as many as 20% of all HIV-infected people do not develop AIDS. Called long-term nonprogressors, these individuals are believed to have genetic and immune response characteristics that slow or halt the course of disease progression. Much research centers on these people, because an understanding of the physiological characteristics that allow them to suppress the infection could be invaluable for treating the disease in other patients.

After HIV infection is established, the immune system regenerates cells only up to a certain point, which would explain a gradual progression to AIDS. The early regulatory functions of the immune system limit viral replication until a certain threshold is reached. When the number of different viral mutants becomes too large, the regulatory system is overwhelmed and shuts down, opening the door to opportunistic infections.

When the total CD4+ T cell count falls from the normal 500 to 1,600 per cubic millimeter of blood to 200 per cubic millimeter, the rate of immune decline accelerates and the HIV-positive person becomes prone to the opportunistic infections and other illnesses that are characteristic of AIDS.

SOME INCONSISTENCIES WITH CURRENT THEORIES. Most scientists agree that there are still gaps and inconsistencies in the knowledge of how HIV causes AIDS. One inconsistency concerns the infection and killing of the helper T cells. Initially, researchers thought that the main tactic of HIV was to infect and destroy the T cells. As these cells died, the numerical strength of the helper

T cell force was depleted, thus causing the immune deficiency associated with AIDS patients.

Other scientists, however, consider this theory too simplistic, because so few T cells—no more than one infected cell in 500—are infected. Rather, two studies published in 2001 in the *Journal of Experimental Medicine*—Hiroshi Mohri et al.'s "Increased Turnover of T Lymphocytes in HIV-1 Infection and Its Reduction by Antiretroviral Therapy" (vol. 194, no. 9, November 5, 2001) and Joseph A. Kovacs et al.'s "Identification of Dynamically Distinct Subpopulations of T Lymphocytes That Are Differentially Affected by HIV" (vol. 194, no. 12, December 17, 2001)—support the idea that HIV does not block the production of T cells but instead accelerates the division of existing T cells. This causes the existing T cells to die off more quickly than normal.

Another inconsistency involves the observation that the rapid decline in the number of T cells comes relatively late in the infection, even though there are clear indications that the immune system has been impaired much earlier.

OPPORTUNISTIC INFECTIONS

Once HIV has destroyed the immune system, the body can no longer protect itself against bacterial, fungal, protozoal, and other viral agents that take advantage of the compromised condition and cause infections. These infections, which would not otherwise occur but for an impaired immune system, are known as opportunistic infections (OIs). In the non-AIDS community, OIs occur in hospitals, where ill, newborn, or older patients may also have less than adequately functioning immune systems. Because patients are considered to have AIDS if at least one OI appears, OIs are also referred to as "AIDS-defining events," even though OIs are not the only AIDS-defining events.

By 1997 the leading OI for Americans suffering from HIV/AIDS was *Pneumocystis carinii* pneumonia (PCP), a lung disease caused by a fungus. Before the discovery of HIV/AIDS, PCP was found almost exclusively in cancer and transplant patients with weakened immune systems. During the 1980s PCP was the AIDS-defining illness for two-thirds of people diagnosed with AIDS in the United States, and it was estimated that 75% of HIV-infected people would develop PCP during their lifetime. According to Laurence Huang et al., in "An Official ATS Workshop Summary: Recent Advances and Future Directions in Pneumocystis Pneumonia (PCP)" (*Proceedings of the American Thoracic Society*, vol. 3, no. 8, November 2006), the incidence of PCP decreased 3.4% per year between 1992 and 1995 and then declined 21.5% annually between 1996 and 1998, when powerful combinations of antiretroviral therapy (ART) were beginning to be used. NAM, a charitable organization that produces and distributes information about HIV/AIDS, explains in "PCP" (2013, http://www.aidsmap.com/PCP/

page/1044747/) that effective HIV treatment and improved treatment for PCP, including the use of antibiotics to prevent its occurrence, have made PCP infection uncommon among people with HIV in the United States. However, PCP remains the most frequently occurring serious OI among HIV-infected people in developing countries.

Although prescription drugs such as trimethoprim-sulfamethoxazole were found to be effective at preventing PCP during the late 1980s, and their widespread use along with the addition of ART a decade later markedly reduced the cases of PCP, researchers find that people who do not adhere to treatment remain at risk of developing the disease. In "Primary Relationships, HIV Treatment Adherence, and Virologic Control" (*AIDS and Behavior*, vol. 16, no. 6, August 2012), Mallory O. Johnson et al. find that patients' positive appraisals of their relationships and positive beliefs about the effectiveness of treatment are associated with greater adherence, whereas concerns about partners and medication are associated with less adherence. In addition, HIV-positive people who smoke are three times more likely to develop PCP than nonsmokers.

Esophageal candidiasis, an infection of the esophagus, and extrapulmonary cryptococcosis, a systemic fungus that enters the body through the lungs and may invade any organ, are also OIs frequently diagnosed in AIDS patients.

Other illnesses such as Burkitt's lymphoma, cervical cancer, and primary brain lymphoma are also considered AIDS-defining events. Wasting syndrome (which is characterized by drastic weight loss and lethargy) is another illness that may be considered an AIDS-defining event. Other examples of AIDS-defining events include diagnosis of *Mycobacterium avium* complex, a serious bacterial infection that may occur in the liver, bone marrow, and spleen or spread throughout the body; cytomegalovirus disease, a member of the herpesvirus group; Kaposi's sarcoma, a once-rare cancer of the blood vessel walls that causes purple lesions on the skin; and toxoplasmic encephalitis, an inflammation of the brain. Patients may experience more than one OI or AIDS-defining event.

In 2006 NIAID researchers identified a critical human cell surface molecule—protein xCT—as the receptor that can make cells vulnerable to infection with Kaposi's sarcoma herpesvirus (KSHV). Although Kaposi's sarcoma was less common in the United States in 2013 than it had been during the early years of the AIDS pandemic; it was the second most-common cancer associated with HIV infection. Figure 1.6 shows how KSHV fuses to and enters a human cell after binding to the protein xCT.

HIV and Tuberculosis

Tuberculosis (TB) is a communicable infection caused by the bacterium *Mycobacterium tuberculosis*. TB was a widespread pandemic in North America during the late 19th and early 20th centuries, and then it faded from

FIGURE 1.6

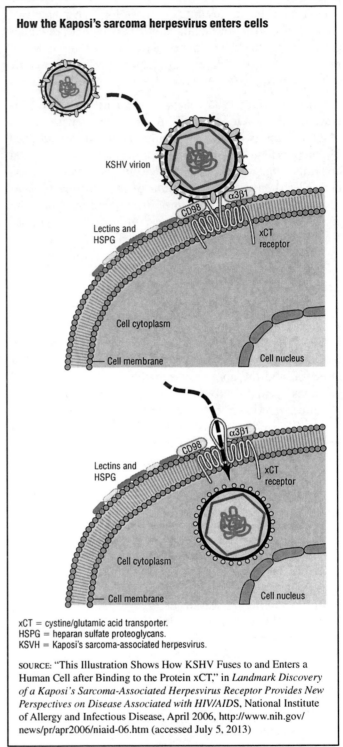

How the Kaposi's sarcoma herpesvirus enters cells

xCT = cystine/glutamic acid transporter.
HSPG = heparan sulfate proteoglycans.
KSVH = Kaposi's sarcoma-associated herpesvirus.

SOURCE: "This Illustration Shows How KSHV Fuses to and Enters a Human Cell after Binding to the Protein xCT," in *Landmark Discovery of a Kaposi's Sarcoma-Associated Herpesvirus Receptor Provides New Perspectives on Disease Associated with HIV/AIDS*, National Institute of Allergy and Infectious Disease, April 2006, http://www.nih.gov/news/pr/apr2006/niaid-06.htm (accessed July 5, 2013)

prominence. However, TB regained a foothold during the 1990s, with the number of cases increasing in the United States. Part of this increase is the parallel increase in the occurrence of the infection in HIV-positive individuals. HIV infection has become one of the strongest known risk factors for the progression of TB from infection to disease.

TB is spread from person to person through the inhalation of airborne particles containing *M. tuberculosis*. The particles, called droplet nuclei, are produced when a person with infectious TB forcefully exhales, such as when coughing, sneezing, speaking, or singing. These infectious particles remain suspended in the air and may be inhaled by someone sharing the same air. The risk of transmission is increased when ventilation is poor and when susceptible people share air for prolonged periods with a person who has untreated TB.

Approximately 85% of TB infections occur in the lungs. This infection is called pulmonary TB. However, TB may occur at any site of the body, such as the larynx, lymph nodes, brain, kidneys, or bones. These cases are called extrapulmonary TB. Except for laryngeal TB, people with extrapulmonary TB are usually not considered infectious.

According to the CDC, in "Tuberculosis (TB)" (September 16, 2012, http://www.cdc.gov/tb/statistics/default.htm), the number of TB cases in the United States declined 5.4% between 2010 and 2011; however, TB remains one of the leading causes of death of people who are HIV infected. This is because people who are not HIV infected can usually defend themselves successfully against TB infection. The risk that TB will develop in people infected only with *M. tuberculosis* is 10% within their lifetime. People with HIV, who have weakened immune systems, are less able to resist infection and are more likely to develop active TB. HIV-infected people with either latent TB infection or active TB disease can be effectively treated with prescription drugs that kill the bacteria.

Extensively drug-resistant TB (XDR-TB), which does not respond to the conventional drugs that are used to combat the disease, poses a new threat to public health initiatives aimed at reducing TB infections. Jason R. Andrews et al. report in "Predictors of Multidrug- and Extensively Drug-Resistant Tuberculosis in a High HIV Prevalence Community" (*PLoS One*, vol. 5, no. 12, December 29, 2010) that multidrug-resistant TB (MDR-TB; this type of TB does not respond to two first-line anti-TB drugs—rifampicin and isoniazid) and XDR-TB continue to appear in places with high HIV prevalence, where the death rate for HIV-coinfected patients remains high. In the developing world, where many cases are undetected, delays in diagnosis and treatment serve to increase the death rate.

In "Treatment Outcomes for Extensively Drug-Resistant Tuberculosis and HIV Co-infection" (*Emerging Infectious Diseases*, vol. 19, no. 3, March 2013), Max R. O'Donnell et al. report that even when treated, many MDR-TB and XDR-TB patients do not fare well. In a study of 6,127 patients with either MDR-TB or XDR-TB, the researchers find a high mortality rate (48%) and a low rate of successful treatment (22%). O'Donnell et al. call for more rapid HIV and TB testing to enable prompt treatment and ongoing drug susceptibility testing to ensure

that patients are receiving effective medication and development of more potent anti-TB drugs.

HIV and Cancer

People with AIDS are susceptible to cancer. Some malignant tumors, such as Kaposi's sarcoma and cancers of the lymph system, have been common among AIDS patients since the disease was first discovered in 1981. More recently, however, physicians and researchers have found that certain forms of cancer are more prevalent among HIV/AIDS patients who are living longer.

Most AIDS-related cancers are believed to be caused by viruses. These cancers are more common among HIV-infected people because HIV suppresses the immune system, enabling cancer-causing viruses to attack more successfully. These cancers include non-Hodgkin's lymphoma (found in lymph tissues) and primary lymphoma of the brain. People infected with HIV are also at greater risk of anal, cervical, liver, lung, oral, and skin cancers as well as myeloma (malignant tumors of the bone marrow), brain tumors, testicular cancers, and leukemia (cancer of the blood cells).

Because anti-HIV-combination drug therapies, such as ART, have become widely used, researchers report a decline in Kaposi's sarcoma and primary lymphoma of the brain. One possible explanation for the decline may be that the combination drug therapies enable the body to recover partial immunity, which in turn helps prevent the development of cancer.

Lung cancer is the third most commonly diagnosed cancer among people with HIV, after non-Hodgkin's lymphoma and Kaposi's sarcoma. In the past, it was assumed that the high rate of lung cancer in HIV-infected people was solely attributable to smoking, but research refutes this assumption. Gregory D. Kirk et al. find in "HIV Infection Is Associated with an Increased Risk for Lung Cancer, Independent of Smoking" (*Clinical Infectious Diseases*, vol. 45, no. 1, July 1, 2007) strong evidence that HIV infection contributes to lung cancer, independent of smoking, and conclude that HIV infection alone increases the risk of developing lung cancer. HIV also increases the lung cancer risk among smokers. Although it is not known how HIV influences the development of lung cancer, Kirk et al. speculate that it might be directly involved in promoting the development of cancer or might increase susceptibility by compromising immune function. HIV might also increase susceptibility to the cancer-causing effects of tobacco.

Other researchers document an association between HIV and lung cancer, independent of smoking. Allison A. Lambert, Christian A. Merlo, and Gregory D. Kirk of the Johns Hopkins School of Medicine observe in "Human Immunodeficiency Virus–Associated Lung Malignancies" (*Clinics in Chest Medicine*, vol. 34, no. 2, June 2013) that lung cancer in HIV-positive patients is diagnosed at younger ages than it is in the general population.

In "Cancer Burden in the HIV-Infected Population in the United States" (*Journal of the National Cancer Institute*, vol. 103, no. 9, May 4, 2011), Meredith S. Shiels et al. explain that since the introduction of ART, the incidence of AIDS-defining infections and cancers, including Kaposi's sarcoma, non-Hodgkin's lymphoma, and invasive cervical carcinoma, have decreased significantly. However, the incidence and numbers of deaths that are attributable to non-AIDS-related malignancies and other diseases have increased. This shift is the result of increased life expectancy and the reduction of competing causes of death.

TOWARD A VACCINE: THE HOPE AND THE REALITIES

The different routes of attack of HIV on the immune system and the ability of the virus to mutate has prompted some observers to opine that an effective vaccine will be difficult to achieve. This sentiment is contrary to the 1984 prediction made by Margaret M. Heckler (1931–), the U.S. secretary of the Department of Health and Human Services, that the identification of HIV would lead to a vaccine within two years.

The intervening years have made many AIDS researchers realize that developing a vaccine to prevent AIDS (confer immunity on the person receiving the vaccine) is challenging. Testing the effectiveness of an AIDS vaccine is also difficult, because deliberate contamination of people with HIV is unethical and illegal. For example, recent studies, including the RV 144 HIV vaccine study conducted in Thailand in 2009, overcome ethical concerns by offering vaccine trials in regions such as Thailand provinces that have some of the highest prevalence rates of HIV infection. These studies also advise their subjects to practice safe sex and supply condoms to help prevent infection.

The Thai study involved the use of two vaccines. When these vaccines were combined, they reduced the risk of infection by 30%. Analysis of the results of the RV 144 HIV vaccine study, which conferred protection in some study subjects but not in other others, continued in 2013. The National Institutes of Health (NIH) reports that the results of this study are being used to plan future studies aimed at creating stronger and more enduring protection against HIV infection.

According to the NIH, in the press release "HIV Vaccine Awareness Day, May 18, 2013" (May 17, 2013, http://www.niaid.nih.gov/news/newsreleases/2013/Pages/HVAD 2013.aspx), vaccine efforts continue despite unfavorable results from two recent studies. The HVTN 505 clinical trial was halted in April 2013, when it was found that HIV infections occurred as often among the vaccine recipients as they did in subjects who received the placebo vaccine (which contained no active drug) and that the vaccine failed to reduce viral load among volunteers who acquired HIV infection. An analysis of the results of the HVTN 503 "Phambili" vaccine clinical trial in South Africa was also disappointing: more subjects who received the investigational vaccine became HIV infected than those who had received the placebo vaccine.

Despite these setbacks, there has been some progress. Researchers have identified antibodies that are capable of neutralizing a wide range of HIV strains when tested in laboratory settings. They have mapped the path of an antibody response in a subject who is one of the 20% of long-term nonprogressors—people who are HIV infected and naturally develop neutralizing antibodies to the virus after several years of infection. Neutralizing antibodies act by binding to the surface of HIV and prevent it from attaching itself to a cell and infecting it. This map may help scientists create a vaccine that could neutralize antibodies the same way this subject does.

Despite the challenges that HIV provides, clinical trials of HIV vaccines continue. In "HIV/AIDS Clinical Trials" (September 30, 2013, http://aidsinfo.nih.gov/clinical-trials), AIDSinfo, a service of the U.S. Department of Health and Human Services, notes that 147 clinical trials of HIV preventive vaccines were planned, under way, or completed in 2013.

Antiretroviral Therapy Is Effective

Although an effective vaccine remains elusive, great strides have been made in treating people infected with HIV. During the mid-1990s a "hit-hard-early" strategy gained favor. In this strategy a cocktail of anti-HIV drugs was given to patients shortly after they were diagnosed. The idea of ART is to suppress the reproduction of the virus as much as possible. Some of the drugs target the virus's reverse transcriptase. By inhibiting the enzyme's activity, the ability of HIV to reproduce is thwarted. However, ART has a downside. Although it is able to suppress the viral load, it is unable to eradicate it, and once ART is initiated, treatment must be ongoing. The therapy is expensive and hard to maintain, and its long-term use is associated with a number of serious side effects. If patients do not adhere to the treatment, then they may not adequately suppress the virus.

Historically, ART was initiated when CD4 cell counts fell below 350 cells per cubic millimeter, and in many countries with limited resources, treatment was deferred until CD4 counts dropped below 200 cells per cubic millimeter. However, Emma Hitt reports in "Starting HAART at Higher T-Cell Counts Improves Survival in Early-Stage HIV" (Medscape.com, June 10, 2009) that early treatment, when CD4 cell counts are between 200 and 350 cells per cubic millimeter, improves survival. Early treatment may also improve tolerability of antiviral drugs and reduce HIV transmission to other uninfected people.

ART MAY INCREASE RISK FOR HEART DISEASE.
Because ART has reduced AIDS-related deaths, people with HIV infections are living longer and suffering from many of the same diseases, such as heart disease, as their uninfected age peers. However, Leslie Modrich et al. suggest in "Association of HIV Infection, Demographic and Cardiovascular Risk Factors with All-Cause Mortality in the Recent HAART Era" (*Journal of Acquired Immune Deficiency Syndrome*, vol. 53, no. 1, January 1, 2010) that HIV-infected patients taking ART are as much as three times more likely to suffer from heart disease than people not infected with HIV and HIV-infected people who have not taken ART.

Promise and Progress

Although recent HIV vaccine trials have not yet produced uniformly favorable results, other research and treatment have yielded promising findings. According to Richard Knox, in "HIV Cure Is Closer as Patient's Full Recovery Inspires New Research" (NPR.org, July 18, 2012), German researchers reported in July 2012 that a 46-year-old American man who had been diagnosed with HIV infection in 1995 was cured by a bone marrow transplant that he received in 2007. The donor for the transplant was genetically resistant to HIV infection. After the transplant, the patient stopped taking the ART he had taken for 11 years and, as of 2012, was still disease free.

In "Absence of Detectable HIV-1 Viremia after Treatment Cessation in an Infant" (*New England Journal of Medicine*, October 23, 2013), Deborah Persaud et al. report that a baby born to an HIV-infected mother was treated with antiretroviral drugs within 30 hours of birth. By the time the baby was one month old, virus levels were undetectable. The baby's mother decided to discontinue the drug treatment after the baby turned 18 months old. When the child was 24 months old, the doctors expected to find high virus levels; instead, they found very small amounts of viral genetic material but no virus that was able to replicate. After 30 months without treatment and with no detectable plasma HIV levels, the child was considered cured of HIV infection. In the editorial "Baby Steps on the Road to HIV Eradication" (*New England Journal of Medicine*, October 23, 2013), Scott M. Hammer comments about this case, "The big question, of course, is, 'Is the child cured of HIV infection?' The best answer at this moment is a definitive 'maybe.' This uncertainty is due to the need for long-term follow-up."

Asier Sáez-Cirión et al. report in "Post-Treatment HIV-1 Controllers with a Long-Term Virological Remission after the Interruption of Early Initiated Antiretroviral Therapy ANRS VISCONTI Study" (*PLoS Pathogens*, vol. 9, no. 3, March 2013) that when early treatment was given to 14 HIV-infected adults, the treatment produced a "functional cure," meaning the virus was still present in the body but at very low levels. The patients were treated within 35 days to 10 weeks of infection and after about two years they discontinued treatment and remained in remission (with barely detectable virus) thereafter.

In "Stem-Cell Therapy Wipes out HIV in Two Patients" (Reuters.com, July 3, 2013), Ben Hirschler reports that Timothy Henrich of Harvard Medical School told attendees at the International AIDS Society conference in Kuala Lumpur that two men with HIV infection who had been on drug treatment were able to discontinue their treatment after receiving a stem cell transplant for lymphoma. Stem cells are very early blood cells and stem cell transplants use stem cells collected from the patient's own blood. A sibling or other matching donor may also donate stem cells. After chemotherapy (drug treatment for cancer) or radiation therapy the stored stem cells are transfused (returned) to the patient, enabling them to make the blood cells the patient needs.

CHAPTER 2
DEFINITION, SYMPTOMS, AND TRANSMITTAL

A DEFINITION OF AIDS

The Centers for Disease Control and Prevention (CDC) is the federal government's clearinghouse, research center, and monitoring agency for all infectious diseases, including HIV/AIDS. The CDC tracks the diseases in the United States and notifies health officials of their occurrence via *Morbidity and Mortality Weekly Report* notices and a website that is updated frequently.

The CDC defines AIDS as a disease caused by infection with HIV that weakens the immune system and increases the risk of certain infections and cancers. The CDC first outlined a surveillance (a constant observation of a process) case definition in 1982, and then revised it in 1983, 1985, 1987, 1993, 2000, and again in 2008 as knowledge about HIV infection increased and additional symptoms were included in the definitions. The 1993 definition emphasized the clinical importance of the CD4+ T cell count and included the addition of three clinical conditions. CD4+ T helper cells are white blood cells that also are called CD4 cells, T-helper cells, or T4 cells because one of their key functions is to send signals to other types of immune cells, including cells that kill viruses or other infectious agents.

THE 1993 AND 2008 CLASSIFICATION REVISIONS AND EXPANDED SURVEILLANCE CASE DEFINITIONS

The "1993 Revised Classification System for HIV Infection and Expanded Surveillance Case Definition for AIDS among Adolescents and Adults" (*Morbidity and Mortality Weekly Report*, vol. 41, no. RR-17, December 18, 1992), by Kenneth G. Castro et al. of the CDC, was revised in 2008 and published as "Revised Surveillance Case Definitions for HIV Infection among Adults, Adolescents, and Children Aged <18 Months and for HIV Infection and AIDS among Children Aged 18 Months to <13 Years—United States, 2008" (*Morbidity and Mortality Weekly Report*, vol. 57, no. RR-10,

December 5, 2008), by Eileen Schneider et al. of the CDC. As of October 2013, it was the. standard surveillance case definition.

The 1993 revision addressed the concerns of many women and physicians, who strongly advocated the inclusion of diseases such as pelvic inflammatory disease (inflammation of the female reproductive organs by microorganisms) and vaginal candidiasis (a fungal infection, commonly called a yeast infection or thrush) as conditions that could precede the development of AIDS, so that women infected with HIV would be included in the revised definition. Advocates cautioned that if the CDC omitted such inclusive criteria, many women would be denied access to treatment, education, and disability benefits.

The 2008 revision combined surveillance case definitions for adults and adolescents by offering a single definition for people aged 13 years and older. It also revised the HIV infection case definition for children under the age of 13 years and the AIDS case definition for children aged 18 months to 13 years old. The case definition for HIV infection includes AIDS and incorporates the HIV infection classification system in which AIDS is called stage 3 infection. Laboratory-confirmed evidence of HIV infection, as opposed to simply the diagnosis of an AIDS-defining condition without confirmation from laboratory tests, is now required to meet the surveillance case definition.

Although reporting criteria include recommendations for diagnosing HIV infection, the primary purpose of the original and updated case definitions for HIV and AIDS is public health surveillance as opposed to the diagnosis of individual patients.

The 2008 Revised Definition and Classification: Tied to CD4+ Cells

The 2008 surveillance case definition emphasizes the central role of the CD4+ T cell counts and percentages, which are objective measures of immunosuppression that are routinely used in the care of HIV-infected people and are available to surveillance programs. As shown in Table 2.1, the 2008 classification system is based on three ranges of CD4+ T-lymphocyte counts and does not require the presence of an AIDS-defining condition. Table 2.2 lists a number of AIDS-defining conditions.

Historically, one of the difficulties researchers faced when making international comparisons were varying case definitions and reporting practices. World Health Organization (WHO) and CDC surveillance case definitions both require laboratory confirmation to establish HIV infection; however, their staging systems are slightly different. In addition, because there is no universal method for measuring CD4+ T-lymphocyte counts and percentages, the WHO advises using clinical and immunologic criteria for staging. Table 2.3 compares the WHO and CDC case definitions.

The Impact of the 1993 Definition on Case Reporting

CDC data indicate that expansion of the AIDS surveillance criteria changed both the process of AIDS surveillance and the number of reported cases. In "Current Trends Update: Impact of the Expanded AIDS Surveillance Case Definition for Adolescents and Adults on Case Reporting—United States, 1993" (*Morbidity and Mortality Weekly Report*, vol. 43, no. 9, March 11, 1994), the CDC reports that in 1993, 103,500 AIDS cases were reported in the United States among adults and adolescents aged 13 years and older. This number was just over twice the 49,016 cases reported in 1992 and likely represented a one-time effect of the 1993 expansion of the AIDS definition. The steep

increase represented the reporting of people who were diagnosed with the newly added conditions before 1993. New reported AIDS cases declined again beginning in 1996 in response to antiretroviral therapy (ART), which slowed the progression from HIV infection to AIDS. Between 1998 and 1999 the decline in the incidence of AIDS began to level. (See Figure 2.1.) Between 1999 and 2010 the number of diagnoses declined and the number of deaths remained fairly stable.

Table 2.4 shows the estimated numbers and rates of people living with HIV infection in 2008, 2009, and 2010. The number and rate of people living with diagnosed HIV infection increased each year during this period.

DIAGNOSIS AND SYMPTOMS OF HIV INFECTION AND AIDS

Only a qualified health professional can diagnose AIDS. To evaluate a patient with a positive HIV test, the health care practitioner performs a complete physical examination and collects the patient's social and family history. Diagnostic laboratory tests are also performed. These tests typically include complete blood count and routine chemistry; CD4+ T cell count; assays (analyses) that measure the amount of HIV-1 ribonucleic acid (RNA) in plasma; tuberculin skin tests to detect the presence of the bacterium that causes tuberculosis; and assays for the microbial agents that cause syphilis, toxoplasmosis, and hepatitis B and C. Female patients are screened for cervical cancer using the *Papanicolaou* smear.

TABLE 2.1

Surveillance case definition for (HIV) infection among adults and adolescents, 2008

[Aged >13 years. United States.]

Stage	Laboratory evidence[a]	Clinical evidence
Stage 1	Laboratory confirmation of HIV infection and CD4+ T-lymphocyte count of ≥500 cells/μL or CD4+ T-lymphocyte percentage of ≥29	None required (but no AIDS-defining condition)
Stage 2	Laboratory confirmation of HIV infection and CD4+ T-lymphocyte count of 200–499 cells/μL or CD4+ T-lymphocyte percentage of 14–28	None required (but no AIDS-defining condition)
Stage 3 (AIDS)	Laboratory confirmation of HIV infection and CD4+ T-lymphocyte count of <200 cells/μL or CD4+ T-lymphocyte percentage of <14[b]	Or documentation of an AIDS-defining condition (with laboratory confirmation of HIV infection)[b]
Stage unknown[c]	Laboratory confirmation of HIV infection and no information on CD4+ T-lymphocyte count or percentage	And no information on presence of AIDS-defining conditions

μL = microliter.
[a]The CD4+ T-lymphocyte percentage is the percentage of total lymphocytes. If the CD4+ T-lymphocyte count and percentage do not correspond to the same HIV infection stage, select the more severe stage.
[b]Documentation of an AIDS-defining condition supersedes a CD4= T-lymphocyte count of ≥200 cells/μL and a CD4+ T-lymphocyte percentage of total lymphocytes of ≥14.
[c]Although cases with no information on CD4+ T-lymphocyte count or percentage or on the presence of AIDS-defining conditions can be classified as stage unknown, every effort should be made to report CD4+ T-lymphocyte counts or percentages and the presence of AIDS-defining conditions at the time of diagnosis. Additional CD4+ T-lymphocyte counts or percentages and any identified AIDS-defining conditions can be reported as recommended.

SOURCE: Eileen Schneider et al., "Table. Surveillance Case Definition for Human Immunodeficiency Virus (HIV) Infection among Adults and Adolescents (Aged >13 years)—United States, 2008," in "Revised Surveillance Case Definitions for HIV Infection among Adults, Adolescents, and Children Aged <18 Months and for HIV Infection and AIDS among Children Aged 18 Months to <13 Years—United States, 2008," *MMWR*, vol. 57, no. RR-10, December 5, 2008, http://www.cdc.gov/mmwr/pdf/rr/rr5710.pdf (accessed July 7, 2013)

TABLE 2.2

AIDS-defining conditions

- Bacterial infections, multiple or recurrent[a]
- Candidiasis of bronchi, trachea, or lungs
- Candidiasis of esophagus[b]
- Cervical cancer, invasive[c]
- Coccidioidomycosis, disseminated or extrapulmonary
- Cryptococcosis, extrapulmonary
- Cryptosporidiosis, chronic intestinal (>1 month's duration)
- Cytomegalovirus disease (other than liver, spleen, or nodes), onset at age >1 month
- Cytomegalovirus retinitis (with loss of vision)[b]
- Encephalopathy, HIV related
- Herpes simplex: chronic ulcers (>1 month's duration) or bronchitis, pneumonitis, or esophagitis (onset at age >1 month)
- Histoplasmosis, disseminated or extrapulmonary
- Isosporiasis, chronic intestinal (>1 month's duration)
- Kaposi sarcoma[b]
- Lymphoid interstitial pneumonia or pulmonary lymphoid hyperplasia complex[a, b]
- Lymphoma, Burkitt (or equivalent term)
- Lymphoma, immunoblastic (or equivalent term)
- Lymphoma, primary, of brain
- *Mycobacterium avium* complex or *Mycobacterium kansasii*, disseminated or extrapulmonary[b]
- *Mycobacterium tuberculosis* of any site, pulmonary,[b, c] disseminated,[b] or extrapulmonary[b]
- *Mycobacterium*, other species or unidentified species, disseminated[b] or extrapulmonary[b]
- *Pneumocystis jirovecii* pneumonia[b]
- Pneumonia, recurrent[b, c]
- Progressive multifocal leukoencephalopathy
- *Salmonella* septicemia, recurrent
- Toxoplasmosis of brain, onset at age >1 month[b]
- Wasting syndrome attributed to HIV

HIV = Human immunodeficiency virus.
[a]Only among children aged <13 years.
[b]Condition that might be diagnosed presumptively.
[c]Only among adults and adolescents aged >13 years.

SOURCE: Eileen Schneider et al., "Appendix A. AIDS-Defining Conditions," in "Revised Surveillance Case Definitions for HIV Infection among Adults, Adolescents, and Children Aged <18 Months and for HIV Infection and AIDS among Children Aged 18 Months to <13 Years—United States, 2008," *MMWR*, vol. 57, no. RR-10, December 5, 2008, http://www.cdc.gov/mmwr/pdf/rr/rr5710.pdf (accessed July 7, 2013)

From HIV to AIDS

Through 2013, among people who were not treated with ART, the average time from initial HIV infection to the development of AIDS was about 10 years. However, advances in treatment have significantly increased the life expectancy of AIDS patients.

Ard van Sighem et al. indicate in "Life Expectancy of Recently Diagnosed Asymptomatic HIV-Infected Patients Approaches That of Uninfected Individuals" (*AIDS*, vol. 24, no. 10, June 19, 2010) that many people diagnosed with HIV infection in the 21st century will have normal life expectancies. Research involving more than 80,000 HIV-infected people from 30 European countries confirms that people who maintain CD4 cell counts of over 500 per cubic millimeter of blood for three years or more and who abstain from illicit drug use can anticipate a life span that is comparable in length to their uninfected peers.

In "Updates of Lifetime Costs of Care and Quality-of-Life Estimates for HIV-Infected Persons in the United States: Late versus Early Diagnosis and Entry into Care" (*Journal of Acquired Immune Deficiency Syndrome*, vol. 64, no. 2, October 1, 2013), Paul G. Farnham et al. observe that quality-of-life estimates for HIV-infected people depend on when people are diagnosed (the stage of the infection) and when they begin ART. An analysis of 10,000 HIV-infected patients in four categories of CD4 counts at diagnosis reveals that early diagnosis and treatment of HIV infection improves both length and quality of life.

THE EARLY STAGE. Although the timing and progression of HIV infection vary, the disease follows a basic pattern. In the beginning of the early stage, shortly after the virus has entered the bloodstream, the T4 cell count is normal (around 1,000 per cubic millimeter) and the virus

TABLE 2.3

Comparison of World Health Organization (WHO) and Centers for Disease Control and Prevention (CDC) stages of HIV infection

[For reporting purposes only. By CD4+ T-lymphocyte count and percentage of total lymphocytes.]

WHO stage[a]	WHO T-lymphocyte count and percentage[b]	CDC stage[c]	CDC T-lymphocyte count and percentage
Stage 1 (HIV infection)	CD4+ T-lymphocyte count of ≥500 cells/μL	Stage 1 (HIV infection)	CD4+ T-lymphocyte count of ≥500 cells/μL or CD4+ T-lymphocyte percentage of ≥29
Stage 2 (HIV infection)	CD4+ T-lymphocyte count of 350–499 cells/μL	Stage 2 (HIV infection)	CD4+ T-lymphocyte count of 200–499 cells/μL or CD4+ T-lymphocyte percentage of 14–28
Stage 3 (advanced HIV disease [AHD])	CD4+ T-lymphocyte count of 200–349 cells/μL	Stage 2 (HIV infection)	CD4+ T-lymphocyte count of 200–499 cells/μL or CD4+ T-lymphocyte percentage of 14–28
Stage 4 (acquired immunodeficiency syndrome [AIDS])	CD4+ T-lymphocyte count of <200 cells/μL or CD4+ T-lymphocyte percentage of <15	Stage 3 (AIDS)	CD4+ T-lymphocyte count of <200 cells/μL or CD4+ T-lymphocyte percentage of <14

HIV = Human immunodeficiency virus.
μL = microliter.
[a]Among adults and children aged ≥5 years.
[b]Percentage applicable for stage 4 only.
[c]Among adults and adolescents (aged ≥13 years). CDC also includes a fourth stage, stage unknown: laboratory confirmation of HIV infection but no information on CD4+ T-lymphocyte count or percentage and no information on AIDS-defining conditions.

SOURCE: Eileen Schneider et al., "Table. Comparison of World Health Organization (WHO) and CDC Stages of Human Immunodeficiency Virus (HIV) Infection, by CD4+ T-Lymphocyte Count and Percentage of Total Lymphocytes," in "Revised Surveillance Case Definitions for HIV Infection among Adults, Adolescents, and Children Aged <18 Months and for HIV Infection and AIDS among Children Aged 18 Months to <13 Years—United States, 2008," *MMWR*, vol. 57, no. RR-10, December 5, 2008, http://www.cdc.gov/mmwr/pdf/rr/rr5710.pdf (accessed July 7, 2013)

FIGURE 2.1

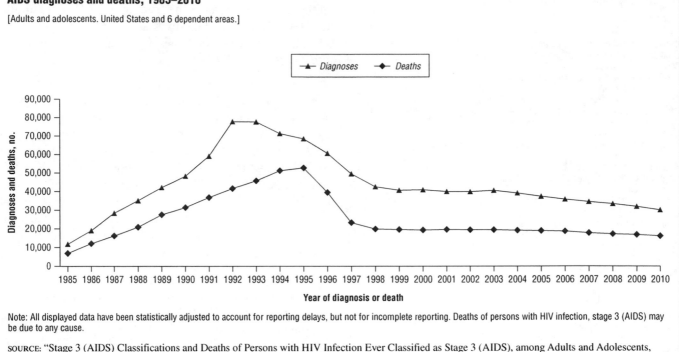

AIDS diagnoses and deaths, 1985–2010

[Adults and adolescents. United States and 6 dependent areas.]

Note: All displayed data have been statistically adjusted to account for reporting delays, but not for incomplete reporting. Deaths of persons with HIV infection, stage 3 (AIDS) may be due to any cause.

SOURCE: "Stage 3 (AIDS) Classifications and Deaths of Persons with HIV Infection Ever Classified as Stage 3 (AIDS), among Adults and Adolescents, 1985–2010—United States and 6 Dependent Areas," in *Epidemiology of HIV Infection through 2011*, Centers for Disease Control and Prevention, National Center for HIV/AIDS, Viral Hepatitis, STD, and TB Prevention, Division of HIV/AIDS Prevention, June 28, 2013, http://www.cdc.gov/hiv/pdf/statistics_epidemiology_of_infection_through_2011.pdf (accessed July 7, 2013)

is undetectable using assays that detect the presence of anti-HIV antibodies. Antibody assays can remain negative for up to six weeks. In unusual cases antibodies may remain undetectable for a year or more. Even after testing positive for the virus or for the presence of the antiviral antibodies, many people remain asymptomatic for years. During this period, which is known as acute retroviral syndrome or primary HIV infection, the virus uses immune system cells called CD4 cells to make copies of itself and destroys these cells in the process. Because of this, the CD4 count can fall quickly.

HIV is most readily transmitted during this stage because the amount of virus in the blood is very high. Over time, the immune response reduces the amount of virus in the body and the CD4 count increases, but generally does not return to pre-infection levels. Some people may develop symptoms like those of infectious mononucleosis—fatigue, fever, swollen glands, and a rash. Often, these symptoms disappear within weeks, and a connection with an HIV infection is not made. Throughout this stage, however, the virus is multiplying and destroying healthy cells. Most people continue to feel fine, although some may have chronically swollen lymph nodes. This stage lasts about five years.

THE MIDDLE STAGE. During a period known as clinical latency (because the virus is relatively inactive or dormant) HIV is still active, but reproduces at very low

levels and often produces no symptoms. Toward the end of this stage, the viral load rises, the CD4 cell count decreases, and the T4 cell count is reduced by half, to around 500 per cubic millimeter. Even with this physiological change, many people are still asymptomatic. As the infection advances, skin tests will likely show that cell-mediated immunity, a form of immunological defense, is disintegrating. The deterioration of the immune system has begun.

People on ART may live in this phase for decades. For those who are not on ART, this stage can last up to a decade. Although ART greatly reduces the risk of transmitting HIV during this phase, it is still very possible that HIV can be transmitted to others. Symptoms of HIV infection—including weight loss; profound, unexplained fatigue; nausea; fever; night sweats; swollen lymph glands; a persistent, dry cough; easy bruising or unexplained bleeding; watery diarrhea; loss of memory; balance problems; mood changes; blurring or loss of vision; and oral lesions, such as thrush (a fungal infection caused by *Candida albicans*, which produces a white coating on the tongue and throat)—appear as the immune system weakens and is unable to defend against them.

ART involves taking a combination of three or more anti-HIV medications from at least two different drug classes daily. ART prevents HIV from reproducing, which helps people infected with HIV live longer, healthier lives and

TABLE 2.4

Number of people living with HIV infection by year and selected characteristics, 2008–10

	2008 No.	2008 Estimated[a] No.	2008 Estimated[a] Rate	2009 No.	2009 Estimated[a] No.	2009 Estimated[a] Rate	2010 No.	2010 Estimated[a] No.	2010 Estimated[a] Rate
Age at end of year									
<13	3,639	3,669	6.8	3,225	3,260	6.0	2,891	2,936	5.5
13–14	1,534	1,541	18.5	1,346	1,354	16.4	1,188	1,199	14.3
15–19	7,707	7,779	35.4	7,666	7,771	35.5	7,277	7,432	33.3
20–24	25,043	25,389	117.4	27,384	27,918	127.8	29,506	30,404	138.2
25–29	48,134	48,609	223.4	49,548	50,206	228.3	50,805	51,819	242.0
30–34	67,679	68,073	343.5	68,887	69,416	343.8	71,031	71,810	353.0
35–39	105,695	105,850	500.6	99,938	100,146	480.7	93,532	93,872	461.4
40–44	155,148	154,765	713.5	148,359	147,983	695.2	143,160	142,807	674.4
45–49	165,594	164,475	712.3	173,544	172,203	744.7	177,283	175,591	766.4
50–54	122,078	120,708	556.2	131,863	130,116	590.4	142,663	140,356	620.6
55–59	74,105	72,950	388.2	83,454	81,886	425.9	92,170	89,948	448.9
60–64	36,674	35,959	234.8	42,161	41,153	256.4	49,446	47,929	278.3
≥65	28,242	27,378	69.5	32,574	31,338	78.0	37,577	35,755	87.1
Race/ethnicity									
American Indian/Alaska Native	2,959	2,946	—	3,079	3,063	—	3,216	3,195	—
Asian[b]	8,340	8,380	—	8,989	9,055	—	9,641	9,746	—
Black/African American	361,001	358,437	—	374,350	371,192	—	387,688	383,712	—
Hispanic/Latino[c]	170,123	170,245	—	176,847	176,935	—	183,414	183,486	—
Native Hawaiian/other Pacific Islander	780	779	—	853	854	—	905	910	—
White	282,664	280,971	—	290,473	288,458	—	298,089	295,545	—
Multiple races	14,634	14,614	—	14,590	14,424	—	14,811	14,499	—
Transmission category									
Male adult or adolescent									
Male-to-male sexual contact	353,275	403,302	—	369,496	423,577	—	385,867	444,092	—
Injection drug use	78,809	94,031	—	77,670	92,994	—	76,708	91,868	—
Male-to-male sexual contact and injection drug use	44,609	49,696	—	44,502	49,662	—	44,520	49,672	—
Heterosexual contact[d]	53,903	67,896	—	55,770	70,653	—	57,428	73,121	—
Perinatal	3,520	3,514	—	3,759	3,752	—	3,960	3,955	—
Other[e]	91,034	3,268	—	96,813	3,219	—	102,494	3,164	—
Subtotal	**625,150**	**621,707**	**499.4**	**648,010**	**643,857**	**512.2**	**670,985**	**665,872**	**525.7**
Female adult or adolescent									
Injection drug use	42,935	56,505	—	42,405	56,160	—	41,982	55,738	—
Heterosexual contact[d]	107,262	149,539	—	110,090	155,490	—	112,784	161,091	—
Perinatal	3,799	3,791	—	4,054	4,041	—	4,290	4,268	—
Other[e]	58,483	1,928	—	62,161	1,937	—	65,593	1,947	—
Subtotal	**212,479**	**211,764**	**162.8**	**218,710**	**217,628**	**165.9**	**224,649**	**223,045**	**167.5**
Child (<13 yrs at end of year)									
Perinatal	3,277	3,303	—	2,876	2,905	—	2,539	2,574	—
Other[e]	362	366	—	349	355	—	352	362	—
Subtotal	**3,639**	**3,669**	**6.8**	**3,225**	**3,260**	**6.0**	**2,891**	**2,936**	**5.5**
Region of residence									
Northeast	222,453	225,059	408.8	226,717	229,603	415.3	230,835	233,770	422.2
Midwest	94,558	93,351	140.2	98,859	97,455	145.8	103,048	101,393	151.4
South	348,765	344,382	307.4	362,778	357,346	315.3	376,988	370,381	322.5
West	156,862	155,845	220.4	162,686	161,660	225.9	168,464	167,446	232.1
U.S. dependent areas	18,634	18,507	422.4	18,909	18,683	425.3	19,194	18,867	458.2
Total[f]	**841,272**	**837,145**	**271.1**	**869,949**	**864,748**	**277.7**	**898,529**	**891,857**	**284.5**

[a]Estimated numbers resulted from statistical adjustment that accounted for reporting delays and missing transmission category, but not for incomplete reporting. Rates are per 100,000 population. Rates by race/ethnicity are not provided because U.S. census information for U.S. dependent areas is limited. Rates are not calculated by transmission category because of the lack of denominator data.
[b]Includes Asian/Pacific Islander legacy cases.
[c]Hispanics/Latinos can be of any race.
[d]Heterosexual contact with a person known to have, or to be at high risk for, HIV infection.
[e]Includes hemophilia, blood transfusion, and risk factor not reported or not identified.
[f]Includes persons of unknown race/ethnicity. Because column totals for estimated numbers were calculated independently of the values for the subpopulations, the values in each column may not sum to the column total.
Note: Data include persons with a diagnosis of HIV infection regardless of stage of disease at diagnosis.

SOURCE: "Table 15b. Persons Living with Diagnosed HIV Infection, by Year and Selected Characteristics, 2008–2010—United States and 6 Dependent Areas," in *HIV Surveillance Report: Diagnoses of HIV Infection in the United States and Dependent Areas, 2011*, vol. 23, Centers for Disease Control and Prevention, National Center for HIV/AIDS, Viral Hepatitis, STD, and TB Prevention, Division of HIV/AIDS Prevention, February 2013, http://www.cdc.gov/hiv/pdf/statistics_2011_HIV_Surveillance_Report_vol_23.pdf (accessed July 7, 2013) may reduce the risk of HIV transmission. The U.S. Food and Drug Administration (FDA) indicates in "Antiretroviral Drugs Used in the Treatment of HIV Infection" (http://www.fda.gov/ForConsumers/byAudience/ForPatient Advocates/HIVandAIDSActivities/ucm118915.htm) that as of August 2013 there were 31 anti-HIV medications available, including eight that were combination drugs containing two or more anti-HIV medications. Because HIV mutates, it can become resistant to some of these drugs, necessitating a change of drug regimen.

Structured treatment interruptions (STIs), initially proposed during the late 1990s, in which the multiple drug therapy that patients receive is stopped for short periods of time, were once thought to be a promising treatment strategy. The idea was that STIs could minimize treatment side effects and possibly decrease drug resistance without losing protection afforded by ART. However, considerable research indicates that STIs may be associated with worse health outcomes in terms of immune function, viral load, and ability to defend against infections than continuous ART. In "HIV Reservoirs and Immune Surveillance Evasion Cause the Failure of Structured Treatment Interruptions: A Computational Study" (*PLoS One*, vol. 7, no. 4, April 27, 2012), Emiliano Mancini et al. explain that STIs are unsuccessful because despite ART there are HIV reservoirs in the body that successfully evade immune surveillance and ART.

THE FINAL STAGE. AIDS is the stage of infection that occurs when the immune system is so damaged that it cannot fend off infections and infection-related cancers. The third and final stage of HIV infection is reached when the CD4+ T cell count drops to 200 per cubic millimeter or below. (Normal CD4 counts are between 500 and 1,600 cells per cubic millimeter.) The appearance of one or more opportunistic infections (OIs), regardless of the CD4 count, is also considered to be diagnostic for AIDS. Without treatment, people diagnosed with AIDS typically survive about three years.

Although many patients are still asymptomatic at the beginning of this stage, the functioning of the immune system is now markedly weakened. The body is far less able to defend itself from invasion. As a consequence, the risk of infection due to opportunistic bacteria, viruses, fungi, and parasites and the possibility of cancer increase dramatically. To prevent *Pneumocystis carinii* pneumonia, a lung disease that is caused by a fungus and one of the most common OIs, patients are usually treated with antibiotics during this stage.

At the onset of the late stage, patients may experience weight loss, diarrhea, lethargy, and recurring fever. Skin and mucous membrane infections increase. Oral fungal infections such as thrush and chronic infection caused by the herpes simplex virus are also common.

As the late stage progresses, the immune system collapses. OIs move deeper into the body. It is not uncommon for a parasitic infection called toxoplasmosis to attack the brain, while the cryptococcosis fungus attacks the nervous system, liver, bones, and skin. Cytomegalovirus can cause pneumonia, encephalitis, and retinitis. The latter, an inflammation of the retina, can cause blindness. Many other infections can occur. The consequences and complications of compromised immune function are many, and death is usually the result of the OIs and cancers that arise due to the impaired immune system—not HIV. Once a dangerous OI develops, life expectancy is about one year without treatment.

Dementia

HIV-associated dementia (also called HIV-associated neurocognitive disorders) is now recognized as a declining cognitive (thinking) function that generally occurs during the late stages of HIV infection. The dementia is caused by HIV infection of the central nervous system, which includes the brain, and is different from the forgetfulness and difficulty in concentrating that can be the consequences of depression and fatigue. Lewis John Haddow et al. estimate in "A Systematic Review of the Screening Accuracy of the HIV Dementia Scale and International HIV Dementia Scale" (*PLoS One*, vol. 8, no. 4, April 16, 2013) that up to 50% of people infected with HIV will develop a neurological disorder, such as dementia.

Selected Cancers

Historically, the diagnosis of specific AIDS-defining cancers—non-Hodgkin's lymphoma, Kaposi's sarcoma, and cervical cancer—was attributed to compromised immune systems, and the occurrence of other cancers was thought to result from the fact that people with HIV/AIDS were living longer because of the widespread use of ART. In "Incidence and Timing of Cancer in HIV-Infected Individuals Following Initiation of Combination Antiretroviral Therapy" (*Clinical Infectious Diseases*, vol. 57, no. 5, September 2013), Elizabeth L. Yanik et al. discuss the results of their study, which considered the incidence and timing of cancer diagnoses among 11,485 patients beginning combination ART between 1996 and 2011. The researchers find that Kaposi's sarcoma and lymphoma rates were highest immediately following ART initiation, especially among patients with low CD4 cell counts. By contrast, other cancers increased with time on ART, which Yanik et al. posit may reflect increased cancer risk with advancing age.

Although investigators do not yet know exactly why the rates of the cancers are higher among people with HIV infection, they hypothesize that:

• HIV or another as yet undetected virus may increase the risk of developing cancer

- ART may increase the risk of developing cancer

- People with HIV may have lifestyle or other environmental exposures that increase their risk for cancer, such as smoking or excessive alcohol consumption

Anouk Kesselring et al. opine in "Immunodeficiency as a Risk Factor for Non-AIDS-Defining Malignancies in HIV-1-Infected Patients Receiving Combination Antiretroviral Therapy" (*Clinical Infectious Diseases*, vol. 52, no. 12, June 15, 2011) that HIV itself may play a role in the development of cancer, either by a direct effect or as an effect of immune suppression.

TRANSMISSION OF HIV

When AIDS was first identified, it was compared with the Black Death of the 14th century, in terms of the public panic surrounding the disease and its possible spread. The comparison is not a good one. The bacterium that caused the Black Death (and that still causes bubonic plague) is highly contagious, largely because it is readily transmitted via food, water, and air. HIV is not nearly as contagious. Moreover, by observing precautions that prevent the sharing of bodily fluids, the transmission of HIV can be almost entirely prevented.

The accumulated knowledge of 30 years of research has definitively established that HIV can only be transmitted by the following routes:

- Oral, anal, or vaginal sex with an infected person. Sexual intercourse—particularly heterosexual sex—is the most common mode of HIV transmission worldwide.

- Sharing drug needles or syringes with an infected person.

- Maternal transmission to a baby at the time of birth and through breast milk. Paul J. Weidle and Steven Nesheim report in "HIV Drug Resistance and Mother-to-Child Transmission of HIV" (*Clinics in Perinatology*, vol. 37, no. 4, December 2010) that pregnant women who develop HIV drug resistance may transmit this resistance to their infants via breastfeeding. Although breastfeeding is a known source of HIV transmission, in many developing countries where alternative sources of nutrition are unavailable, the benefits of breastfeeding outweigh the risks. For this reason, the WHO recommends in *HIV Transmission through Breastfeeding: A Review of Available Evidence, 2007 Update* (2008, http://whqlibdoc.who.int/publications/2008/9789241596596_eng.pdf) that HIV-infected women "breastfeed their infants exclusively for the first six months of life, unless replacement feeding is acceptable, feasible, affordable, sustainable and safe for them and their infants before that time. When those conditions are met,

WHO recommends avoidance of all breastfeeding by HIV-infected women."

- Transplantation of HIV-infected organs or transfusion of infected bodily fluids, such as blood or blood products. During the mid-1980s the transfusion of HIV-infected blood caused thousands of cases of AIDS and led to many deaths in Europe, the United States, and Canada. The blood agencies of the affected countries have revamped their blood-testing policies so that molecular assay techniques, which detect HIV genetic material, are used to screen donated blood.

Confirming the involvement of bodily fluids in HIV transmission, high concentrations of HIV have been found in blood, semen, and cerebrospinal fluid. Not all bodily fluids seem to be involved equally, because HIV concentrations 1,000 times less have been found in saliva, tears, vaginal secretions, breast milk, and feces. However, there have been no reports of HIV transmission from tears or human bites. In fact, Diane C. Shugars et al. report in "Endogenous Salivary Inhibitors of Human Immunodeficiency Virus" (*Archives of Oral Biology*, vol. 44, no. 6, June 1999) that HIV is rarely transmitted through salivary secretions because a protein found in human saliva actually blocks the virus from entering the system.

Figure 2.2 shows the number of AIDS cases in adolescents and adults by year of diagnosis and transmission category in the United States between 1985 and 2011.

Casual Contact

Although HIV is an infectious, contagious disease, it is not spread in the same manner as a common cold. It is not spread by sneezing or coughing, as are airborne illnesses. HIV is not spread by sharing a bathroom, by swimming in a pool, or by hugging or shaking hands. Studies of family members who lived with and cared for AIDS patients have not found definitive evidence that anyone has become infected through casual contact. Still, myths abound. To combat misinformation, the U.S. surgeon general and public health education initiatives continue to stress that HIV is not spread by:

- Bites from mosquitoes or other insects

- Bites from animals

- Food handled, prepared, or served by HIV-infected people

- Forks, spoons, knives, or drinking glasses used by HIV-infected people

- Casual contact such as touching, hugging, or kissing a person who is HIV positive (open-mouth kissing with a person who is HIV positive is not recommended because of potential exposure to blood)

FIGURE 2.2

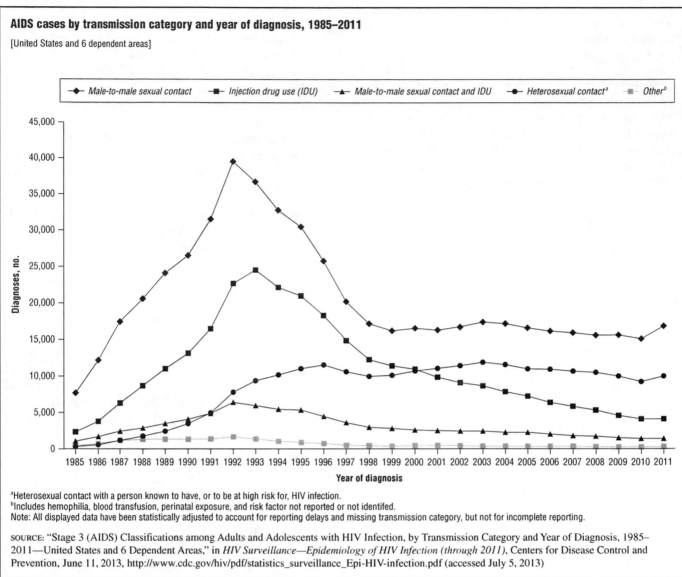

AIDS cases by transmission category and year of diagnosis, 1985–2011

[United States and 6 dependent areas]

Legend: ◆ Male-to-male sexual contact ■ Injection drug use (IDU) ▲ Male-to-male sexual contact and IDU ● Heterosexual contact[a] ▨ Other[b]

[a]Heterosexual contact with a person known to have, or to be at high risk for, HIV infection.
[b]Includes hemophilia, blood transfusion, perinatal exposure, and risk factor not reported or not identifed.
Note: All displayed data have been statistically adjusted to account for reporting delays and missing transmission category, but not for incomplete reporting.

SOURCE: "Stage 3 (AIDS) Classifications among Adults and Adolescents with HIV Infection, by Transmission Category and Year of Diagnosis, 1985–2011—United States and 6 Dependent Areas," in *HIV Surveillance—Epidemiology of HIV Infection (through 2011)*, Centers for Disease Control and Prevention, June 11, 2013, http://www.cdc.gov/hiv/pdf/statistics_surveillance_Epi-HIV-infection.pdf (accessed July 5, 2013)

Donating Blood

Health officials agree that donating blood poses no danger of HIV infection for blood donors. The needles used to draw blood from donors are new and are thrown away after one use. Therefore, contact with HIV from donating blood is impossible.

SAFETY OF BLOOD AND TRANSPLANT PROCEDURES

To safeguard the nation's transplant recipients, the CDC suggests that all donors of blood products, tissues, and organs be screened and tested. The recommendations include screening for behaviors (risk factors) associated with the acquisition of HIV infection, a physical examination for signs and symptoms related to HIV infection, and laboratory screening for antibodies to HIV. It is important to remember that the CDC does not regulate medical protocol; its main function is to offer health care

guidelines and information to the nation and its health care providers.

The U.S. Blood Supply

Before HIV-antibody testing began in 1985, it is estimated that 70% of hemophiliacs (people with inherited bleeding disorders) who received blood products were given tainted blood-clotting factor (a concentrate of blood used to stem bleeding) and were therefore infected with HIV. According to Steve Sternberg, in "A Legacy of Tainted Blood" (USAToday.com, July 11, 2006), approximately 10,000 of these patients developed AIDS and approximately 5,000 have died.

The widespread use of two blood-screening tests, both of which are also used on plasma and other blood products, has strengthened the safety of the U.S. blood and plasma supply. Since 1992 the U.S. Public Health Service, an arm of the U.S. Department of Health and

Human Services, has required that all blood and plasma donations be screened for the rare HIV-2 antibody, as well as for the more common HIV-1 antibody.

In 2001 the FDA approved the first nucleic acid test (NAT) system to screen plasma donors for HIV. Rather than relying on the identification of antigens or antibodies, the NAT provides extremely sensitive detection of RNA from HIV-1. Even with this system, however, there is still some risk due to the "window period," during which a person who has acquired the HIV-1 infection may still test negative. For HIV-1 antigen and antibody detection, the window period is 16 and 21 days, respectively, following infection. NAT systems reduce the window period to 12 days. Put another way, anyone who is infected with HIV and who donates blood more than 12 days after exposure to the virus will register HIV positive.

There are many measures in place to ensure the safety of the U.S. blood supply; however, the FDA admits that it is impossible to ensure zero risk of transmitting infectious disease. So even though the U.S. blood supply is considered safe, blood banks across the country nonetheless encourage individuals concerned about tainted blood to bank their own blood for possible future use.

In "New Technologies Promise to Improve Blood Supply Safety" (*Nature Medicine*, vol. 17, no. 5, May 5, 2011), Michelle Pflumm explains that to further improve the safety of the blood supply, U.S. blood banks have introduced new technologies that use deoxyribonucleic acid–based screening to detect previously undetectable levels of HIV and other pathogens in blood. Although officials assert that the U.S. blood supply is "safer than it's ever been," they concede that "transfusion is still associated with [a] risk of transmission."

Foreign Blood Supplies

Historically, HIV infection from contaminated blood has been much more common in other countries. According to Craig R. Whitney, in "Top French Officials Cleared over Blood with AIDS Virus" (NYTimes.com, March 10, 1999), a French court ruled in 1998 that a former prime minister and two former cabinet members would be tried on charges that they allowed HIV-contaminated blood to be used for transfusions between 1984 and 1985. Relatives of the patients argued that the French government had refused U.S. technology that would have detected antibodies in the tainted blood in favor of a French procedure that was in development. Approximately 4,400 people acquired HIV as a result of this action. Many of the victims were hemophiliacs, and about 40% of the total number infected had died of AIDS. The former French officials, Prime Minister Laurent Fabius (1946–), Minister of Social Affairs Georgina Dufoix (1942–), and Minister of Health Edmond Hervé (1942–), faced charges of involuntary homicide and went

to trial in 1999. Hervé was convicted without a penalty and Dufoix and Fabius were acquitted. The tragedy resulted in the overhaul of the blood supply and donation networks in France.

Jane Perlez notes in "Parents Sue Romania over Child's H.I.V. Infection" (NYTimes.com, August 31, 1995) that the WHO reported in 1995 that 3,000 children in Romania—home to thousands of abandoned babies left in squalid institutions after the fall of the Romanian dictator Nicolae Ceausescu (1918–1989)—were infected by contaminated blood and syringes during the late 1980s. The WHO estimated that 1,000 of those children had died. According to Perlez, "Romania has more than half of the juvenile AIDS cases in Europe. More than 90 percent of the country's reported AIDS cases are among children, most of whom were infected by contaminated needles and syringes." The Romanian Health Ministry faced litigation for causing the spread of HIV.

According to the article "Another German Trial for H.I.V.-Tainted Blood" (Reuters, November 30, 1995), Gunter Kurt Eckert, the owner of a German drug laboratory, was charged in 1995 with nearly 6,000 counts of murder or attempted murder for selling HIV-tainted blood products to German hospitals in 1987. Nearly 90% of the 6,000 batches had not been tested for HIV. Testing has been mandatory in Germany since 1986. Eckert was found guilty and sentenced to six and a half years in prison.

The article "Canada's Tainted Blood Scandal: A Timeline" (CBC.ca, October 1, 2007) notes that the Canadian blood collection, testing, and distribution system was completely overhauled in the wake of the distribution of blood that was contaminated with HIV and the hepatitis C virus. In 1989 Ottawa established a $150 million fund to compensate the 1,250 Canadians who were infected with HIV as a result of contact with infected blood. It was discovered that 95% of hemophiliacs who received blood products prior to 1990 had been infected with hepatitis C. In 2001 the Canadian Supreme Court ruled that the negligence of the blood agency during the early years of the AIDS crisis entitled several thousand affected Canadians to a $1.2 billion federal-provincial government compensation offer. Legal wrangling in the intervening years delayed the implementation of the court's ruling.

Although the WHO has examined blood safety and all developed countries have strengthened their screening efforts, problems persist in developing countries. The WHO notes in the fact sheet "Blood Safety and Availability" (June 2013, http://www.who.int/mediacentre/factsheets/fs279/en/) that 25 of the 151 countries reporting blood-screening data in 2011 were unable to screen all donated blood for one or more transmissible infections, including HIV.

Organ and Tissue Transplants

There are cases of HIV transmission through organ (kidney, liver, heart, lung, and pancreas) and other tissue transplants. However, the risk of such transmission is low simply because there are far fewer transplant cases than blood transfusions.

In 1994 the FDA began regulating the sale of bone, skin, corneas, cartilage, tendons, and similar nonblood vessel–bearing tissues that are used for transplants. The FDA requires that all procurement agencies conduct behavioral screening and infectious-disease (HIV-1, HIV-2, hepatitis B virus, and hepatitis C virus) testing of donors.

In "HIV Transmitted from a Living Organ Donor— New York City, 2009" (*Morbidity and Mortality Weekly Report*, vol. 60, no. 10, March 18, 2011), the CDC reports the first documented case in the United States of HIV transmission through the transplantation of an organ from a living donor, despite screening. The recipient of the kidney tested negative for HIV 12 days before the transplant. One year after the transplant, the recipient was hospitalized with candidiasis, and HIV infection was confirmed with a positive Western blot. Because the recipient had not engaged in any behaviors that would increase the risk for acquiring HIV, the donor was investigated. The donor was an adult male with a previous diagnosis of syphilis (a sexually transmitted infection) and a history of sex with male partners; however, he tested negative for HIV 79 days before the transplant. During the public health investigation, the donor reported unprotected sex with one male partner during the year before the transplant, including the time between his initial evaluation and organ donation. When advanced deoxyribonucleic acid testing was performed on a sample of the donor's blood that was drawn 11 days before the transplant, three HIV genes were identified.

TESTING PEOPLE FOR HIV

A person who is infected with HIV produces antibodies specific to the virus as part of the body's immune response. Although the antibodies are not enough to successfully fight HIV, they are of diagnostic value, as they indicate the presence of the virus.

Antibody-based HIV testing is done, rather than a direct test for the virus itself, because it is too difficult to isolate the virus from the blood. Testing serves to determine if there is a viral infection in donated blood, tissues, or organs. This protects the recipients of the donated material and can be used to identify HIV-infected donors.

An antibody-based test cannot detect all HIV-positive blood. It typically takes between four and 12 weeks following HIV infection for antibodies to appear, although in rare cases this period can be up to one year. The introduction of tests that detect the viral nucleic acid rather than the HIV antibodies has markedly increased the detection sensitivity of blood screening. Still, even nucleic acid detection has a window period, albeit a shorter one, of about 12 days.

The fact that detection is not absolute from the moment of HIV infection means that the possibility exists that some HIV-infected donors may not be diagnosed and their blood may enter the nation's blood supply. However, the number of predicted contaminated blood samples is extremely small. To further reduce the chances of contaminated blood entering the blood supply, blood banks routinely question potential donors about high-risk behaviors. Any donor whose behavior might indicate an increased risk of HIV infection (such as injection drug use or unsafe sex) is automatically excluded from donating blood.

Diagnostic Tools for HIV Antibodies

Two tests commonly used to detect HIV antibodies are believed to be about 99% reliable. These tests are the enzyme-linked immunosorbent assay (ELISA) and the Western blot.

Introduced in 1985, ELISA is a test that was designed for screening rather than for diagnosing. The assay uses purified HIV antigens to probe for the presence of complimentary antibodies in a sample such as blood. If anti-HIV antibodies are present in the sample, they attach themselves to the viral proteins that have been immobilized on a plastic surface. A second antibody that has been raised against the anti-HIV antibody (antibodies are proteins, too, so they can function as antigens, stimulating the formation of antibodies) is bound to the anti-HIV antibodies. The second antibody contains a chemical that can be made to change color. The color change reveals the presence of the anti-HIV antibody. If no color change appears, no anti-HIV antibody is present in the blood sample. This test is reliable, simple to conduct, and inexpensive.

The Western blot, introduced in 1987, is a confirmatory test. This means it is commonly used to verify the results of the less-specific assays. The Western blot technique separates the various HIV proteins from one another, based on their speed of movement through a gel under the influence of electricity. The separated proteins are transferred from the gel to a membrane made of a material such as nitrocellulose. When the nitrocellulose is exposed to a blood sample, antibodies that recognize one of the proteins on the nitrocellulose will bind to the particular protein. As with ELISA, a color reaction can be induced to indicate the site of the bound antibodies. The Western blot provides a positive, negative, or intermediate result. The presence of three or more of the color bands confirms an HIV infection. If fewer—one or two—bands appear, the test is considered intermediate and retesting is performed six months later. If no color bands appear, the test is considered negative with no HIV present, although many people who test negative also repeat the test six months later.

The FDA ensures that diagnostic and blood-screening assays for HIV accurately detect and/or measure HIV in blood and other bodily fluids, including urine and saliva. The ELISA and Western blot antibody tests diagnose HIV exposure or infection in individuals. Other tests, such as polymerase chain reaction (PCR) viral load and HIV genotyping, are used to monitor patients' progress. PCR uses a heat-resistant bacterial enzyme to amplify the copies of target stretches of genetic material to detectable amounts. HIV genotyping tests blood from HIV-infected people for HIV strains associated with certain patterns of resistance. A variety of screening tests, including NAT, ELISA, and PCR, are used to prevent infected blood from entering blood banks.

Bodily Fluid Tests

In June 1998 the FDA approved a urine-based diagnostic kit for HIV marketed by Calypte Biomedical Corporation that does not require confirmation by a blood test. Urine tests are easier to use and cost less than blood tests. According to the National Institutes of Health, there is no evidence that HIV is spread through urine. Therefore, the chances of accidental infection through needle sticks or the handling of samples are lessened. The urine test and its urine-based confirmation test, like most blood tests, recognize the existence of antibodies, not the actual virus.

The test is marketed to life insurance companies, clinical laboratories, public health agencies, the military, immigration authorities, and the criminal justice system. In July 2005 Calypte began marketing its products in developing countries; however, as of October 2013, Calypte rapid test products, which detect HIV-1 and HIV-2 antibodies in the blood, saliva, and urine, were not yet available in the United States. Calypte also manufactures an enzyme immunoassay developed by the CDC that can distinguish between recent and established HIV-1 infections.

According to the press release "Calypte Biomedical Announces Successful Conclusion of Internal Trials" (March 2, 2011, http://globenewswire.com), Calypte announced in March 2011 the successful completion of studies of its saliva rapid test, which indicated that the test is 100% accurate.

In 2013 Calypte (http://www.calypte.com/product.html) was developing a rapid test for professional use at its Portland, Oregon, facility. An over-the-counter version for consumers was slated to follow. In September 2007 the U.S. Agency for International Development (USAID) placed the Calypte oral test on its rapid HIV test waiver list, which, under the U.S. Acquisition and Assistance Policy Directive,

permits the test to be used in USAID-funded projects. The USAID decision allows countries whose governments have approved the test to purchase it with funds from the President's Emergency Plan for AIDS Relief (this program was launched in 2003 to combat global HIV/AIDS).

Home Testing

The FDA notes in "Testing for HIV" (http://www.fda.gov/biologicsbloodvaccines/safetyavailability/hivhometestkits/ucm126460.htm) that as of August 2013, it had approved only one method of home testing for HIV-1: the Home Access Express HIV-1 Test System, produced by the Home Access Health Corporation. The FDA warned that the more than one dozen unapproved home HIV tests advertised could produce inaccurate results. Users mail an anonymous blood sample to a laboratory and receive results seven days after the sample arrives at the laboratory, or if they choose the "express" option, results are available the same day the sample arrives at the laboratory. Proponents of home testing state that it offers the advantages of privacy and ease of use. Critics of home testing point out that it is expensive; a kit costs as much as $65 and may be prohibitively expensive for poorer populations—for whom such a test is most needed. Critics also question the impersonal practice of relaying HIV-positive results and follow-up counseling by telephone.

In July 2012 the FDA approved the first rapid-response test for home use. The OraQuick In-Home HIV Test does not require sending a sample to a laboratory for analysis. Using a sample of saliva, the kit provides a test result in 20 to 40 minutes and is approved for over-the-counter sale in stores and online. The FDA observes that positive test results using this home test must be confirmed by follow-up laboratory-based testing. It also cautions that the test can give a false negative result (reporting no infection when HIV infection is present) for a number of reasons, including HIV infection within three months or less before testing.

Rapid-Response Tests for Use in Clinics

The FDA has approved a number of rapid-response tests that are designed for use in clinics. The first test to be approved is manufactured by Murex Diagnostics Inc. This test detects the presence of HIV antibodies in about 10 minutes. The test is as accurate as the standard Western blot test. However, because the Western blot test also looks for protein bands, this test remains the absolute antibody-based indicator of HIV.

Another similar rapid-response test kit, developed and manufactured by the Canadian-based MedMira Inc., was granted FDA approval in April 2003 for sale in the United States. The kit is also approved in China, where HIV infection rates dramatically increased during the first decade of the 21st century.

TABLE 2.5

FDA-approved rapid HIV tests, 2013

	FDA approval received	Specimen type	Sensitivity*	Specificity*	Manufacturer	Approved for HIV-2 detection?
OraQuick Advance Rapid HIV-1/2 Antibody Test	Nov 2002	Oral fluid	99.3%	99.80%	OraSure Technologies, Inc. www.orasure.com	Yes
		Whole blood (finger stick or venipuncture)	99.6%	100.00%		
		Plasma	99.6%	99.90%		
Uni-Gold Recombigen HIV	Dec 2003	Whole blood (finger stick or venipuncture)	100.0%	99.70%	Trinity Biotech www.unigoldhiv.com	No
		Serum & plasma	100.0%	99.80%		
Reveal G-3 Rapid HIV-1	Apr 2003	Serum	99.8%	99.10%	MedMira, Inc. www.medmira.com	No
		Plasma	99.8%	98.60%		
MultiSpot HIV-1/HIV-2 Rapid Test	Nov 2004	Serum	100.0%	99.93%	BioRad Laboratories www.biorad.com	Yes-differentiates HIV-1 from HIV-2
		Plasma	100.0%	99.91%		
Clearview HIV 1/2 STAT-PAK	May 2006	Whole blood (finger stick or venipuncture)	99.7%	99.90%	Inverness Medical Professional Diagnostics www.invernessmedicalpd.com	Yes
		Serum & plasma	99.7%	99.90%		
Clearview COMPLETE HIV 1/2	May 2006	Whole blood (finger stick or venipuncture)	99.7%	99.90%	Inverness Medical Professional Diagnostics www.invernessmedicalpd.com	Yes
		Serum & plasma	99.7%	99.90%		
Alere Determine HIV-1/2	Aug 2013	Serum, plasma or whole blood	100.0%	99.75%	Alere	Yes-differentiates HIV-1 from HIV-2

FDA = U.S. Food and Drug Administration.
*Sensitivity is the probability that the test result will be reactive if the specimen is a true positive; specificity is the probability that the test result will be nonreactive if the specimen is a true negative. Data are from the FDA summary basis of approval, for HIV-1 only.
Note: Trade names are for identification purposes only and do not imply endorsement. This information was compiled from package inserts and direct calls to manufacturers.

SOURCE: Adapted from "FDA-Approved Rapid HIV Antibody Screening Tests, February 4, 2008," in *Rapid HIV Testing*, Centers for Disease Control and Prevention, February 15, 2008, http://www.cdc.gov/hiv/topics/testing/rapid/pdf/RT_Comparison-Chart_2-4-08.pdf (accessed July 9, 2013)

Table 2.5 lists the rapid HIV tests that had been approved by the FDA as of 2008. It also shows the bodily fluids that can be used and the sensitivity and specificity of each of the rapid HIV tests. Sensitivity is the ability or extent to which a diagnostic test detects a disease when it is truly present. Specificity is the ability or extent to which a diagnostic test excludes the presence of a disease when it is truly not present. In other words, a sensitive test will produce a positive test result when the patient has the disease, whereas a specific test will give a negative result when the patient does not have the disease.

In August 2013 the FDA approved another rapid test, the Alere Determine HIV-1/2 Ag/Ab Combo test, which is the first test to detect antigens to both HIV-1 and HIV-2 simultaneously. HIV-1 is responsible for the majority of HIV infections worldwide. HIV-2 is largely reported in West Africa; however, cases of HIV-2 infection have occurred in North America and Europe.

Rapid HIV tests are used more frequently in other countries, such as China. In developing countries quick-response tests are used to screen blood before transfusions and to screen pregnant women so medical interventions can be given to prevent mother-to-child transmission of the virus. They are also used in rural clinics.

Promoting HIV Testing

National HIV Testing Day (2013, http://aids.gov/news-and-events/awareness-days/hiv-testing-day/) has been celebrated on June 27 of each year since 1995. AIDS.gov describes how to plan the HIV/AIDS awareness activities and directs people to HIV information and resources, including testing sites and other services. The CDC also has an information and referral website (http://hivtest.cdc.gov/) that answers frequently asked questions about HIV infection and AIDS and locates test centers by zip code.

Choosing Not to Be Tested

Despite efforts to encourage HIV testing, the CDC reports in "HIV in the United States: At a Glance" (April 23, 2013, http://www.cdc.gov/hiv/statistics/basics/ataglance.html) that one out of five people living with HIV infection are unaware of their status because they have not been tested. The reasons for not being tested include denial of HIV risk factors, stigma and fear of testing positive, and lack of access to testing. In "Why Youths Aren't Getting Tested for HIV" (CNN.com, February 19, 2013), Sari Zeidler offers another reason: physicians' difficulty talking about sexually transmitted infections, especially with gay, bisexual, and transgendered men. This discomfort may result in missed opportunities to test people who are at risk for HIV infection.

Revised Recommendations for HIV Testing

In 2006 the CDC revised its recommendations for HIV testing, which were published by Bernard M. Branson et al. in "Revised Recommendations for HIV Testing of Adults, Adolescents, and Pregnant Women in Health-Care

Settings" (*Morbidity and Mortality Weekly Report*, vol. 55, no. RR-14, September 22, 2006). The 2006 recommendations updated and replaced guidelines issued in 1993. The major revisions from the 1993 guidelines are to advise routine HIV screening of adults, adolescents, and pregnant women in health care settings in the United States; to screen people who are at high risk for HIV infection at least annually; to eliminate the requirement for separate written consent for HIV testing, making general consent sufficient to permit HIV testing; and to remove the requirement to provide prevention counseling as part of HIV screening and testing in health care settings. The 2006 guidelines also advise that HIV screening be part of routine prenatal screening for all pregnant women and that repeat screening during the third trimester of pregnancy be performed in areas where there are high rates of HIV infection among pregnant women.

In 2013 the CDC urged community health centers (CHCs) to implement routine HIV testing consistent with the 2006 recommendations. In *Implementation of Routine HIV Testing in Health Care Settings: Issues for Community Health Centers* (January 2011, http://www.cdc.gov/hiv/topics/testing/resources/guidelines/pdf/routinehivtestng.pdf), the CDC explains that CHCs provide primary care for more than 16 million people, including vulnerable populations that may be at high risk of HIV infection. The CDC developed a plan as well as tools and resources that CHCs can use to institute routine HIV screening. Figure 2.3 shows a roadmap for implementing routine HIV testing and following up on test results.

Test Tracks HIV/AIDS Progression

In June 1996 the FDA approved a test to help determine how fast an HIV infection will progress to full-blown AIDS. Developed by Roche Diagnostic Systems Inc., the Amplicor HIV-1 monitor test is not intended to screen for HIV or to confirm an HIV diagnosis. Instead, the test detects the amount of HIV in the blood (the viral load) by measuring HIV genetic material. An increased viral load indicates the advancement of the infection toward AIDS and an increasing predisposition to develop OIs. The test is based on a technique developed in 1984 called the polymerase chain reaction, which can be completed in less than one hour. This test was the first PCR-based test to be approved.

FDA approval was granted in 1997 to expand the use of the test as an aid in managing HIV in patients undergoing ART. In 1999 a more sensitive version of the test became available, and this test has been widely used since then—to help evaluate and track the progression of HIV infection and disease and to predict the risk of complications and OIs.

In "Detection of Drug Resistance Mutations at Low Plasma HIV-1 RNA Load in a European Multicentre

FIGURE 2.3

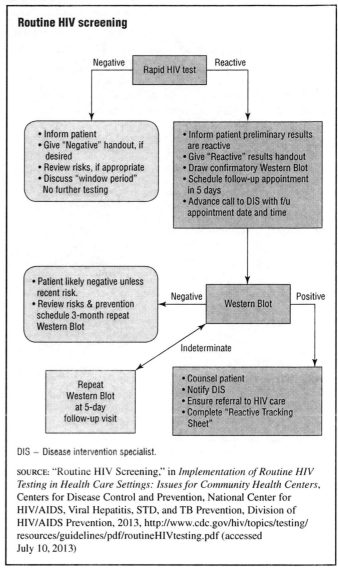

Routine HIV screening

DIS – Disease intervention specialist.

SOURCE: "Routine HIV Screening," in *Implementation of Routine HIV Testing in Health Care Settings: Issues for Community Health Centers*, Centers for Disease Control and Prevention, National Center for HIV/AIDS, Viral Hepatitis, STD, and TB Prevention, Division of HIV/AIDS Prevention, 2013, http://www.cdc.gov/hiv/topics/testing/resources/guidelines/pdf/routineHIVtesting.pdf (accessed July 10, 2013)

Cohort Study" (*Journal of Antimicrobial Chemotherapy*, vol. 66, no. 8, August 2011), Mattia C. F. Prosperi et al. report that although there are not yet conclusive data to support the clinical utility of this approach, "testing at low viral load may identify emerging antiretroviral drug resistance at an early stage," when prompt treatment changes may most effectively reduce the accumulation of resistance and viral adaptive changes.

World Health Organization and U.S. Preventive Services Task Force Guidelines

In 2013 the WHO issued new guidelines for preventing and treating HIV infection. Gottfried Hirnschall et al. detail in "The Next Generation of the World Health Organization's Global Antiretroviral Guidance" (*Journal of the International AIDS Society*, vol. 16, June 30, 2013) the more than 50 new recommendations, including guidelines for HIV testing, using ART for prevention, linking individuals to HIV care and treatment services, and initiating, maintaining, and monitoring ART. The updated guidelines are based on new evidence of the benefits of earlier ART and new testing approaches and technologies, such as CD4 point-of-care tests, which enable easier access to HIV testing and care.

The U.S. Preventive Services Task Force (USPSTF) also updated its HIV screening guidelines in 2013. In "Screening for HIV" (April 2013, http://www.uspreventive servicestaskforce.org/uspstf13/hiv/hivfinalrs.htm), the USPSTF recommends that clinicians screen all adolescents and adults aged 15 to 65 years for HIV infection. Younger adolescents and older adults who are at increased risk should also be screened. Furthermore, the USPSTF advises clinicians to screen all pregnant women for HIV.

CHAPTER 3
PATTERNS AND TRENDS IN HIV/AIDS SURVEILLANCE

DETERMINING THE NUMBER OF PEOPLE INFECTED WITH HIV

The Centers for Disease Control and Prevention (CDC) keeps track of the number of people in the United States who are infected with HIV, the virus that causes AIDS. These CDC figures, which have always been acknowledged as estimates, have been criticized as being inaccurate—either too high or too low. Nonetheless, the historical continuity of CDC data permits trend analyses. Therefore, when viewed over a number of years, the figures provide a reasonable indication of the progress of the disease in the United States.

Estimates of HIV infection are important because they directly influence public health and medical resource allocation as well as political and economic decisions. Definitive figures are difficult to obtain because laws prevent testing for HIV without consent and permission. Furthermore, many people are understandably reluctant to participate in community or household surveys because of confidentiality concerns and fear of losing or failing to obtain insurance coverage.

Health officials contend that knowing the prevalence of HIV infections (prevalence is a measure of all cases of illness existing at a given point in time) is not as crucial as knowing whether the number of HIV infections is rising or falling. The rate at which people develop HIV/AIDS during a specified period is known as the incidence rate. The CDC explains in "HIV Surveillance Supported by the Division of HIV/AIDS Prevention" (June 21, 2013, http://www.cdc.gov/hiv/statistics/recommendations/publications.html) that before April 2008 estimates were based on reports from states that mandated confidential reporting of HIV cases, along with other small studies and surveys. Beginning in April 2008 all jurisdictions implemented universal confidential name-based HIV infection reporting, and *HIV Surveillance Report: Diagnoses of HIV Infection in the United States and Dependent Areas,*

2011 (February 2013, http://www.cdc.gov/hiv/surveillance/resources/reports/2011report/pdf/2011_HIV_Surveillance_Report_vol_23.pdf) was the first of the CDC's annual reports to include data on the diagnoses of HIV from all 50 states and six U.S. dependent areas.

CDC data through 2010 indicate that an estimated 888,921 adults and adolescents were living with HIV infection. (See Figure 3.1.) During this same period, 2,936 children under the age of 13 years were living with HIV infection. (See Figure 3.2.)

The prevalence rate of HIV infection among adults and adolescents was estimated at 342.2 per 100,000 population at the end of 2010. Figure 3.1 shows that the rates of HIV infection varied widely from state to state, from 32.7 per 100,000 in North Dakota to 810 per 100,000 in New York.

The CDC also compiles figures on the numbers of people living with AIDS. Figure 3.3 shows that 498,704 adults and adolescents were living with AIDS at the end of 2010. According to the CDC, in *Epidemiology of HIV Infection through 2011* (January 14, 2013, http://www.cdc.gov/hiv/pdf/statistics_surveillance_Epi-HIV-infection.pdf), 463 children under the age of 13 years were living with AIDS at the end of 2010.

AIDS CASE NUMBERS

The first cases of what came to be recognized as AIDS were reported in the United States in June 1981. Five young, homosexual males in California were diagnosed with *Pneumocystis carinii* pneumonia and other opportunistic infections. The CDC notes in *HIV/AIDS Surveillance Report: U.S. HIV and AIDS Cases Reported through December 1997* (1997, http://www.cdc.gov/hiv/topics/surveillance/resources/reports/pdf/hivsur92.pdf) that by August 1989 approximately 100,000 cases of AIDS had been reported to the agency. By December 1997 that

FIGURE 3.1

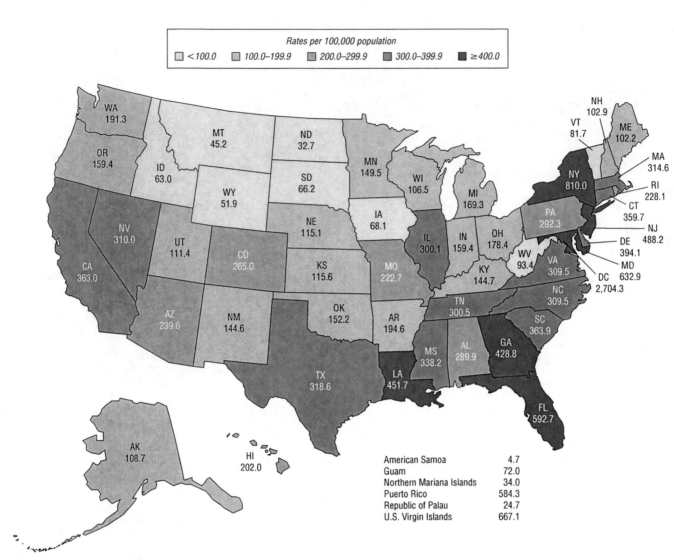

Adults and adolescents living with diagnosed HIV infection, yearend 2010

[United States and 6 dependent areas. Population = 888,921.]

Total rate = 342.2

Rates per 100,000 population

☐ <100.0   ☐ 100.0–199.9   ☐ 200.0–299.9   ☐ 300.0–399.9   ■ ≥400.0

American Samoa	4.7
Guam	72.0
Northern Mariana Islands	34.0
Puerto Rico	584.3
Republic of Palau	24.7
U.S. Virgin Islands	667.1

Note: Data include persons with a diagnosis of HIV infection regardless of stage of disease at diagnosis. All displayed data have been statistically adjusted to account for reporting delays, but not for incomplete reporting.

SOURCE: "Adults and Adolescents Living with Diagnosed HIV Infection, Year-end 2010—United States and 6 Dependent Areas," in *Epidemiology of HIV Infection through 2011*, Centers for Disease Control and Prevention, National Center for HIV/AIDS, Viral Hepatitis, STD, and TB Prevention, Division of HIV/AIDS Prevention, June 28, 2013, http://www.cdc.gov/hiv/pdf/statistics_epidemiology_of_infection_through_2011.pdf (accessed July 7, 2013)

number had risen to 641,086; of these, 390,692 people had died. Cumulatively, through 2011 there were 1,155,792 reported cases of AIDS in the United States—1,146,271 among adults and adolescents and 9,521 among children under the age of 13 years. (See Table 3.1.) According to the CDC, in *HIV Surveillance Report: Diagnoses of HIV Infection in the United States and Dependent Areas, 2011,* as of 2010, 658,992 people had died of the disease.

During the mid-1990s the number of AIDS cases rose dramatically. This surge was not an actual numerical increase, but was due to the expanded 1993 AIDS surveillance definition, which added diseases and conditions that had not been part of the previous definition of AIDS. By the late 1990s the number of AIDS cases leveled off and began to decline, probably as a result of the increasing use of antiretroviral therapy, which delays the progression of HIV infection. Between 2008 and 2011 the number of cases diagnosed each year decreased, from 50,501 in 2008 to 49,273 in 2011, and the rate per 100,000 population decreased slightly from 16.6 in 2008

FIGURE 3.2

Children under 13 years of age living with diagnosed HIV infection, yearend 2010

[United States and 6 dependent areas. Population = 2,936.]

Total rate = 5.5

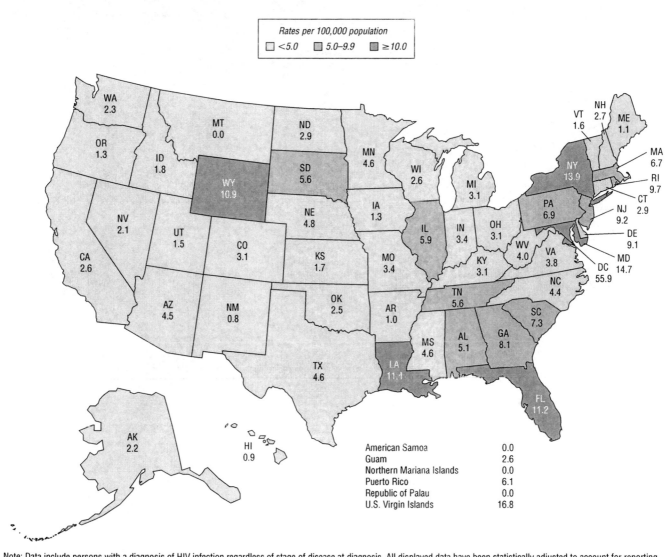

Rates per 100,000 population

□ <5.0   ▨ 5.0–9.9   ■ ≥10.0

American Samoa	0.0
Guam	2.6
Northern Mariana Islands	0.0
Puerto Rico	6.1
Republic of Palau	0.0
U.S. Virgin Islands	16.8

Note: Data include persons with a diagnosis of HIV infection regardless of stage of disease at diagnosis. All displayed data have been statistically adjusted to account for reporting delays, but not for incomplete reporting.

SOURCE: "Rates of Children Aged <13 Years Living with Diagnosed HIV Infection, Year-end 2010—United States and 6 Dependent Areas," in *Epidemiology of HIV Infection through 2011*, Centers for Disease Control and Prevention, National Center for HIV/AIDS, Viral Hepatitis, STD, and TB Prevention, Division of HIV/AIDS Prevention, June 28, 2013, http://www.cdc.gov/hiv/pdf/statistics_epidemiology_of_infection_through_2011.pdf (accessed July 7, 2013)

to 15.8 in 2011. (See Table 3.2.) The numbers of AIDS diagnoses also decreased during this same period, with the rate per 100,000 population falling from 10.7 in 2008 to 10.3 in 2011. (See Table 3.1.)

THE NATURE OF THE EPIDEMIC

Changes in the distribution of HIV infection illustrate the increasing diversity of those affected by the epidemic. The CDC notes in "Current Trends Update: Acquired Immunodeficiency Syndrome—United States, 1981–1990"

(*Morbidity and Mortality Weekly Report*, vol. 40, no. 22, June 7, 1991) that all the 189 AIDS cases reported in 1981 in the United States were males. Three-fourths (76%) of them were men who had sex with men (MSM) living in New York and California. In 1990, of the 43,339 AIDS cases reported by all states, approximately 30% were from New York and California, 11.5% were women, and about 2% were children. In 1999 the proportions of reported cases among women, African Americans, Hispanics, and people exposed through heterosexual contact all increased. By contrast, the

FIGURE 3.3

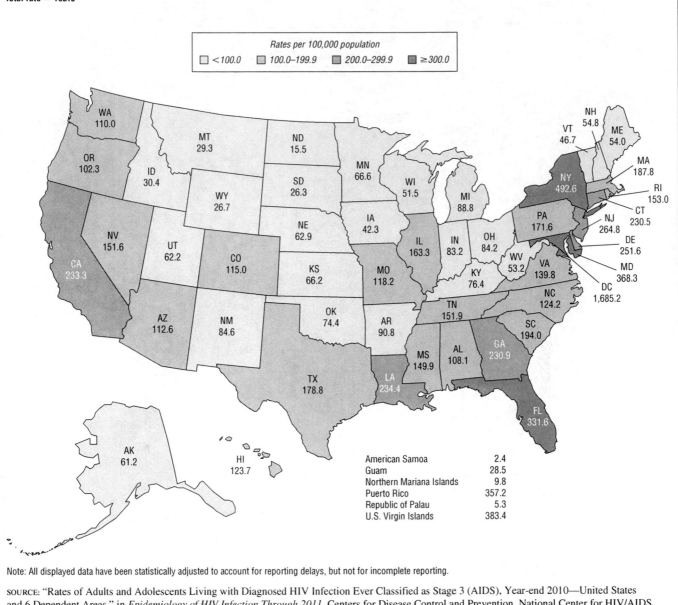

Adults and adolescents living with diagnosed AIDS, yearend 2010

[United States and 6 dependent areas. Population = 498,704.]

Total rate = 192.0

Rates per 100,000 population

☐ <100.0 ▨ 100.0–199.9 ▨ 200.0–299.9 ▨ ≥300.0

American Samoa	2.4
Guam	28.5
Northern Mariana Islands	9.8
Puerto Rico	357.2
Republic of Palau	5.3
U.S. Virgin Islands	383.4

Note: All displayed data have been statistically adjusted to account for reporting delays, but not for incomplete reporting.

SOURCE: "Rates of Adults and Adolescents Living with Diagnosed HIV Infection Ever Classified as Stage 3 (AIDS), Year-end 2010—United States and 6 Dependent Areas," in *Epidemiology of HIV Infection Through 2011*, Centers for Disease Control and Prevention, National Center for HIV/AIDS, Viral Hepatitis, STD, and TB Prevention, Division of HIV/AIDS Prevention, June 28, 2013, http://www.cdc.gov/hiv/pdf/statistics_epidemiology_of_infection_through_2011.pdf (accessed July 7, 2013)

percentage of reported cases among whites and MSM declined somewhat.

Table 3.1 and Table 3.2 show that between 2008 and 2011 MSM sexual contact continued to account for the largest proportion of diagnosed cases; however, there were still substantial numbers of HIV and AIDS diagnoses attributable to injection drug use, and high-risk heterosexual contact also grew among males and females. By contrast, the number of cases diagnosed in children under the age of 13 years declined during this period.

Regional Differences

AIDS cases have been reported in all 50 states, the District of Columbia, and dependent areas. The distribution of cases, however, is far from even. In 2011 the highest rate by far was in the District of Columbia, where the rate was 82.5 per 100,000 population. (See Figure 3.4.) Rates were highest in Georgia, Maryland, Louisiana, New York, and Florida, with respective rates of 22.8, 20.1, 18.4, 18.4, and 18.1, and lowest in North Dakota (0.6), Montana (1.2), and Idaho (1.4). Figure 3.5 shows the corresponding AIDS rates for children under the age

TABLE 3.1

AIDS diagnoses by selected characteristics, 2008–11 and cumulative

	2008 No.	2008 Estimated[a] No.	2008 Rate	2009 No.	2009 Estimated[a] No.	2009 Rate	2010 No.	2010 Estimated[a] No.	2010 Rate	2011 No.	2011 Estimated[a] No.	2011 Rate	Cumulative[b] No.	Cumulative Est. No.[a]
Age at diagnosis (yr)														
<13	36	37	0.1	13	14	0.0	22	24	0.0	12	15	0.0	9,483	9,521
13–14	59	62	0.8	44	48	0.6	45	49	0.6	39	49	0.6	1,417	1,452
15–19	442	458	2.1	433	456	2.1	443	479	2.2	397	510	2.4	7,890	8,129
20–24	1,720	1,776	8.3	1,886	1,975	9.2	1,910	2,072	9.5	1,915	2,425	10.9	45,917	46,957
25–29	3,130	3,232	15.1	3,047	3,189	14.7	2,853	3,099	14.7	2,692	3,433	16.1	133,343	135,135
30–34	3,801	3,923	20.1	3,566	3,732	18.8	3,269	3,555	17.7	3,162	4,001	19.5	217,408	219,784
35–39	4,863	5,028	24.1	4,239	4,436	21.6	3,671	3,975	19.8	3,218	4,071	20.8	236,996	239,749
40–44	5,582	5,776	27.0	4,887	5,130	24.4	4,255	4,630	22.1	3,785	4,783	22.7	196,730	199,727
45–49	4,960	5,136	22.5	4,719	4,949	21.7	4,223	4,592	20.3	3,978	4,994	22.5	130,981	133,612
50–54	3,349	3,463	16.2	3,397	3,566	16.4	3,116	3,387	15.2	2,862	3,567	15.8	76,080	77,843
55–59	1,923	1,990	10.7	1,884	1,978	10.4	1,705	1,854	9.4	1,761	2,198	10.9	41,364	42,372
60–64	967	998	6.6	902	947	6.0	890	967	5.7	892	1,107	6.2	21,871	22,369
≥65	742	767	2.0	752	791	2.0	720	781	1.9	722	899	2.2	18,731	19,143
Race/ethnicity														
American Indian/Alaska Native	153	156	6.7	123	126	5.4	134	142	6.2	128	146	6.4	3,741	3,787
Asian[c]	457	478	3.6	386	408	3.0	363	404	2.7	382	492	3.3	8,789	9,054
Black/African American	15,213	15,711	42.1	14,198	14,861	39.4	13,438	14,558	38.3	12,685	15,958	41.6	477,971	486,282
Hispanic/Latino[d]	6,220	6,482	13.8	6,129	6,476	13.4	5,370	5,902	11.6	4,912	6,355	12.2	198,218	202,182
Native Hawaiian/other Pacific Islander	38	39	9.0	45	48	10.7	34	36	7.3	40	47	9.3	883	901
White	8,676	8,929	4.5	8,094	8,452	4.2	7,135	7,712	3.9	6,698	8,304	4.2	431,084	435,613
Multiple races	817	849	19.2	794	840	18.4	648	708	12.5	590	750	12.9	17,357	17,804
Transmission category														
Male adult or adolescent														
Male-to-male sexual contact	12,279	15,427	—	12,140	15,458	—	11,207	14,934	—	10,654	16,694	—	499,157	555,032
Injection drug use	2,102	2,985	—	1,719	2,563	—	1,466	2,323	—	1,221	2,346	—	163,203	187,938
Male-to-male sexual contact and injection drug use	1,425	1,714	—	1,188	1,491	—	1,050	1,393	—	856	1,392	—	74,468	80,902
Heterosexual contact[e]	2,709	3,724	—	2,562	3,581	—	2,149	3,256	—	1,982	3,526	—	60,901	77,521
Other[f]	4,713	165	—	4,532	134	—	4,400	123	—	4,364	131	—	102,366	11,975
Subtotal	**23,228**	**24,015**	**19.6**	**22,141**	**23,226**	**18.7**	**20,272**	**22,030**	**17.6**	**19,077**	**24,088**	**19.1**	**900,185**	**913,368**
Female adult or adolescent														
Injection drug use	1,310	2,041	—	1,101	1,776	—	931	1,582	—	782	1,615	—	73,382	89,800
Heterosexual contact[e]	4,154	6,432	—	3,849	6,073	—	3,365	5,697	—	2,947	6,206	—	104,037	136,675
Other[f]	2,846	119	—	2,665	122	—	2,532	130	—	2,617	129	—	51,122	6,427
Subtotal	**8,310**	**8,593**	**6.7**	**7,615**	**7,971**	**6.2**	**6,828**	**7,410**	**5.6**	**6,346**	**7,949**	**6.0**	**228,541**	**232,902**
Child (<13 yrs at diagnosis)														
Perinatal	31	32	—	12	13	—	17	19	—	10	12	—	8,623	8,658
Other[g]	5	5	—	1	1	—	5	5	—	2	2	—	860	863
Subtotal	**36**	**37**	**0.1**	**13**	**14**	**0.0**	**22**	**24**	**0.0**	**12**	**15**	**0.0**	**9,483**	**9,521**
Region of residence														
Northeast	7,188	7,701	14.0	6,641	7,255	13.1	5,787	6,610	11.9	5,117	6,849	12.3	342,363	349,250
Midwest	3,743	3,796	5.7	3,695	3,797	5.7	3,383	3,590	5.4	3,221	3,876	5.8	119,496	120,772
South	14,972	15,272	13.6	13,899	14,324	12.6	13,150	13,985	12.2	12,867	15,855	13.7	447,686	453,737
West	5,671	5,875	8.3	5,534	5,835	8.2	4,802	5,278	7.3	4,230	5,472	7.5	228,666	232,033
Total[h]	**31,574**	**32,645**	**10.7**	**29,769**	**31,211**	**10.2**	**27,122**	**29,463**	**9.5**	**25,435**	**32,052**	**10.3**	**1,138,211[i]**	**1,155,792**

[a]Estimated numbers resulted from statistical adjustment that accounted for reporting delays and missing transmission category, but not for incomplete reporting. Rates are per 100,000 population. Rates are not calculated by transmission category because of the lack of denominator data.
[b]From the beginning of the epidemic through 2011.
[c]Includes Asian/Pacific Islander legacy cases.
[d]Hispanics/Latinos can be of any race.
[e]Heterosexual contact with a person known to have, or to be at high risk for, HIV infection.
[f]Includes hemophilia, blood transfusion, perinatal exposure, and risk factor not reported or not identified.
[g]Includes hemophilia, blood transfusion, and risk factor not reported or not identified.
[h]Because column totals for estimated numbers were calculated independently of the values for the subpopulations, the values in each column may not sum to the column total.
[i]Includes persons of unknown race/ethnicity.

SOURCE: "Table 2a. Stage 3 (AIDS), by Year of Diagnosis and Selected Characteristics, 2008–2011 and Cumulative—United States," in *HIV Surveillance Report: Diagnoses of HIV Infection in the United States and Dependent Areas, 2011*, vol. 23, Centers for Disease Control and Prevention, National Center for HIV/AIDS, Viral Hepatitis, STD, and TB Prevention, Division of HIV/AIDS Prevention, February 2013, http://www.cdc.gov/hiv/pdf/statistics_2011_HIV_Surveillance_Report_vol_23.pdf (accessed July 7, 2013)

TABLE 3.2

HIV infection by year of diagnosis and selected characteristics, 2008–11

| | 2008 | | | 2009 | | | 2010 | | | 2011 | | |
| | No. | Estimated[a] | | No. | Estimated[a] | | No. | Estimated[a] | | No. | Estimated[a] | |
		No.	Rate		No.	Rate		No.	Rate		No.	Rate
Age at diagnosis (yr)												
<13	245	252	0.5	204	213	0.4	209	226	0.4	165	192	0.4
13–14	42	43	0.5	29	30	0.4	41	45	0.5	44	53	0.6
15–19	2,195	2,252	10.4	2,148	2,234	10.4	2,051	2,185	9.9	1,936	2,240	10.4
20–24	6,530	6,696	31.4	6,675	6,950	32.3	6,977	7,472	34.4	6,943	8,054	36.4
25–29	6,890	7,073	33.0	6,490	6,764	31.2	6,250	6,713	31.7	6,397	7,484	35.2
30–34	6,093	6,260	32.1	5,676	5,913	29.7	5,401	5,800	28.9	5,311	6,209	30.3
35–39	6,434	6,596	31.6	5,603	5,844	28.5	4,990	5,373	26.8	4,515	5,285	27.0
40–44	6,785	6,966	32.6	5,936	6,200	29.5	5,157	5,560	26.6	4,909	5,753	27.4
45–49	5,921	6,071	26.6	5,195	5,418	23.7	4,741	5,112	22.6	4,734	5,564	25.1
50–54	3,804	3,900	18.2	3,600	3,757	17.3	3,411	3,664	16.4	3,383	3,951	17.5
55–59	2,254	2,311	12.5	2,111	2,202	11.6	2,024	2,180	11.0	1,979	2,312	11.4
60–64	1,132	1,158	7.7	992	1,034	6.5	1,037	1,121	6.6	1,057	1,229	6.9
≥65	901	926	2.4	811	850	2.1	762	818	2.0	808	948	2.3
Race/ethnicity												
American Indian/Alaska Native	217	225	9.6	195	205	8.7	208	222	9.8	188	212	9.3
Asian	791	816	6.1	717	753	5.5	721	780	5.3	821	982	6.5
Black/African American	23,848	24,419	65.4	21,727	22,618	60.0	20,525	22,030	58.0	19,846	23,168	60.4
Hispanic/Latino[b]	9,405	9,691	20.6	9,061	9,495	19.6	8,548	9,225	18.2	8,555	10,159	19.5
Native Hawaiian/other Pacific Islander	77	79	17.9	78	80	17.9	58	62	12.4	68	78	15.3
White	13,923	14,277	7.2	12,846	13,371	6.7	12,172	13,069	6.6	11,996	13,846	7.0
Multiple races	965	994	22.5	846	886	19.4	819	879	15.6	707	827	14.2
Transmission category												
Male adult or adolescent												
Male-to-male sexual contact	21,891	28,077	—	21,219	27,545	—	20,813	27,725	—	21,005	30,573	—
Injection drug use	1,916	3,039	—	1,474	2,570	—	1,252	2,305	—	1,052	2,220	—
Male-to-male sexual contact and injection drug use	1,307	1,731	—	1,125	1,547	—	1,045	1,466	—	916	1,407	—
Heterosexual contact[c]	3,458	5,200	—	3,035	4,691	—	2,710	4,391	—	2,600	4,588	—
Other[d]	8,565	55	—	8,042	38	—	7,611	31	—	7,648	36	—
Subtotal	**37,137**	**38,104**	**31.0**	**34,895**	**36,392**	**29.4**	**33,431**	**35,918**	**28.7**	**33,221**	**38,825**	**30.8**
Female adult or adolescent												
Injection drug use	1,143	2,035	—	890	1,700	—	721	1,449	—	613	1,428	—
Heterosexual contact[c]	5,567	10,078	—	4,672	9,084	—	4,285	8,659	—	3,703	8,814	—
Other[d]	5,134	33	—	4,809	20	—	4,405	17	—	4,479	15	—
Subtotal	**11,844**	**12,146**	**9.5**	**10,371**	**10,804**	**8.4**	**9,411**	**10,125**	**7.7**	**8,795**	**10,257**	**7.7**
Child (<13 yrs at diagnosis)												
Perinatal	196	201	—	164	171	—	164	174	—	110	127	—
Other[e]	49	50	—	40	42	—	45	51	—	55	65	—
Subtotal	**245**	**252**	**0.5**	**204**	**213**	**0.4**	**209**	**226**	**0.4**	**165**	**192**	**0.4**
Region of residence												
Northeast	9,936	10,711	19.5	9,088	10,061	18.2	8,431	9,725	17.6	7,989	10,024	18.1
Midwest	5,851	5,902	8.9	5,826	5,933	8.9	5,540	5,774	8.6	5,573	6,237	9.3
South	24,771	25,091	22.4	22,410	22,992	20.3	21,252	22,379	19.5	21,326	24,296	20.9
West	8,668	8,797	12.4	8,146	8,423	11.8	7,828	8,390	11.6	7,293	8,717	12.0
Total[f]	**49,226**	**50,501**	**16.6**	**45,470**	**47,408**	**15.4**	**43,051**	**46,268**	**15.0**	**42,181**	**49,273**	**15.8**

Note: Data include persons with a diagnosis of HIV infection regardless of stage of disease at diagnosis.

[a]Estimated numbers resulted from statistical adjustment that accounted for reporting delays and missing transmission category, but not for incomplete reporting. Rates are per 100,000 population. Rates are not calculated by transmission category because of the lack of denominator data.

[b]Hispanics/Latinos can be of any race.

[c]Heterosexual contact with a person known to have, or to be at high risk for, HIV infection.

[d]Includes hemophilia, blood transfusion, perinatal exposure, and risk factor not reported or not identified.

[e]Includes hemophilia, blood transfusion, and risk factor not reported or not identified.

[f]Because column totals for estimated numbers were calculated independently of the values for the subpopulations, the values in each column may not sum to the column total.

SOURCE: "Table 1a. Diagnoses of HIV Infection, by Year of Diagnosis and Selected Characteristics, 2008–2011—United States," in *HIV Surveillance Report: Diagnoses of HIV Infection in the United States and Dependent Areas, 2011*, vol. 23, Centers for Disease Control and Prevention, National Center for HIV/AIDS, Viral Hepatitis, STD, and TB Prevention, Division of HIV/AIDS Prevention, February 2013, http://www.cdc.gov/hiv/pdf/statistics_2011_HIV_Surveillance_Report_vol_23.pdf (accessed July 7, 2013)

FIGURE 3.4

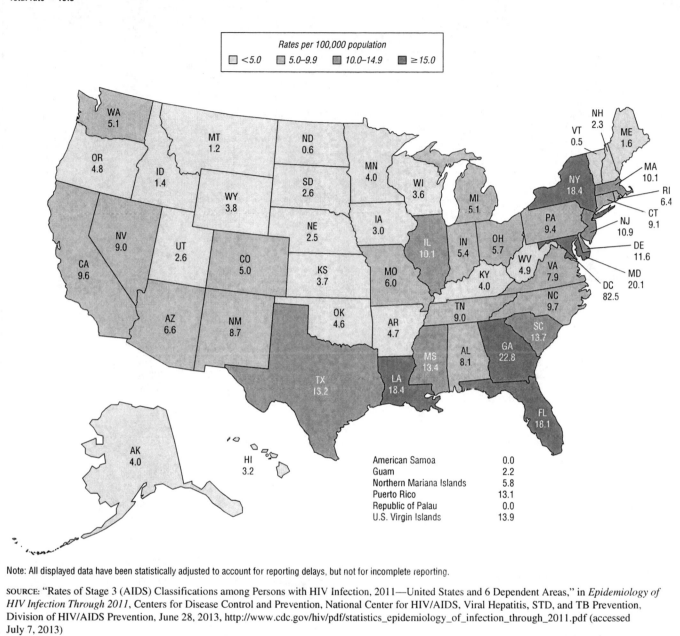

Rates of AIDS in adults and adolescents by state, 2011

[United States and 6 dependent areas. Population = 32,561.]

Total rate = 10.3

Rates per 100,000 population

☐ <5.0   ▨ 5.0–9.9   ▨ 10.0–14.9   ▨ ≥15.0

WA 5.1
MT 1.2
ND 0.6
OR 4.8
ID 1.4
WY 3.8
SD 2.6
MN 4.0
NV 9.0
UT 2.6
CO 5.0
NE 2.5
IA 3.0
WI 3.6
MI 5.1
CA 9.6
AZ 6.6
NM 8.7
KS 3.7
OK 4.6
MO 6.0
IL 10.1
IN 5.4
OH 5.7
KY 4.0
AR 4.7
TN 9.0
MS 13.4
AL 8.1
GA 22.8
SC 13.7
TX 13.2
LA 18.4
FL 18.1
WV 4.9
VA 7.9
NC 9.7
PA 9.4
NY 18.4
VT 0.5
NH 2.3
ME 1.6
MA 10.1
RI 6.4
CT 9.1
NJ 10.9
DE 11.6
MD 20.1
DC 82.5
AK 4.0
HI 3.2

American Samoa   0.0
Guam   2.2
Northern Mariana Islands 5.8
Puerto Rico   13.1
Republic of Palau   0.0
U.S. Virgin Islands   13.9

Note: All displayed data have been statistically adjusted to account for reporting delays, but not for incomplete reporting.

SOURCE: "Rates of Stage 3 (AIDS) Classifications among Persons with HIV Infection, 2011—United States and 6 Dependent Areas," in *Epidemiology of HIV Infection Through 2011*, Centers for Disease Control and Prevention, National Center for HIV/AIDS, Viral Hepatitis, STD, and TB Prevention, Division of HIV/AIDS Prevention, June 28, 2013, http://www.cdc.gov/hiv/pdf/statistics_epidemiology_of_infection_through_2011.pdf (accessed July 7, 2013)

of 13 years at the end of 2010. The estimated rates for children living with AIDS ranged from 0 per 100,000 population in Maine, Montana, Utah, Vermont, Washington, and Wyoming to 19.5 per 100,000 population in the District of Columbia.

RATES IN MAJOR METROPOLITAN AREAS. Most AIDS cases are concentrated in larger metropolitan regions (the city and surrounding suburbs). In 2011 the annual metropolitan AIDS diagnosis rates per 100,000 people were highest on the coasts, such as in the Fort Lauderdale, Florida, division (34.1); the Miami, Florida, division (29.1); the New York–White Plains–Wayne, New York, division (25.1); Baltimore–Towson, Maryland (24.3); the Washington division (22); and the San Francisco, California, division (20.1). (See Table 3.3.) By contrast, the midwestern metropolitan areas displayed some of the lowest rates: Akron, Ohio (2.5), Grand Rapids, Michigan (3.9), and Toledo, Ohio (4.4). Provo–Orem, Utah, had the lowest overall rate (0.9), followed by Boise City–Nampa, Idaho (2.4).

There are several reasons for the higher rates in urban areas. First, metropolitan areas are often more tolerant of

FIGURE 3.5

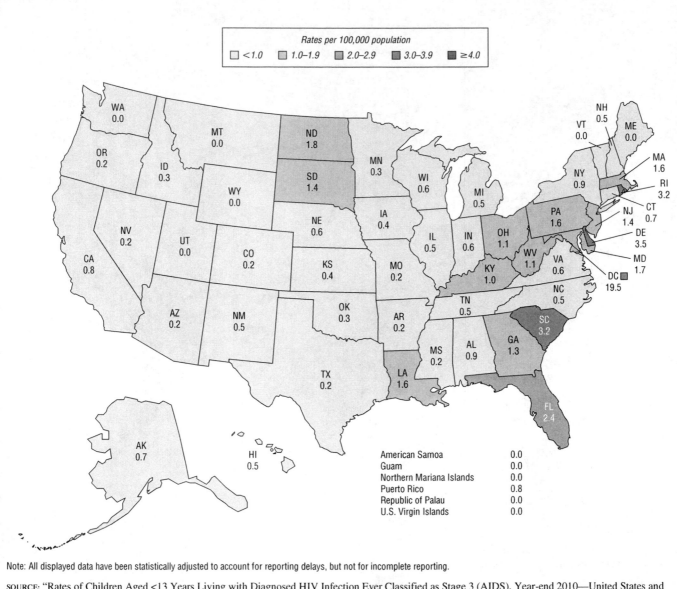

Rates of AIDS in children, by state, 2010

[United States and 6 dependent areas. Population = 463.]

Total rate = 0.9

Rates per 100,000 population

☐ <1.0   ☐ 1.0–1.9   ☐ 2.0–2.9   ☐ 3.0–3.9   ☐ ≥4.0

WA 0.0
MT 0.0
ND 1.8
MN 0.3
NH 0.5
VT 0.0
ME 0.0
OR 0.2
ID 0.3
SD 1.4
WI 0.6
NY 0.9
MA 1.6
RI 3.2
WY 0.0
IA 0.4
MI 0.5
PA 1.6
NJ 1.4
CT 0.7
NV 0.2
NE 0.6
IL 0.5
IN 0.6
OH 1.1
DE 3.5
UT 0.0
CO 0.2
KS 0.4
MO 0.2
WV 1.1
VA 0.6
MD 1.7
CA 0.8
KY 1.0
DC 19.5
AZ 0.2
NM 0.5
OK 0.3
AR 0.2
TN 0.5
NC 0.5
SC 3.2
MS 0.2
AL 0.9
GA 1.3
TX 0.2
LA 1.6
FL 2.4
AK 0.7
HI 0.5

American Samoa	0.0
Guam	0.0
Northern Mariana Islands	0.0
Puerto Rico	0.8
Republic of Palau	0.0
U.S. Virgin Islands	0.0

Note: All displayed data have been statistically adjusted to account for reporting delays, but not for incomplete reporting.

SOURCE: "Rates of Children Aged <13 Years Living with Diagnosed HIV Infection Ever Classified as Stage 3 (AIDS), Year-end 2010—United States and 6 Dependent," in *Epidemiology of HIV Infection through 2011*, Centers for Disease Control and Prevention, National Center for HIV/AIDS, Viral Hepatitis, STD, and TB Prevention, Division of HIV/AIDS Prevention, June 28, 2013, http://www.cdc.gov/hiv/pdf/statistics_epidemiology_of_infection_through_2011.pdf (accessed July 7, 2013)

alternative lifestyles such as those of MSM, a group with high-risk sexual behaviors. Second, large metropolitan areas have greater numbers of people who use injection drugs, which is another risk factor for HIV infection. Third, although HIV infection and transmission are not restricted to more populated areas, people seeking treatment may migrate to these areas for access to medical care and social services.

AIDS Transmission Categories Have Changed

The distribution of AIDS diagnoses by transmission category has changed since the beginning of the epidemic.

In 1985 MSM accounted for about two-thirds of all AIDS diagnoses, but in 1999 it accounted for 40% of diagnoses. (See Figure 3.6.) Beginning in 2001 the percentage of AIDS diagnoses attributable to MSM began to increase and by 2011 it accounted for about half (52%) of all AIDS diagnoses.

AIDS diagnoses attributable to injection drug use grew from 20% to 32% between 1985 and 1993 and subsequently decreased to 13% in 2011. AIDS diagnoses attributable to MSM and injection drug use declined from 9% in 1985 to 4% in 2011. In contrast, the percentage of

TABLE 3.3

Reported AIDS cases and annual rates, by metropolitan area of residence and age category, 2011, and cumulative

Area of residence	Diagnosis, 2011				Diagnosis, cumulative[a]			Prevalence of stage 3 (AIDS) year-end 2010		
					Adults or adolescents	Children	Total			
	No.	Estimated[b]		Rank[d]	Estimated[b]			No.	Estimated[b]	
		No.	Rate[c]		No.	No.	No.		No.	Rate[c]
Akron, OH	16	18	2.5	100	873	1	874	390	375	53.4
Albany–Schenectady–Troy, NY	48	64	7.4	60	2,623	26	2,649	1,170	1,164	133.7
Albuquerque, NM	96	105	11.6	30	1,753	3	1,756	740	722	81.1
Allentown–Bethlehem–Easton, PA–NJ	38	52	6.3	74	1,685	20	1,705	849	848	103.1
Atlanta–Sandy Springs–Marietta, GA	1,001	1,463	27.3	3	28,855	142	28,997	12,888	12,679	239.8
Augusta–Richmond County, GA–SC	90	132	23.4	6	2,311	23	2,334	945	907	162.5
Austin–Round Rock, TX	163	241	13.5	23	5,865	26	5,891	2,666	2,632	152.3
Bakersfield, CA	71	99	11.6	31	2,112	9	2,121	1,276	1,307	155.1
Baltimore–Towson, MD	460	663	24.3	5	24,772	227	24,999	10,925	10,790	397.5
Baton Rouge, LA	230	238	29.4	1	5,002	23	5,025	2,215	2,087	259.4
Birmingham–Hoover, AL	68	78	6.9	66	3,029	25	3,054	1,248	1,192	105.5
Boise City–Nampa, ID	14	15	2.4	101	395	0	395	203	200	32.4
Boston, MA–NH[e]	267	486	10.6	37	16,379	163	16,542	7,129	7,358	161.4
Boston Division	146	268	14.1	—	10,144	100	10,244	4,252	4,385	232.0
Cambridge Division	79	144	9.5	—	3,902	38	3,941	1,812	1,878	124.8
Peabody Division	38	70	9.4	—	1,964	24	1,989	903	937	125.8
Bridgeport–Stamford–Norwalk, CT	74	82	8.9	44	4,215	57	4,272	1,901	1,847	201.1
Buffalo–Niagara Falls, NY	81	105	9.3	41	2,924	21	2,945	1,180	1,170	103.1
Cape Coral–Fort Myers, FL	67	73	11.5	32	2,109	26	2,135	940	919	148.2
Charleston–North Charleston, SC	97	103	15.0	17	2,557	23	2,580	1,143	1,091	163.3
Charlotte–Gastonia–Concord, NC–SC	218	240	13.4	24	4,404	22	4,426	2,112	2,037	115.5
Chattanooga, TN–GA	36	44	8.3	50	1,222	3	1,225	611	598	113.0
Chicago, IL–IN–WI	812	1,162	12.2	27	36,260	266	36,526	15,604	15,390	162.5
Chicago Division	747	1,082	13.7	—	33,985	253	34,238	14,555	14,370	182.1
Gary Division	38	42	6.0	—	1,296	8	1,304	558	534	75.3
Lake Division	27	37	4.3	—	979	5	984	491	486	55.8
Cincinnati–Middletown, OH–KY–IN	136	155	7.3	62	3,531	20	3,551	1,667	1,626	76.2
Cleveland–Elyria–Mentor, OH	108	117	5.6	80	4,941	49	4,990	2,250	2,177	104.9
Colorado Springs, CO	24	26	3.9	91	682	5	687	305	299	45.9
Columbia, SC	149	154	19.9	10	4,135	25	4,160	2,131	2,044	265.5
Columbus, OH	188	206	11.1	35	4,172	22	4,194	1,819	1,761	95.7
Dallas, TX	728	977	15.0	18	24,757	62	24,819	11,039	10,857	169.6
Dallas Division	590	783	18.0	—	19,651	37	19,688	8,835	8,693	204.3
Fort Worth Division	138	194	8.9	—	5,106	25	5,131	2,204	2,163	100.9
Dayton, OH	32	35	4.1	90	1,488	15	1,503	701	679	80.7
Denver–Aurora, CO	176	191	7.4	59	8,122	23	8,145	3,723	3,665	143.5
Des Moines, IA	29	32	5.5	81	676	4	680	332	327	57.1
Detroit, MI	312	343	8.0	53	12,422	77	12,499	5,063	4,863	113.3
Detroit Division	229	249	13.8	—	9,781	60	9,841	3,810	3,645	200.8
Warren Division	83	93	3.8	—	2,641	17	2,658	1,253	1,218	49.2
Durham–Chapel Hill, NC	34	40	7.9	56	1,487	10	1,497	637	617	121.9
El Paso, TX	53	71	8.6	47	1,891	10	1,901	985	972	121.0
Fresno, CA	74	101	10.7	36	2,010	11	2,022	950	979	104.9
Grand Rapids–Wyoming, MI	28	30	3.9	92	1,001	6	1,007	495	484	62.6
Greensboro–High Point, NC	66	73	10.0	39	1,645	19	1,664	735	711	98.0
Greenville, SC	54	55	8.5	49	1,553	4	1,557	718	689	107.9
Harrisburg–Carlisle, PA	46	64	11.5	33	1,544	9	1,553	740	738	134.0
Hartford–West Hartford–East Hartford, CT	92	100	8.2	51	5,753	47	5,800	2,421	2,324	191.7
Honolulu, HI	32	35	3.6	95	2,469	14	2,483	995	975	102.0
Houston–Baytown–Sugar Land, TX	893	1,176	19.3	12	31,644	174	31,818	12,757	12,487	208.9
Indianapolis, IN	151	164	9.2	42	4,653	25	4,678	2,217	2,141	121.6
Jackson, MS	104	114	20.9	8	3,040	30	3,070	1,425	1,363	252.3
Jacksonville, FL	243	272	20.0	9	7,541	78	7,619	3,413	3,317	246.0
Kansas City, MO–KS	143	163	7.9	54	5,791	16	5,807	2,641	2,588	126.9
Knoxville, TN	36	40	5.7	79	1,116	5	1,121	566	551	78.8
Lakeland, FL	74	83	13.6	22	2,332	21	2,353	1,056	1,026	170.1
Lancaster, PA	20	27	5.1	85	885	21	906	413	412	79.2
Las Vegas–Paradise, NV	200	220	11.2	34	5,861	28	5,889	2,889	2,820	144.3
Little Rock–North Little Rock, AR	43	45	6.3	73	1,653	14	1,667	826	796	113.4
Los Angeles, CA	1,098	1,665	12.9	25	68,572	306	68,878	29,388	29,150	226.9
Los Angeles Division	922	1,425	14.4	—	60,344	262	60,606	25,545	25,231	256.8
Santa Ana Division	176	240	7.8	—	8,228	45	8,273	3,843	3,919	129.9
Louisville, KY–IN	78	87	6.7	68	2,899	28	2,927	1,383	1,326	103.1
Madison, WI	14	15	2.6	99	629	5	634	309	300	52.6
McAllen–Edinburg–Pharr, TX	55	72	9.0	43	896	12	908	491	485	62.2
Memphis, TN–MS–AR	270	306	23.1	7	6,504	20	6,524	3,326	3,258	247.1

TABLE 3.3

Reported AIDS cases and annual rates, by metropolitan area of residence and age category, 2011, and cumulative [CONTINUED]

	Diagnosis, 2011				Diagnosis, cumulative[a]			Prevalence of stage 3 (AIDS) year-end 2010		
					Adults or adolescents	Children	Total			
		Estimated[b]				Estimated[b]			Estimated[b]	
Area of residence	No.	No.	Rate[c]	Rank[d]	No.	No.	No.	No.	No.	Rate[c]
Miami, FL	1,453	1,599	28.2	2	65,460	1,008	66,468	27,433	26,692	478.5
Fort Lauderdale Division	551	607	34.1	—	20,046	265	20,311	8,837	8,615	491.7
Miami Division	674	743	29.1	—	34,217	518	34,735	13,819	13,428	536.5
West Palm Beach Division	228	249	18.6	—	11,197	225	11,422	4,777	4,649	351.4
Milwaukee–Waukesha–West Allis, WI	102	114	7.3	61	3,020	19	3,039	1,381	1,337	85.9
Minneapolis–St. Paul–Bloomington, MN–WI	158	176	5.3	83	5,312	23	5,335	2,633	2,590	78.8
Modesto, CA	12	16	3.0	97	831	6	837	415	425	82.5
Nashville–Davidson–Murfreesboro, TN	115	128	7.9	55	4,668	21	4,689	2,590	2,529	158.6
New Haven–Milford, CT	90	102	11.9	29	5,074	76	5,150	2,228	2,157	250.1
New Orleans–Metairie–Kenner, LA	287	301	25.3	4	10,439	71	10,510	4,091	3,888	331.3
New York, NY–NJ–PA	2,785	3,631	19.1	13	225,131	3,034	228,165	84,427	85,741	453.2
Edison Division	85	111	4.7	—	7,650	145	7,796	2,788	2,793	119.2
Nassau Division	156	202	7.1	—	9,305	118	9,422	3,563	3,539	124.8
New York–White Plains—Wayne Division	2,228	2,931	25.1	—	185,376	2,417	187,793	70,708	72,041	621.5
Newark Division	316	387	18.0	—	22,800	354	23,154	7,368	7,368	342.8
North Port–Bradenton–Sarasota, FL	42	48	6.8	67	2,334	29	2,363	1,028	996	141.6
Ogden–Clearfield, UT	3	3	0.6	103	291	4	295	151	149	27.1
Oklahoma City, OK	77	79	6.2	75	2,710	5	2,715	1,113	1,069	85.0
Omaha–Council Bluffs, NE–IA	31	34	3.9	93	1,300	5	1,305	675	665	76.6
Orlando, FL	333	369	17.0	14	10,894	99	10,993	5,240	5,114	239.0
Oxnard–Thousand Oaks–Ventura, CA	19	25	3.0	96	1,207	3	1,210	541	551	66.8
Palm Bay–Melbourne–Titusville, FL	33	35	6.5	70	1,760	11	1,771	801	781	143.7
Philadelphia, PA–NJ–DE–MD	668	904	15.1	16	33,641	323	33,963	15,133	15,051	252.0
Camden Division	68	86	6.9	—	3,733	44	3,777	1,544	1,550	123.9
Philadelphia Division	530	726	18.0	—	26,315	256	26,571	12,078	11,993	298.8
Wilmington Division	70	91	12.9	—	3,593	22	3,615	1,511	1,507	213.4
Phoenix–Mesa–Scottsdale, AZ	273	307	7.2	64	9,432	32	9,464	4,441	4,349	103.3
Pittsburgh, PA	89	117	5.0	87	3,795	20	3,815	1,599	1,592	67.5
Portland–South Portland, ME	14	15	2.9	98	679	1	680	327	322	62.7
Portland–Vancouver–Beaverton, OR–WA	132	145	6.4	72	5,685	10	5,695	2,640	2,596	116.3
Poughkeepsie–Newburgh–Middletown, NY	38	51	7.5	58	3,460	25	3,485	1,347	1,332	198.5
Providence–New Bedford–Fall River, RI–MA	77	107	6.7	69	4,599	44	4,643	2,059	2,040	127.4
Provo–Orem, UT	4	5	0.9	102	141	3	144	77	76	14.3
Raleigh–Cary, NC	98	111	9.5	40	2,787	16	2,803	1,540	1,491	131.1
Richmond, VA	182	203	16.0	15	4,196	36	4,232	1,859	1,797	142.6
Riverside–San Bernardino–Ontario, CA	177	235	5.5	82	10,538	62	10,601	5,320	5,429	127.9
Rochester, NY	98	127	12.0	28	3,676	16	3,692	1,656	1,649	156.4
Sacramento–Arden–Arcade–Roseville, CA	83	109	5.0	86	4,815	29	4,845	2,187	2,233	103.6
St. Louis, MO–IL	196	231	8.1	52	7,252	41	7,293	3,312	3,255	114.6
Salt Lake City, UT	48	55	4.8	88	2,007	10	2,017	1,006	992	87.9
San Antonio, TX	195	274	12.5	26	6,338	31	6,369	2,832	2,790	129.5
San Diego–Carlsbad–San Marcos, CA	253	331	10.5	38	15,220	72	15,292	7,190	7,344	236.5
San Francisco, CA	460	601	13.7	20	45,614	103	45,717	16,139	16,422	378.1
Oakland Division	183	240	9.2	—	11,626	52	11,678	4,973	5,062	197.3
San Francisco Division	277	362	20.1	—	33,988	50	34,038	11,166	11,360	639.0
San Jose–Sunnyvale–Santa Clara, CA	122	160	8.6	48	4,726	15	4,741	2,274	2,336	126.8
San Juan–Caguas–Guaynabo, PR	279	359	14.5	19	24,294	281	24,575	7,755	7,857	317.2
Scranton–Wilkes–Barre, PA	20	29	5.2	84	697	6	703	335	334	59.3
Seattle, WA	213	241	6.9	65	10,576	28	10,604	4,757	4,673	135.5
Seattle Division	177	200	7.4	—	9,376	19	9,395	4,235	4,163	157.0
Tacoma Division	36	41	5.1	—	1,200	9	1,209	522	510	64.1
Springfield, MA	35	61	8.8	45	2,521	30	2,551	1,014	1,044	150.6
Stockton, CA	37	50	7.2	63	1,402	14	1,416	712	729	106.1
Syracuse, NY	40	51	7.8	57	1,559	9	1,568	658	651	98.2
Tampa–St. Petersburg–Clearwater, FL	345	385	13.6	21	13,517	121	13,639	5,857	5,696	204.3
Toledo, OH	26	29	4.4	89	1,013	15	1,028	463	448	68.8
Tucson, AZ	57	64	6.5	71	2,369	10	2,379	1,008	982	99.9
Tulsa, OK	52	55	5.8	77	1,815	10	1,825	783	751	79.9
Virginia Beach–Norfolk–Newport News, VA–NC	132	148	8.8	46	5,624	66	5,690	2,522	2,415	144.2
Washington, DC–VA–MD–WV	758	1,111	19.5	11	39,244	335	39,579	18,371	18,321	326.6
Bethesda Division	78	127	10.4	—	3,808	27	3,835	2,126	2,166	179.0
Washington Division	680	984	22.0	—	35,436	308	35,744	16,245	16,155	367.2
Wichita, KS	21	23	3.6	94	997	2	999	456	445	71.3
Worcester, MA	26	49	6.1	76	2,171	21	2,192	1,000	1,031	129.0
Youngstown–Warren–Boardman, OH–PA	28	32	5.7	78	685	0	685	294	283	50.1
Subtotal for MSAs (population ≥500,000)	**20,546**	**26,152**	**12.6**	**—**	**995,155**	**8,575**	**1,003,730**	**420,611**	**417,561**	**203.0**

TABLE 3.3

Reported AIDS cases and annual rates, by metropolitan area of residence and age category, 2011, and cumulative [CONTINUED]

	Diagnosis, 2011				Diagnosis, cumulative[a]			Prevalence of stage 3 (AIDS) year-end 2010		
					Adults or adolescents	Children	Total			
		Estimated[b]				Estimated[b]			Estimated[b]	
Area of residence	No.	No.	Rate[c]	Rank[d]	No.	No.	No.	No.	No.	Rate[c]
Metropolitan areas (population of 50,000–499,999)	3,148	3,795	6.7	—	112,641	835	113,475	49,958	48,882	86.2
Nonmetropolitan areas	1,935	2,295	4.5	—	66,804	471	67,275	30,587	29,709	58.7
Total[f]	**25,813**	**32,539**	**10.3**	**—**	**1,179,925**	**9,926**	**1,189,851**	**503,685**	**498,788**	**159.3**

MSA = Metropolitan statistical area.
[a]From the beginning of the epidemic through 2011.
[b]Estimated numbers resulted from statistical adjustment that accounted for reporting delays, but not for incomplete reporting.
[c]Rates are per 100,000 population.
[d]Based on estimated rate.
[e]Counts of stage 3 (AIDS) classifications for the metropolitan divisions do not sum to the MSA total. MSA total includes data from 1 metropolitan division with population of <500,000.
[f]Includes persons whose county of residence is unknown. Because column totals for estimated numbers were calculated independently of the values for the subpopulations, the values in each column may not sum to the column total.
Note: Because of the lack of U.S. census information for all U.S. dependent areas, table includes data for only the 50 states, the District of Columbia, and Puerto Rico.

SOURCE: "Table 24. Stage 3 (AIDS), 2011 and Cumulative, and Persons Living with Diagnosed HIV Infection Ever Classified As Stage 3 (AIDS) (Prevalence), Year-end 2010, by Metropolitan Statistical Area of Residence—United States and Puerto Rico," in *HIV Surveillance Report: Diagnoses of HIV Infection in the United States and Dependent Areas, 2011*, vol. 23, Centers for Disease Control and Prevention, National Center for HIV/AIDS, Viral Hepatitis, STD, and TB Prevention, Division of HIV/AIDS Prevention, February 2013, http://www.cdc.gov/hiv/pdf/statistics_2011_HIV_Surveillance_Report_vol_23.pdf (accessed July 7, 2013)

AIDS diagnoses attributable to heterosexual contact skyrocketed from 3% in 1985 to nearly 31% in 2011.

Rates among Women

In 2011 reported AIDS cases among women that were attributable to injection drug use (1,615) accounted for 20% of the total number of cases (7,949). (See Table 3.1.) When considering the role of heterosexual contact in the acquisition of AIDS, the proportion was far higher for women in 2011 (an estimated 6,206 cases, representing 78% of the total of 7,949) than for men (an estimated 3,526, representing 15% of the total of 24,088). (See Table 3.1.)

Decline in AIDS Due to Blood Transfusions

As a result of screening procedures for blood and blood products that began in 1985, the CDC indicates that the number of AIDS cases among adult and adolescent transfusion recipients decreased between 1995 (664 cases) and 1997 (409 cases). A pronounced decrease in 1999 (256 cases) was followed by a steady decline after an initial slight increase to 282 cases in 2000: 218 cases in 2001, 219 in 2003, 160 in 2005, and 109 in 2007. By 2008 the numbers had dropped so low that the CDC began reporting cases attributable to blood transfusion along with hemophilia, perinatal exposure, and other unidentified risk factors in a category called "Other." This category has declined steadily, from an estimated 289 cases in 2008 to 262 cases in 2011. (See Table 3.1.)

Current Age and Sex Distribution

Of the 1,155,792 estimated cumulative total reported cases of AIDS in 2011, 1,146,271 (99% of the cumulative total) were among adults and adolescents. (See Table 3.1.) The remaining 9,521 cases (1%) were children under the age of 13 years. According to the CDC, in 2010 more people between the ages of 45 to 49 years (108,877) and 50 to 54 years (90,646) were living with AIDS (199,523, or 40% of all cases) than in any other age category. (See Table 3.4.)

Cumulatively, the total number of AIDS cases that were reported in adults and adolescents at the end of 2011 occurred predominantly in males (913,368 cases, or 79% of the cumulative total). (See Table 3.1.) Females accounted for 232,902 cumulative cases (21% of the cumulative total).

Race and Ethnicity Influence Risk

The changing racial and ethnic profile and characteristics of Americans with HIV/AIDS between 1993 and 2011 reflect a shift in the population at risk for HIV/AIDS. In *HIV/AIDS Surveillance Report: U.S. HIV and AIDS Cases Reported through December 2001* (2001, http://www.cdc.gov/hiv/topics/surveillance/resources/reports/2001report/pdf/2001surveillance-report_year-end.pdf), the CDC indicates that in 1993 there were 60,587 cases reported among African Americans. By 2011 the number of cases had reached 486,282, far outpacing all other races. (See Table 3.1.)

In 1999 African Americans accounted for 41% (127,169) of people estimated to be living with HIV/AIDS. By 2010 this figure had risen to 42% (209,707). (See Table 3.4.) In contrast, the proportion of whites

FIGURE 3.6

AIDS diagnoses by transmission category, 1985–2011

[United States and 6 dependent areas]

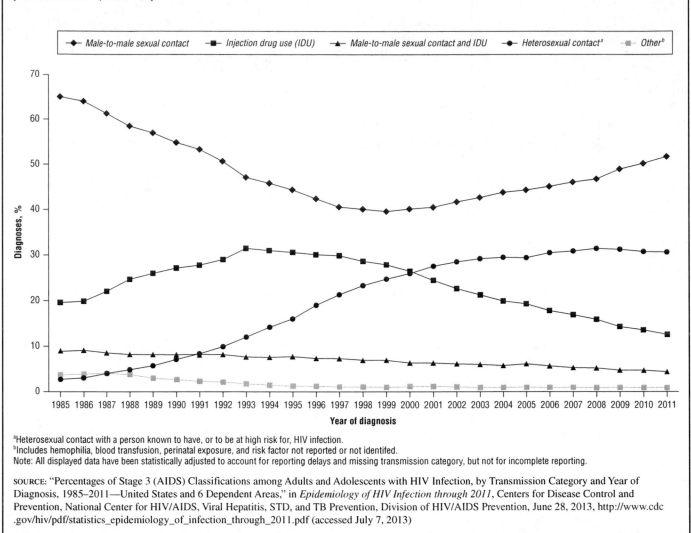

[a] Heterosexual contact with a person known to have, or to be at high risk for, HIV infection.
[b] Includes hemophilia, blood transfusion, perinatal exposure, and risk factor not reported or not identifed.
Note: All displayed data have been statistically adjusted to account for reporting delays and missing transmission category, but not for incomplete reporting.

SOURCE: "Percentages of Stage 3 (AIDS) Classifications among Adults and Adolescents with HIV Infection, by Transmission Category and Year of Diagnosis, 1985–2011—United States and 6 Dependent Areas," in *Epidemiology of HIV Infection through 2011*, Centers for Disease Control and Prevention, National Center for HIV/AIDS, Viral Hepatitis, STD, and TB Prevention, Division of HIV/AIDS Prevention, June 28, 2013, http://www.cdc.gov/hiv/pdf/statistics_epidemiology_of_infection_through_2011.pdf (accessed July 7, 2013)

living with HIV/AIDS in 1999 was 38% (120,731), and by 2010 it was 32% (162,308).

In 2011 Hispanics accounted for an estimated 6,355 new reported AIDS cases. (See Table 3.1.) The corresponding figures for whites and African Americans were 8,304 and 15,958, respectively. The total number of male and female adult and adolescent reported AIDS cases in native Hawaiians and other Pacific Islanders (47) and Asian Americans (492) were the lowest of all the racial and ethnic groups in the United States.

The racial and ethnic difference is particularly alarming among children under the age of 13 years. As shown in Table 3.5, in 2011 the rate of HIV infection per 100,000 population for African American children (1.7) was about seven times the rate for Hispanic (0.2) and Asian American children (0.3). The other racial and ethnic categories were negligible.

The racial disparity is also reflected in the acquisition of HIV infection by infants born to HIV-infected mothers. Between 1994 and 2011 the number of reported cases of HIV/AIDS among African American infants was significantly greater than the reported cases for white and Hispanic infants born to HIV-infected mothers. In 2011 nearly eight times as many African American infants were HIV infected (85) through perinatal exposure (before, during, or immediately after birth) than were white infants (11). (See Table 3.5.)

Causes of Racial Disparities

In "HIV among African Americans" (May 15, 2013, http://www.cdc.gov/hiv/risk/racialethnic/aa/facts/index.html), the CDC notes that African Americans accounted for an estimated 44% of all new HIV infections in 2010, even though they accounted for just 12% to 14% of the U.S. population. That same year more new

TABLE 3.4

Numbers of persons living with AIDS, by year and selected characteristics, 2008–10

| | 2008 | | | 2009 | | | 2010 | | |
	No.	Estimated[a] No.	Rate	No.	Estimated[a] No.	Rate	No.	Estimated[a] No.	Rate
Age at end of year									
<13	709	713	1.3	550	554	1.0	457	463	0.9
13–14	628	631	7.6	487	492	6.0	330	334	4.0
15–19	2,824	2,847	13.0	2,738	2,770	12.7	2,574	2,619	11.7
20–24	6,408	6,500	30.0	7,021	7,155	32.8	7,574	7,808	35.5
25–29	15,388	15,559	71.5	15,721	15,962	72.6	16,075	16,465	76.9
30–34	28,208	28,402	143.3	28,251	28,510	141.2	28,417	28,807	141.6
35–39	53,837	53,968	255.3	50,238	50,389	241.9	46,309	46,546	228.8
40–44	90,141	89,959	414.7	85,264	85,121	399.9	80,961	80,857	381.9
45–49	103,220	102,555	444.1	107,885	107,100	463.1	109,867	108,877	475.2
50–54	79,219	78,329	360.9	85,233	84,117	381.7	92,088	90,646	400.8
55–59	49,055	48,286	257.0	55,398	54,367	282.8	60,963	59,512	297.0
60–64	24,581	24,101	157.4	28,266	27,602	172.0	33,084	32,085	186.3
≥65	18,907	18,292	46.5	21,926	21,081	52.5	25,359	24,147	58.8
Race/ethnicity									
American Indian/Alaska Native	1,591	1,566	—	1,654	1,624	—	1,732	1,697	—
Asian[b]	4,647	4,690	—	4,980	5,039	—	5,294	5,384	—
Black/African American	197,837	195,963	—	205,154	202,823	—	212,660	209,707	—
Hispanic/Latino[c]	102,733	103,182	—	106,768	107,243	—	110,305	110,778	—
Native Hawaiian/other Pacific Islander	428	428	—	468	470	—	495	499	—
White	157,054	155,471	—	161,096	159,261	—	164,578	162,308	—
Multiple races	8,736	8,745	—	8,762	8,665	—	8,899	8,700	—
Transmission category									
Male adult or adolescent									
Male-to-male sexual contact	198,240	219,782	—	206,071	229,262	—	213,480	238,339	—
Injection drug use	53,466	62,550	—	53,018	62,186	—	52,659	61,745	—
Male-to-male sexual contact and injection drug use	29,562	31,818	—	29,676	31,061	—	29,033	32,120	—
Heterosexual contact[d]	32,724	39,625	—	34,305	41,684	—	35,559	43,401	—
Perinatal	2,075	2,077	—	2,187	2,189	—	2,284	2,288	—
Other[e]	44,655	2,332	—	47,434	2,316	—	50,251	2,272	—
Subtotal	360,722	358,183	287.7	372,690	369,598	294.0	384,066	380,164	300.1
Female adult or adolescent									
Injection drug use	27,059	34,312	—	26,983	34,430	—	26,956	34,481	—
Heterosexual contact[d]	57,372	73,418	—	59,652	76,995	—	61,671	80,289	—
Perinatal	2,148	2,147	—	2,279	2,280	—	2,401	2,402	—
Other[e]	25,113	1,369	—	26,822	1,361	—	28,505	1,365	—
Subtotal	111,692	111,245	85.5	115,736	115,066	87.7	119,533	118,538	89.0
Child (<13 yrs at end of year)									
Perinatal	685	689	—	531	535	—	439	444	—
Other[e]	24	24	—	19	19	—	18	18	—
Subtotal	709	713	1.3	550	554	1.0	457	463	0.9
Region of residence									
Northeast	132,725	133,866	243.1	135,369	136,640	247.2	137,618	138,856	250.8
Midwest	48,927	47,986	72.1	51,357	50,278	75.2	53,605	52,343	78.2
South	186,481	183,167	163.5	193,542	189,395	167.1	200,926	195,879	170.5
West	93,949	93,798	132.7	97,496	97,445	136.2	100,579	100,614	139.5
U.S. dependent areas	11,043	11,326	258.5	11,214	11,462	260.9	11,330	11,475	278.7
Total[f]	473,125	470,144	152.3	488,978	485,220	155.8	504,058	499,167	159.3

[a]Estimated numbers resulted from statistical adjustment that accounted for reporting delays and missing transmission category, but not for incomplete reporting. Rates are per 100,000 population. Rates by race/ethnicity are not provided because U.S. census information for U.S. dependent areas is limited. Rates are not calculated by transmission category because of the lack of denominator data.
[b]Includes Asian/Pacific Islander legacy cases.
[c]Hispanics/Latinos can be of any race.
[d]Heterosexual contact with a person known to have, or to be at high risk for, HIV infection.
[e]Includes hemophilia, blood transfusion, and risk factor not reported or not identified.
[f]Includes persons of unknown race/ethnicity. Because column totals for estimated numbers were calculated independently of the values for the subpopulations, the values in each column may not sum to the column total.

SOURCE: "Table 16b. Persons Living with Diagnosed HIV Infection Ever Classified as Stage 3 (AIDS), by Year and Selected Characteristics, 2008–2010—United States and 6 Dependent Areas," in *HIV Surveillance Report: Diagnoses of HIV Infection in the United States and Dependent Areas, 2011*, vol. 23, Centers for Disease Control and Prevention, National Center for HIV/AIDS, Viral Hepatitis, STD, and TB Prevention, Division of HIV/AIDS Prevention, February 2013, http://www.cdc.gov/hiv/pdf/statistics_2011_HIV_Surveillance_Report_vol_23.pdf (accessed July 7, 2013)

TABLE 3.5

Diagnosed HIV infection, by race/ethnicity and selected characteristics, 2011

	American Indian/Alaska Native			Asian			Black/African American			Hispanic/Latino			Native Hawaiian/other Pacific Islander			White			Multiple races			Total		
	No.	Estimated[b] No.	Rate	No.	Estimated[b] No.	Rate	No.	Estimated[b] No.	Rate	No.	Estimated[b] No.	Rate[a]	No.	Estimated[b] No.	Rate	No.	Estimated[b] No.	Rate	No.	Estimated[b] No.	Rate	No.	Estimated[b] No.[c]	Rate
Age at diagnosis (yr)																								
<13	0	0	0.0	7	8	0.3	107	125	1.7	22	25	0.2	0	0	0.0	25	29	0.1	4	4	0.2	165	192	0.4
13–14	0	0	0.0	0	0	0.0	28	33	2.9	9	11	0.6	0	0	0.0	6	7	0.2	1	1	0.5	44	53	0.6
15–19	10	11	5.8	22	27	2.9	1,294	1,494	46.3	310	370	8.1	2	2	5.9	266	301	2.5	32	35	5.8	1,936	2,240	10.4
20–24	33	38	19.9	100	120	10.7	4,051	4,689	146.9	1,261	1,491	33.3	15	18	36.6	1,356	1,551	12.3	127	148	30.6	6,943	8,054	36.4
25–29	29	33	19.7	133	160	12.8	2,979	3,482	127.2	1,466	1,743	39.9	14	16	33.8	1,659	1,912	15.5	117	139	35.9	6,397	7,484	35.2
30–34	24	26	17.3	133	158	12.4	2,185	2,551	97.0	1,380	1,640	38.7	7	8	19.2	1,479	1,705	14.4	103	121	36.2	5,311	6,209	30.3
35–39	27	31	21.6	141	168	12.9	1,801	2,096	84.7	1,118	1,338	34.0	15	17	47.0	1,342	1,551	13.6	71	84	30.1	4,515	5,285	27.0
40–44	16	18	11.8	109	130	10.7	1,980	2,328	89.1	1,080	1,280	35.8	6	7	19.3	1,645	1,906	14.5	85	85	32.7	4,909	5,753	27.4
45–49	21	24	15.0	81	99	9.0	2,018	2,383	86.9	833	992	31.6	3	3	9.4	1,710	1,984	13.5	68	79	32.5	4,734	5,564	25.1
50–54	9	10	6.1	44	53	5.2	1,549	1,809	67.2	535	637	24.7	3	4	11.5	1,197	1,384	8.7	46	55	24.1	3,383	3,951	17.5
55–59	13	15	10.9	19	23	2.6	968	1,141	50.4	274	320	16.2	2	2	9.2	671	773	5.2	32	37	20.1	1,979	2,312	11.4
60–64	4	4	3.9	20	24	3.2	505	590	32.8	140	162	10.9	1	1	5.3	369	427	3.2	18	21	14.9	1,057	1,229	6.9
≥65	2	2	1.2	12	14	0.9	381	447	12.7	127	152	5.1	0	0	0.0	271	315	1.0	15	18	6.7	808	948	2.3
Transmission category																								
Male adult or adolescent																								
Male-to-male sexual contact	85	120	—	451	705	—	7,676	11,805	—	4,816	6,949	—	47	61	—	7,537	10,375	—	393	558	—	21,005	30,573	—
Injection drug use	13	17	—	11	23	—	381	1,083	—	278	566	—	4	4	—	345	495	—	20	33	—	1,052	2,220	—
Male-to-male sexual contact and injection drug use	8	12	—	18	24	—	202	433	—	181	282	—	0	0	—	484	621	—	23	34	—	916	1,407	—
Heterosexual contact[d]	9	12	—	37	65	—	1,635	3,117	—	520	801	—	2	3	—	362	536	—	35	54	—	2,600	4,588	—
Other[e]	27	1	—	168	4	—	4,184	9	—	1,460	6	—	8	2	—	1,692	14	—	109	0	—	7,648	36	—
Subtotal	142	161	18.0	685	821	13.8	14,078	16,447	112.8	7,255	8,605	43.4	61	70	34.2	10,420	12,041	14.5	580	679	38.5	33,221	38,825	30.8
Female adult or adolescent																								
Injection drug use	14	19	—	4	10	—	221	715	—	84	210	—	0	1	—	278	445	—	12	28	—	613	1,428	—
Heterosexual contact[d]	13	32	—	55	141	—	2,360	5,875	—	582	1,318	—	4	7	—	643	1,325	—	46	116	—	3,703	8,814	—
Other[e]	19	0	—	70	2	—	3,080	5	—	612	2	—	3	0	—	630	6	—	65	0	—	4,479	15	—
Subtotal	46	51	5.5	129	153	2.3	5,661	6,595	40.0	1,278	1,530	7.9	7	8	3.9	1,551	1,776	2.0	123	144	7.5	8,795	10,257	7.7
Child (<13 years at diagnosis)																								
Perinatal	0	0	—	5	6	—	73	85	—	19	21	—	0	0	—	10	11	—	3	3	—	110	127	—
Other[f]	0	0	—	2	2	—	34	40	—	3	4	—	0	0	—	15	18	—	1	1	—	55	65	—
Subtotal	0	0	0.0	7	8	0.3	107	125	1.7	22	25	0.2	0	0	0.0	25	29	0.1	4	4	0.2	165	192	0.4
Region of residence																								
Northeast	5	6	4.8	165	215	6.8	3,588	4,445	71.9	2,053	2,594	36.1	4	5	24.9	2,020	2,572	6.8	154	187	23.2	7,989	10,024	18.1
Midwest	23	26	6.5	81	93	5.2	2,700	3,030	43.9	580	669	13.9	3	3	11.7	2,028	2,234	4.3	158	182	16.3	5,573	6,237	9.3
South	57	62	8.2	212	243	7.3	12,233	14,079	64.1	3,366	3,787	20.0	11	12	15.8	5,154	5,778	8.4	293	336	18.0	21,326	24,296	20.9
West	103	119	11.7	363	431	6.4	1,325	1,614	49.0	2,556	3,110	14.7	50	58	15.0	2,794	3,262	8.5	102	122	5.9	7,293	8,717	12.0
Total[g]	188	212	9.3	821	982	6.5	19,846	23,168	60.4	8,555	10,159	19.5	68	78	15.3	11,996	13,846	7.0	707	827	14.2	42,181	49,273	15.8

TABLE 3.5

Diagnosed HIV infection, by race/ethnicity and selected characteristics, 2011 [CONTINUED]

Reported numbers less than 12, as well as estimated numbers (and accompanying rates and trends) based on these numbers, should be interpreted with caution because the numbers have underlying relative standard errors greater than 30% and are considered unreliable.

aHispanics/Latinos can be of any race.

bEstimated numbers resulted from statistical adjustment that accounted for reporting delays and missing transmission category, but not for incomplete reporting. Rates are per 100,000 population. Rates are not calculated by transmission category because of the lack of denominator data.

cBecause the estimated totals were calculated independently of the corresponding values for each subpopulation, the subpopulation values may not sum to the totals shown here.

dHeterosexual contact with a person known to have, or to be at high risk for, HIV infection.

eIncludes hemophilia, blood transfusion, perinatal exposure, and risk factor not reported or not identified.

fIncludes hemophilia, blood transfusion, and risk factor not reported or not identified.

gBecause column totals for estimated numbers were calculated independently of the values for the subpopulations, the values in each column may not sum to the column total.

Note: Data include persons with a diagnosis of HIV infection regardless of stage of disease at diagnosis.

SOURCE: "Table 3a. Diagnoses of HIV Infection, by Race/Ethnicity and Selected Characteristics, 2011—United States," in *HIV Surveillance Report: Diagnoses of HIV Infection in the United States and Dependent Areas, 2011,* vol. 23, Centers for Disease Control and Prevention, National Center for HIV/AIDS, Viral Hepatitis, STD, and TB Prevention, Division of HIV/AIDS Prevention, February 2013, http://www.cdc.gov/hiv/pdf/statistics_2011_HIV_Surveillance_Report_vol_23.pdf (accessed July 7, 2013)

HIV infections (4,800) were diagnosed in young African American MSM than in any other age or racial group of MSM. According to the CDC, the rate of new HIV infections among African American women (38.1 per100,000 population) "was 20 times as high as the rate for white women, and almost five times as high as that of Latinas." This disparity is attributed to factors such as disproportionately higher prevalence rates of other sexually transmitted infections, housing conditions, lack of education and social support, stigma, fear, and poverty.

To reduce disparities in the incidence and prevalence of HIV infection, the CDC supports prevention and intervention programs for African Americans, such as the Act against AIDS campaign (2013, http://www.cdc.gov/actagainstaids/), which aims to improve knowledge and dispel misperceptions about HIV in the United States. The campaign consists of several programs, including "Take Charge. Take the Test," which encourages African American women to get HIV testing; "Testing Makes Us Stronger," which aims to increase HIV testing among gay and bisexual men; and "Let's Stop HIV Together," which seeks to reduce stigma and increase awareness.

HOW HIV IS TRANSMITTED

HIV can be transmitted by sexual contact with an infected person; by needle sharing among infected injection drug users; through the receipt of infected blood, blood products, or tissue; and directly from an infected mother to her infant during pregnancy, delivery, or breastfeeding.

In the United States MSM remain the majority of HIV carriers, although prevalence among heterosexuals is on the rise. The CDC reports in *HIV/AIDS Surveillance Report: AIDS Cases Reported through December 1988*

(January 1989, http://www.cdc.gov/hiv/topics/surveillance/resources/reports/pdf/surveillance88.pdf) that 70% of adult and adolescent males with AIDS had a single risk factor of a history of high-risk sexual activity in 1987. Although 69% (16,694 of 24,088) of the reported cases of AIDS among adult and adolescent males were attributable to MSM in 2011, cumulatively the percentage of affected MSM was 61% (555,032 of 913,368). (See Table 3.1.) Adult and adolescent males with a history of injection drug use as their only risk factor made up 14% of all cases in 1987. This proportion has remained relatively constant in the intervening years, and although a cumulative of 21% (187,938 of 913,368) of AIDS cases in adult and adolescent males were attributable to injection drug use, they accounted for 10% (2,346 of 24,088) of cases in 2011.

Adult and adolescent females with a history of heterosexual contact as their only risk factor made up 31% of AIDS cases in adult and adolescent females in 1987. By 2011 this percentage had increased to 78% (6,206 of 7,949). (See Table 3.1.) Researchers suggest that one reason for steadily increasing HIV infection and AIDS among heterosexuals is that an increased proportion report multiple sex partners, which is a risk factor for HIV infection.

MORTALITY FROM AIDS

According to the CDC, in *HIV/AIDS Surveillance Report: U.S. HIV and AIDS Cases Reported through December 2001*, the number of deaths due to AIDS peaked at 51,670 in 1995. Since then, the number of deaths each year has been dropping. In 2010 the disease killed 16,093 Americans. (See Table 3.6.) As a result of more effective treatment, fewer people are dying from AIDS. As fewer people become infected with HIV, the death rate in subsequent years will drop proportionally.

TABLE 3.6

AIDS deaths, 2008–10 and cumulative

	2008			2009			2010			Cumulative[b]	
		Estimated[a]			Estimated[a]			Estimated[a]			
	No.	No.	Rate	No.	No.	Rate	No.	No.	Rate	No.	Est. No.[a]
Age at death (yr)											
<13	4	5	0.0	3	4	0.0	0	0	0.0	5,201	5,239
13–14	0	0	0.0	2	2	0.0	1	2	0.0	302	308
15–19	39	43	0.2	27	31	0.1	26	34	0.2	1,309	1,343
20–24	144	161	0.7	150	175	0.8	130	168	0.8	9,892	10,080
25–29	435	485	2.2	404	472	2.1	285	371	1.7	48,021	48,669
30–34	738	824	4.2	690	804	4.0	574	742	3.6	103,822	105,201
35–39	1,467	1,631	7.7	1,264	1,471	7.1	912	1,170	5.8	129,774	131,947
40–44	2,533	2,817	13.0	2,092	2,429	11.4	1,630	2,100	9.9	120,788	123,638
45–49	3,037	3,378	14.6	2,805	3,247	14.0	2,425	3,137	13.7	90,010	93,024
50–54	2,758	3,063	14.1	2,634	3,046	13.8	2,353	3,001	13.3	58,359	60,806
55–59	2,030	2,247	12.0	2,042	2,357	12.3	1,832	2,343	11.7	34,778	36,451
60–64	1,124	1,243	8.1	1,175	1,346	8.4	1,208	1,540	8.9	19,939	20,899
≥65	1,169	1,293	3.3	1,262	1,449	3.6	1,169	1,485	3.6	20,408	21,388
Race/ethnicity											
American Indian/Alaska Native	71	78	—	60	69	—	56	68	—	1,882	1,945
Asian[c]	78	86	—	53	59	—	49	59	—	3,147	3,212
Black/African American	7,714	8,619	—	6,896	8,016	—	5,941	7,684	—	253,089	261,090
Hispanic/Latino[d]	2,845	3,102	—	2,707	3,091	—	2,323	2,928	—	116,215	118,783
Native Hawaiian/other Pacific Islander	13	14	—	6	7	—	9	10	—	363	371
White	4,338	4,828	—	4,057	4,668	—	3,655	4,668	—	259,937	265,132
Multiple races	417	461	—	768	921	—	511	673	—	7,897	8,383
Transmission category											
Male adult or adolescent											
Male-to-male sexual contact	4,649	6,164	—	4,439	6,126	—	3,903	5,980	—	280,571	305,705
Injection drug use	2,479	3,197	—	2,322	3,103	—	1,946	2,907	—	122,194	137,079
Male-to-male sexual contact and injection drug use	1,116	1,338	—	1,105	1,381	—	913	1,258	—	46,268	49,922
Heterosexual contact[e]	1,271	1,785	—	1,086	1,646	—	991	1,654	—	27,147	34,437
Perinatal	21	23	—	20	23	—	20	26	—	297	316
Other[f]	1,822	106	—	1,716	93	—	1,530	97	—	47,829	9,295
Subtotal	**11,358**	**12,614**	**10.1**	**10,688**	**12,372**	**9.8**	**9,303**	**11,923**	**9.4**	**524,306**	**536,754**
Female adult or adolescent											
Injection drug use	1,429	1,903	—	1,221	1,708	—	985	1,563	—	48,553	56,708
Heterosexual contact[e]	1,691	2,565	—	1,715	2,661	—	1,460	2,540	—	44,564	55,533
Perinatal	44	48	—	42	48	—	29	38	—	405	434
Other[f]	952	56	—	881	43	—	768	29	—	19,574	4,324
Subtotal	**4,116**	**4,572**	**3.5**	**3,859**	**4,459**	**3.4**	**3,242**	**4,170**	**3.1**	**113,096**	**116,998**
Child (<13 yrs at death)											
Perinatal	3	3	—	3	4	—	0	0	—	4,721	4,756
Other[f]	1	1	—	0	0	—	0	0	—	480	483
Subtotal	**4**	**5**	**0.0**	**3**	**4**	**0.0**	**0**	**0**	**0.0**	**5,201**	**5,239**
Region of residence											
Northeast	4,232	4,598	8.4	3,997	4,481	8.1	3,538	4,394	7.9	199,628	203,545
Midwest	1,634	1,872	2.8	1,265	1,506	2.3	1,135	1,524	2.3	62,670	64,553
South	7,024	7,918	7.1	6,838	8,096	7.1	5,766	7,501	6.5	233,893	242,002
West	2,090	2,273	3.2	1,987	2,188	3.1	1,719	2,110	2.9	123,857	125,947
U.S. dependent areas	498	530	12.1	463	563	12.8	387	564	13.7	22,555	22,944
Total[g]	**15,478**	**17,191**	**5.6**	**14,550**	**16,834**	**5.4**	**12,545**	**16,093**	**5.1**	**642,603**	**658,992**

[a]Estimated numbers resulted from statistical adjustment that accounted for reporting delays and missing transmission category, but not for incomplete reporting. Rates are per 100,000 population. Rates by race/ethnicity are not provided because U.S. census information for U.S. dependent areas is limited. Rates are not calculated by transmission category because of the lack of denominator data.
[b]From the beginning of the epidemic through 2010.
[c]Includes Asian/Pacific Islander legacy cases.
[d]Hispanics/Latinos can be of any race.
[e]Heterosexual contact with a person known to have, or to be at high risk for, HIV infection.
[f]Includes hemophilia, blood transfusion, and risk factor not reported or not identified.
[g]Includes persons of unknown race/ethnicity. Because column totals for estimated numbers were calculated independently of the values for the subpopulations, the values in each column may not sum to the column total.
Note: Deaths of persons with diagnosed HIV infection may be due to any cause.

SOURCE: "Table 12b. Deaths of Persons with Diagnosed HIV Infection Ever Classified as Stage 3 (AIDS), by Year of Death and Selected Characteristics, 2008–2010 and Cumulative—United States and 6 Dependent Areas," in *HIV Surveillance Report: Diagnoses of HIV Infection in the United States and Dependent Areas, 2011*, vol. 23, Centers for Disease Control and Prevention, National Center for HIV/AIDS, Viral Hepatitis, STD, and TB Prevention, Division of HIV/AIDS Prevention, February 2013, http://www.cdc.gov/hiv/pdf/statistics_2011_HIV_Surveillance_Report_vol_23.pdf (accessed July 7, 2013)

CHAPTER 4
POPULATIONS AT RISK

This chapter examines the prevalence rates of HIV infection—that is, the total number of people with HIV/AIDS in a population at a specified time. Prevalence rates are based on surveys of selected segments of the general population and of people in high-risk groups. They are not absolute numbers. Prevalence rates identify trends such as the geographic distribution of disease or changes in how the disease is transmitted. The Centers for Disease Control and Prevention (CDC) conducts HIV surveillance—collecting, analyzing, and publicizing prevalence rates and other information about new and existing cases of HIV/AIDS.

INCREASE IN HIV INFECTION AND AIDS AMONG HETEROSEXUALS

The increase in the number and proportion of HIV/AIDS cases among heterosexuals signals a major shift in the patterns of the epidemic. In 2011, 49,081 new cases of HIV infection among adults and adolescents were reported to the CDC. (See Table 4.1.) Approximately 27% (13,402) were attributed to heterosexual contact. In comparison, the CDC reports in *Weekly Surveillance Report, 1985* (December 30, 1985, http://www.cdc.gov/hiv/topics/surveillance/resources/reports/pdf/surveillance85.pdf) that 1% of all AIDS cases were attributable to heterosexual transmission in 1985.

The CDC notes that between 1997 and 2001 the number of new AIDS cases dropped significantly and that the proportions of those infected in each exposure category also changed. Cases attributed to male-to-male sexual contact (MSM) represented 35% of all cases in 1997 and 1998; thereafter, they dropped to 34% in 1999, to 32% in 2000, and to 31% in 2001. In 2003 the MSM rate rebounded to 35% and by 2011 it accounted for 62% (30,573) of new cases among adult and adolescent males. (See Table 4.1.) MSM continued to represent in 2011 the largest proportion (48%, or 555,032 of

1,155,792) of cumulative AIDS cases since 1981. (See Table 4.2.)

According to the CDC, in *HIV Surveillance in Women* (June 11, 2013, http://www.cdc.gov/hiv/pdf/statistics_surveillance_Women.pdf), there were 10,257 cases of HIV infection among adult and adolescent females reported by the 50 states, the District of Columbia, and six U.S. dependent areas in 2011. The majority of the cases were attributable to high-risk heterosexual contact, which accounted for between 82.2% and 92.7% of cases in adult and adolescent females. (See Table 4.3.) The percentage of cases attributable to injection drug use increased with advancing age, from 7% of females aged 13 to 19 years to 17.4% of females aged 45 years and older.

The proportion of women who contracted AIDS through heterosexual contact remained relatively constant at 37% in 2001 and 38% in 2002. In 2003, however, the proportion increased to 45%, and in 2011 it had risen to between 51.8% and 85.5% of cases in adult and adolescent females. (See Table 4.4.)

In 2011 the largest number of HIV infections in adult and adolescent females was among African American females—64% (6,595 of 10,257) of HIV diagnoses were in African American females (see Table 4.5), although African Americans accounted for just 12% of the U.S. female population. In contrast, white females made up 66% of the U.S. female adult and adolescent population but accounted for just 17% (1,776) of HIV infection diagnoses among females.

INJECTION DRUG USERS

During the 1990s the proportions of both HIV infection and AIDS deaths that were attributable to injection drug use among adults and adolescents increased. According to the CDC, in 1995 injection drug use was the exposure category for 25% of male and 47% of female AIDS deaths. Since 1995 the percentage of HIV/AIDS cases attributable to injection drug use has been steadily decreasing. By 2011 injection drug use accounted for an estimated 6% of cases of HIV infection in adult and adolescent males and 14% of cases in adult and adolescent females. (See Table 3.2 in Chapter 3.)

How HIV Is Transmitted through Injection Drug Use

HIV can be transmitted through injection drug use when the blood of an HIV-infected drug user is transferred to a drug user who is not yet infected with HIV. This transfer occurs almost exclusively through the sharing of injecting equipment, primarily needles and syringes.

Blood enters and makes contact with the needle and syringe in two ways. The first occurs when blood is drawn into the syringe to verify that the needle is inside a vein, before the injection of the drug. The second occurs following the injection, when the syringe is

TABLE 4.1

HIV infections by transmission category, 2011

Transmission category	Estimated number of diagnoses of HIV infection, 2011		
	Adult and adolescent males	Adult and adolescent females	Total
Male-to-male sexual contact	30,573	NA	30,573
Injection drug use	2,220	1,428	3,648
Male-to-male sexual contact and injection drug use	1,407	NA	1,407
Heterosexual contact[a]	4,588	8,814	13,402
Other[b]	36	15	51

[a]Heterosexual contact with a person known to have, or to be at high risk for, HIV infection.
[b]Includes hemophilia, blood transfusion, perinatal exposure, and risk not reported or not identified.

SOURCE: "Estimated Number of Diagnoses of HIV Infection, 2011," in *HIV/AIDS: Statistics Overview*, Centers for Disease Control and Prevention, National Center for HIV/AIDS, Viral Hepatitis, STD, and TB Prevention, Division of HIV/AIDS Prevention, April 23, 2013, http://www.cdc.gov/hiv/statistics/basics/index.html (accessed July 19, 2013)

TABLE 4.2

AIDS by transmission category, 2011 and cumulative through 2010

Transmission category	Estimated number of AIDS diagnoses, 2011		
	Adult and adolescent males	Adult and adolescent females	Total
Male-to-male sexual contact	16,694	NA	16,694
Injection drug use	2,346	1,615	3,961
Male-to-male sexual contact and injection drug use	1,392	NA	1,392
Heterosexual contact[a]	3,526	6,206	9,732
Other[b]	131	129	260

	Cumulative estimated number of AIDS diagnoses, through 2010[c]		
Male-to-male sexual contact	555,032	NA	555,032
Injection drug use	187,938	89,800	277,738
Male-to-male sexual contact and injection drug use	80,902	NA	80,902
Heterosexual contact[a]	77,521	136,675	214,196
Other[b]	11,975	6,427	18,402

[a]Heterosexual contact with a person known to have, or to be at high risk for, HIV infection.
[b]Includes hemophilia, blood transfusion, perinatal exposure, and risk not reported or not identified.
[c]From the beginning of the epidemic through 2011.

SOURCE: Adapted from "Estimated Number of AIDS Diagnoses, 2011," and "Cumulative Estimated Number of AIDS Diagnoses, through 2010," in *HIV/AIDS: Statistics Overview*, Centers for Disease Control and Prevention, National Center for HIV/AIDS, Viral Hepatitis, STD, and TB Prevention, Division of HIV/AIDS Prevention, April 23, 2013, http://www.cdc.gov/hiv/statistics/basics/index.html (accessed July 19, 2013)

TABLE 4.3

HIV Infection among females, by transmission category and age at diagnosis, 2011

[United States and 6 dependent areas]

	Age at diagnosis (in years)				
Transmission category	13–19 Population = 523	20–24 Population = 1,142	25–34 Population = 2,649	35–44 Population = 2,581	≥45 Population = 3,618
	%	%	%	%	%
Injection drug use	7.0	8.8	12.7	14.2	17.4
Heterosexual contact[a]	92.7	91.2	87.2	85.8	82.2
Other[b]	0.3	0.0	0.0	0.1	0.3
Total	**100.0**	**100.0**	**100.0**	**100.0**	**100.0**

[a]Heterosexual contact with a person known to have, or to be at high risk for, HIV infection.
[b]Includes blood transfusion, perinatal exposure, and risk factor not reported or not identified.
Note: Data include persons with a diagnosis of HIV infection regardless of stage of disease at diagnosis. All displayed data have been statistically adjusted to account for reporting delays and missing transmission category, but not for incomplete reporting.

SOURCE: "Diagnoses of HIV Infection among Adult and Adolescent Females, by Transmission Category and Age at Diagnosis 2011—United States and 6 Dependent Areas," in *HIV Surveillance in Women*, Centers for Disease Control and Prevention, June 11, 2013, http://www.cdc.gov/hiv/pdf/statistics_surveillance_Women.pdf (accessed July 19, 2013)

TABLE 4.4

AIDS diagnoses among females, by transmission category and age at diagnosis, 2011

[United States and 6 dependent areas]

Transmission category	Age at diagnosis (in years)				
	13–19 Population = 187	20–24 Population = 414	25–34 Population = 1,777	35–44 Population = 2,352	≥45 Population = 3,372
	%	%	%	%	%
Injection drug use	5.7	11.9	14.1	18.5	26.6
Heterosexual contact[a]	51.8	82.3	85.5	81.4	72.9
Other[b]	42.5	5.8	0.4	0.1	0.5
Total	**100.0**	**100.0**	**100.0**	**100.0**	**100.0**

[a]Heterosexual contact with a person known to have, or to be at high risk for, HIV infection.
[b]Includes blood transfusion, perinatal exposure, and risk factor not reported or not identified.
Note: All displayed data have been statistically adjusted to account for reporting delays and missing transmission category, but not for incomplete reporting.

SOURCE: "Stage 3 (AIDS) Classifications among Adult and Adolescent Females, by Transmission Category and Age at Diagnosis, 2011—United States and 6 Dependent Areas," in *HIV Surveillance in Women*, Centers for Disease Control and Prevention, June 11, 2013, http://www.cdc.gov/hiv/pdf/statistics_surveillance_Women.pdf (accessed July 19, 2013)

TABLE 4.5

HIV diagnoses among adult and adolescent females by race/ethnicity, 2011

[United States]

Race/ethnicity	No.	Rate
American Indian/Alaska Native	51	5.5
Asian	153	2.3
Black/African American	6,595	40.0
Hispanic/Latino[a]	1,530	7.9
Native Hawaiian/other Pacific Islander	8	3.9
White	1,776	2.0
Multiple races	144	7.5
Total	**10,257**	**7.7**

[a]Hispanics/Latinos can be of any race.
Note: Data include persons with a diagnosis of HIV infection regardless of stage of disease at diagnosis. All displayed data have been statistically adjusted to account for reporting delays, but not for incomplete reporting. Rates are per 100,000 population.

SOURCE: "Diagnoses of HIV Infection among Adult and Adolescent Females, by Race/Ethnicity 2011—United States," in *HIV Surveillance in Women*, Centers for Disease Control and Prevention, June 11, 2013, http://www.cdc.gov/hiv/pdf/statistics_surveillance_Women.pdf (accessed July 19, 2013)

refilled several times with blood from the vein to "wash out" any heroin, cocaine, or other drug left in the syringe after the first injection. Even the smallest amount of HIV-infected blood left in the syringe can cause the virus to be transmitted to the next user of the contaminated syringe and needle.

Among injection drug users (IDUs) the risk of HIV infection increases in proportion to the duration of injection drug use—the longer the drug use, the greater the risk of infection. Diseases such as hepatitis show this same pattern. Risk also increases with the frequency of needle sharing and injection drug use in a geographic area, such as a large city, where there is a high prevalence of HIV infection.

General Trends

Table 4.1 shows that in 2011 injection drug use was responsible for 3,648 HIV infections (7.4% of the 49,081 infections) and an additional 1,407 HIV infections (3%) were attributable to MSM in conjunction with injection drug use.

HIV is also spread among non-IDUs who trade sex for drugs, especially crack cocaine, as well as the partners of these users. Those who trade sex for drugs often engage in unprotected sex and have multiple sex partners. People who exchange sex for drugs and have a sexually transmitted infection (STI) that causes ulcers or sores on the genitals, such as syphilis or herpes simplex, are at a higher risk for HIV infection. Drug and/or alcohol users may also be at greater risk for infection because these substances often lessen inhibitions and reduce the reluctance to have unsafe, unprotected sex.

WOMEN AND HIV/AIDS

The proportion of women among AIDS sufferers increased steadily, from a reported 7% in 1985 to 25% in 2011. (See Figure 4.1.) The CDC indicates that 89,800 cases (39%) of the 232,902 cumulative AIDS cases from 1981 through 2011 among females were associated either directly or indirectly with injection drug use. (See Table 3.1 in Chapter 3.)

The racial and ethnic differences among females with HIV/AIDS are striking. In *HIV Surveillance in Women*, the CDC notes that although African American and Hispanic females made up 12% and 15%, respectively, of all females in the United States in 2011, they accounted for 64% (6,595) and 15% (1,530), respectively, of the 10,257 adult and adolescent females diagnosed with HIV infection

FIGURE 4.1

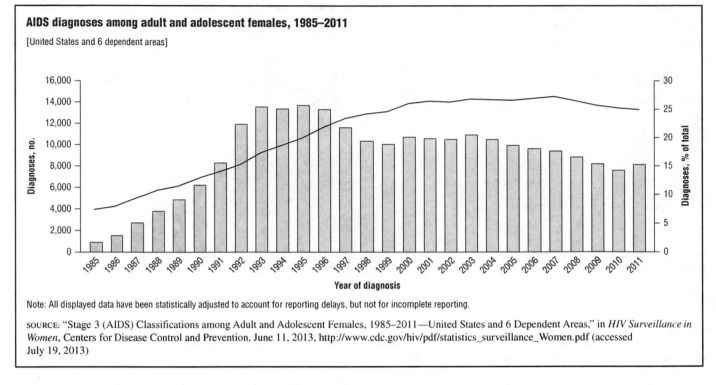

AIDS diagnoses among adult and adolescent females, 1985–2011

[United States and 6 dependent areas]

Note: All displayed data have been statistically adjusted to account for reporting delays, but not for incomplete reporting.

SOURCE: "Stage 3 (AIDS) Classifications among Adult and Adolescent Females, 1985–2011—United States and 6 Dependent Areas," in *HIV Surveillance in Women*, Centers for Disease Control and Prevention, June 11, 2013, http://www.cdc.gov/hiv/pdf/statistics_surveillance_Women.pdf (accessed July 19, 2013)

in 2011. (See Table 4.5.) In contrast, white females made up 66% of the U.S. female population but just 17% (1,776) of adult and adolescent females diagnosed with HIV.

Women can infect their unborn children with HIV during the course of pregnancy, during delivery, or by breastfeeding after birth. The dramatic decrease in the number of women who gave birth to HIV-infected babies during the 1990s was largely attributable to the introduction of antiretroviral therapy (ART). Women of childbearing age can be tested for HIV, and, if they are positive, they have the option of receiving ART before they become pregnant to decrease the chances of transmitting the virus to their unborn children.

Along with ART, which lowers the mother's viral load to undetectable levels, deliveries via elective cesarean section (the surgical delivery of a baby) rather than vaginal births may also help reduce mother-to-child transmission. In "Pregnant Women, Infants, and Children" (May 2, 2013, http://www.cdc.gov/hiv/risk/gender/pregnantwomen/index.html), the CDC states that with treatment perinatal transmission can be reduced to less than 1%.

HIV/AIDS in Women in Small Towns and Rural Areas

Most HIV/AIDS cases occur among women who live in large metropolitan areas with populations of greater than 500,000. However, the number of HIV/AIDS cases is increasing in rural areas, especially through heterosexual transmission. Figure 4.2 reveals that at the end of 2010 the highest rates of women living with AIDS were

reported in the District of Columbia (847.3 cases per 100,000 population), New York (282.4), the U.S. Virgin Islands (262.7), Maryland (244), Puerto Rico (207.5), and Florida (188). In contrast, the lowest rates were reported by states in the Midwest.

Sexually Transmitted Infections

Preventing, identifying, and promptly treating STIs is vitally important for the health of young women. Most HIV in women is spread through heterosexual sex (see Table 4.3), and the increase in STIs parallels that of HIV/AIDS.

In "The Role of STD Detection and Treatment in HIV Prevention—CDC Fact Sheet" (September 1, 2010, http://www.cdc.gov/std/Hiv/STDFact-STD-HIV.htm), the CDC explains that women with STIs are "at least two to five times more likely than uninfected [women] to acquire HIV infection if they are exposed to the virus through sexual contact" because they have an increased number of HIV target cells (CD4+ T cells) present in their cervical secretions. These cells facilitate the entrance of HIV into the body. Furthermore, women with STIs are more likely to shed HIV in both ulcer-forming and inflammatory genital secretions. They are also more likely to shed HIV in greater amounts than people infected with HIV alone, which contributes to the spread of HIV. By treating an STI, the shedding of HIV on sexual contact is lessened, which in turn reduces the spread of HIV infection.

FIGURE 4.2

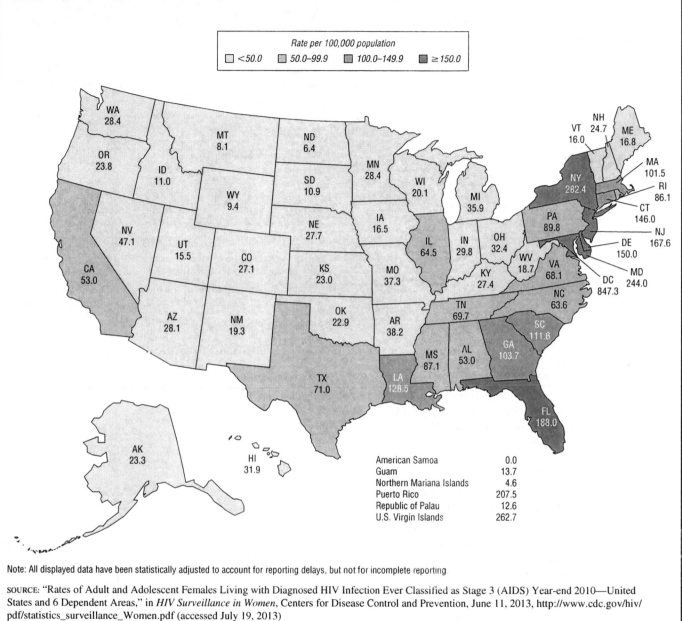

Rates of females living with diagnosed AIDS, 2010

[United States and 6 dependent areas. Population = 118,538.]

Total rate = 89.0

Rate per 100,000 population

□ <50.0   ▨ 50.0–99.9   ▨ 100.0–149.9   ▨ ≥150.0

WA 28.4
OR 23.8
MT 8.1
ND 6.4
MN 28.4
ID 11.0
WY 9.4
SD 10.9
NV 47.1
UT 15.5
CO 27.1
NE 27.7
IA 16.5
CA 53.0
KS 23.0
MO 37.3
AZ 28.1
NM 19.3
OK 22.9
AR 38.2
TX 71.0
WI 20.1
MI 35.9
IL 64.5
IN 29.8
OH 32.4
KY 27.4
TN 69.7
MS 87.1
AL 53.0
GA 103.7
LA 128.5
WV 18.7
VA 68.1
NC 63.6
SC 111.6
FL 188.0
NY 282.4
PA 89.8
VT 16.0
NH 24.7
ME 16.8
MA 101.5
RI 86.1
CT 146.0
NJ 167.6
DE 150.0
MD 244.0
DC 847.3
AK 23.3
HI 31.9

American Samoa   0.0
Guam   13.7
Northern Mariana Islands 4.6
Puerto Rico   207.5
Republic of Palau   12.6
U.S. Virgin Islands   262.7

Note: All displayed data have been statistically adjusted to account for reporting delays, but not for incomplete reporting.

SOURCE: "Rates of Adult and Adolescent Females Living with Diagnosed HIV Infection Ever Classified as Stage 3 (AIDS) Year-end 2010—United States and 6 Dependent Areas," in *HIV Surveillance in Women*, Centers for Disease Control and Prevention, June 11, 2013, http://www.cdc.gov/hiv/pdf/statistics_surveillance_Women.pdf (accessed July 19, 2013)

MSM SEXUAL CONTACT

MSM is still the major risk category for HIV infection, although the increase in the number of cases has slowed in recent years. Epidemiologists (public health researchers who analyze the extent and types of illnesses in a population and the factors that influence their distribution) believe that HIV/AIDS among MSM may have peaked in 1992. As in previous years, in 2011 MSM contact accounted for two-thirds of HIV exposure and transmission for males with or without injection drug use (21,921, or 66%, of the 33,221 cases). (See Table 3.5 in Chapter 3.)

OLDER ADULTS

The National Institute on Drug Abuse (NIDA) reports in "Who Is at Risk for HIV Infection and Which Populations Are Most Affected?" (July 2012, http://www.drugabuse.gov/publications/research-reports/hivaids/who-risk-hiv-infection-which-populations-are-most-affected) that since 1999 new HIV infections have been increasing among adults aged 50 years and older, who accounted for 16% of the new diagnoses of HIV infection in 2010. The institute explains that adults may not feel they are at risk and therefore may engage in unsafe sex. Also, medical

FIGURE 4.3

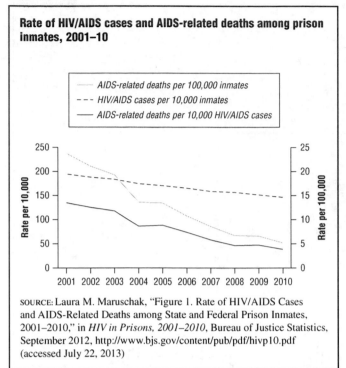

Rate of HIV/AIDS cases and AIDS-related deaths among prison inmates, 2001–10

- AIDS-related deaths per 100,000 inmates
- - - HIV/AIDS cases per 10,000 inmates
- AIDS-related deaths per 10,000 HIV/AIDS cases

SOURCE: Laura M. Maruschak, "Figure 1. Rate of HIV/AIDS Cases and AIDS-Related Deaths among State and Federal Prison Inmates, 2001–2010," in *HIV in Prisons, 2001–2010*, Bureau of Justice Statistics, September 2012, http://www.bjs.gov/content/pub/pdf/hivp10.pdf (accessed July 22, 2013)

practitioners may underestimate older adults' risk for HIV infection. The NIDA predicts that by 2015 half of all new cases of HIV infection will occur in people over the age of 50 years and observes that HIV-infected older adults progress more quickly to AIDS than do younger adults.

PRISONERS AND AIDS

According to Laura M. Maruschak of the Bureau of Justice Statistics, in *HIV in Prisons, 2001–2010* (September 2012, http://www.bjs.gov/content/pub/pdf/hivp10.pdf), the number of HIV-positive state and federal prisoners has declined 3% each year since 2001. Likewise, among inmates with HIV/AIDS the number of AIDS-related deaths has declined an average of 13% per year, and among all inmates it has dropped 16% per year. (See Figure 4.3.) The number of state inmates with HIV/AIDS decreased from 19,290 in 2009 to 18,515 in 2010. The number of federal inmates with HIV/AIDS declined from 1,590 to 1,578 during the same period.

Between 2008 and 2010 the number and rate of AIDS-related deaths in state prisons decreased. (See Table 4.6.) AIDS-related deaths in state prisons decreased from 89 in 2009 to 69 in 2010 among males, from 70 to 43 among non-Hispanic African Americans, and from 87 to 60 among all state inmates aged 35 years and older.

Every year since statistics have been gathered, AIDS-related conditions have been the second-leading cause of death for state prison inmates, behind "illness/natural causes." Nevertheless, the proportion of deaths

attributable to AIDS has declined markedly since 1995. Maruschak notes that the rate of AIDS-related deaths for state prison inmates dropped below the rate for the U.S. general population. (See Figure 4.4.) This sharp drop is likely attributable to effective treatment with combination ART.

Geographic Differences

Maruschak indicates that 20,093 U.S. inmates were confirmed as infected with HIV or diagnosed with AIDS in 2010. (See Table 4.7.) Less than half (47%) of all state prisoners with HIV/AIDS were held in California, Florida, New York, and Texas. Each of these states reported more than 1,000 inmates with HIV/AIDS at the close of 2010.

Sex, Racial, and Age Differences

At year-end 2010, 20,093 U.S. inmates were reported as infected with HIV or had confirmed cases of AIDS, which was a slight decrease from the previous year's estimate of 20,880 HIV/AIDS cases. (See Table 4.7.) The numbers of AIDS-related deaths in U.S. prisons also decreased slightly—from 102 in 2008, to 101 in 2009, to 79 in 2010. (See Table 4.8.)

Male inmates make up the overwhelming majority of HIV-infected or confirmed cases of AIDS among inmates in state and federal prisons. In 2010 an estimated 18,337 male inmates were known to be HIV positive or diagnosed with AIDS, compared with 1,756 female inmates. (See Table 4.9.) However, as a percentage of the U.S. inmate population, a higher percentage of female inmates were reported with HIV/AIDS (1.9% compared with 1.4% of male inmates).

The AIDS-related deaths in state prisons occurred largely among males, who accounted for 96% (69) of such deaths in 2010. (See Table 4.6.) The majority of these deaths (43, or 60%) were among African American inmates. Female inmates accounted for three (4%) of the AIDS-related deaths, and one death was of an inmate who was aged 20 to 24 years.

Drug and Needle Use among Prisoners

Public education campaigns about the "safer" use of drugs and syringes appear to be reducing HIV infection in the general public. However, these measures seem to be having little effect in prisons. Many incarcerated IDUs continue to inject while in prison, often sharing needles because injection equipment is in short supply.

This is a dilemma for prisons, where syringes and needles are prohibited, as are illegal drugs, and chemicals for disinfecting the illicit needles are not readily available. Although state and federal prison officials in the United States want to stop the spread of HIV among inmates, most cannot keep pace with or stem the flow of illegal drugs into

TABLE 4.6

AIDS-related deaths among state prison inmates, 2008–10

	Number of AIDS-related deaths[a]			Rate of AIDS-related deaths per 100,000 inmates[b]		
Characteristics	2008	2009	2010	2008	2009	2010
State total	89	94	72	7	7	5
Sex						
Male	78	89	69	6	7	6
Female	11	5	3	12	5	3
Race/Hispanic[c]						
White[d]	21	15	23	4	3	5
Black[d]	57	70	43	27	33	21
Hispanic	10	8	5	2	1	1
Age						
19 or younger	0	0	0	0	0	0
20–24	0	3	1	0	1	0
25–34	9	4	11	2	1	3
35–44	21	29	22	5	7	5
45–54	43	38	25	23	20	13
55 or older	16	20	13	24	30	20

[a]Based on individual reports submitted to the program.
[b]To calculate the age rates, the number of state prisoners by age was first estimated by applying the age distribution reported in the 2004 Survey of Inmates in State Correctional Facilities to the 2008–2010 midyear custody counts in National Prisoner Statistics Program-1.
[c]Detail does not sum to total because deaths among those of other races are excluded.
[d]Excludes persons of Hispanic/Latino origin.
Note: Includes deaths in a private facilities.

SOURCE: Laura M. Maruschak, "Table 5. AIDS-Related Deaths among State Prison Inmates in Custody, by Demographic Characteristics, 2008–2010," in *HIV in Prisons, 2001–2010*, Bureau of Justice Statistics, September 2012, http://www.bjs.gov/content/pub/pdf/hivp10.pdf (accessed July 22, 2013)

FIGURE 4.4

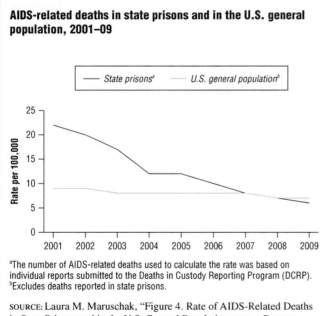

AIDS-related deaths in state prisons and in the U.S. general population, 2001–09

[a]The number of AIDS-related deaths used to calculate the rate was based on individual reports submitted to the Deaths in Custody Reporting Program (DCRP).
[b]Excludes deaths reported in state prisons.

SOURCE: Laura M. Maruschak, "Figure 4. Rate of AIDS-Related Deaths in State Prisons and in the U.S. General Population among Persons Ages 15 to 54, 2001–2009," in *HIV in Prisons, 2001–2010*, Bureau of Justice Statistics, September 2012, http://www.bjs.gov/content/pub/pdf/hivp10.pdf (accessed July 22, 2013)

prisons. To minimize the spread of HIV in prisons, countries such as Switzerland and the United Kingdom provide prisoners with disinfectant or clean needles. U.S. officials believe these actions endorse illegal drug use. Instead, they focus on providing treatment and rehabilitation programs for drug-addicted prisoners.

Nonetheless, many observers feel that prison systems can and should do more to prevent HIV transmission related to injection drug use. They assert that needle and syringe programs and drug substitution therapy, such as methadone maintenance (the use of methadone as treatment for a person who is addicted to heroin), sharply reduce the sharing of injecting equipment and the spread of HIV and other bloodborne pathogens. For example, Sheryl L. Catz et al. describe in "Prevention Needs of HIV-Positive Men and Women Awaiting Release from Prison" (*AIDS and Behavior*, vol.16, no. 1, January 2012) a Wisconsin prison system initiative that offers health education classes to inmates who are HIV negative or positive. Among the topics covered is the transmission of STIs, including HIV. The researchers note that needle exchange programs are crucial for reducing the risk of transmission, that there are not enough of these programs, and that clean needles are neither affordable nor legal.

U.S. Prison Systems Take Action to Prevent HIV Infection

In "Integrated Prevention Services for HIV Infection, Viral Hepatitis, Sexually Transmitted Diseases, and Tuberculosis for Persons Who Use Drugs Illicitly: Summary Guidance from CDC and the U.S. Department of Health and Human Services" (*Morbidity and Mortality*

TABLE 4.7

Inmates infected with HIV or diagnosed with AIDS, by jurisdiction, yearend 2008–10

Jurisdiction	Total HIV/AIDS cases[a]			HIV/AIDS cases as a percent of total custody population[b]		
	2008	2009	2010	2008	2009	2010
U.S. total[c]	21,611	20,880	20,093	1.6%	1.5%	1.5%
Federal	1,538	1,590	1,578	0.9%	0.9%	0.9%
State	20,073	19,290	18,515	1.6%	1.6%	1.5%
Alabama	275	275	252	1.1	1.0	1.0
Alaska	13	28	—	0.4	0.7	—
Arizona	179	154	164	0.6	0.5	0.5
Arkansas	118	112	128	0.9	0.8	0.9
California	1,402	1,235	1,098	0.8	0.7	0.7
Colorado	173	185	181	1.0	1.0	1.0
Connecticut	380	320	301	2.0	1.8	1.7
Delaware	132	71	73	1.9	1.1	1.1
Florida	3,250	3,082	2,920	3.6	3.4	3.2
Georgia	961	951	912	1.8	1.8	1.9
Hawaii	23	24	18	0.7	0.8	0.5
Idaho	28	23	20	0.6	0.4	0.4
Illinois	457	460	487	1.0	1.0	1.0
Indiana	—	—	—	—	—	—
Iowa	41	28	36	0.5	0.3	0.4
Kansas	46	53	33	0.5	0.6	0.4
Kentucky	131	90	87	1.0	0.7	0.7
Louisiana	458	573	665	2.2	2.9	3.5
Maine	9	8	15	0.4	0.4	0.8
Maryland	588	565	722	2.6	2.6	3.2
Massachusetts	264	247	206	2.4	2.2	1.8
Michigan	341	404	233	0.7	0.9	0.5
Minnesota	44	48	47	0.5	0.5	0.5
Mississippi	246	222	254	2.0	1.9	2.3
Missouri	304	313	273	1.0	1.0	0.9
Montana	6	7	7	0.4	0.4	0.4
Nebraska	16	21	20	0.4	0.5	0.4
Nevada	116	132	133	0.9	1.1	1.1
New Hampshire	16	12	12	0.6	0.4	0.5
New Jersey	520	417	420	2.3	2.0	1.9
New Mexico	33	34	27	0.5	0.5	0.4
New York	3,500	3,200	3,080	5.8	5.5	5.5
North Carolina	824	791	720	2.1	2.0	1.8
North Dakota	6	7	9	0.4	0.5	0.6
Ohio	414	379	381	0.8	0.8	0.8
Oklahoma	139	146	155	0.8	0.8	0.9
Oregon[d]	55	66	63	0.4	0.5	0.5
Pennsylvania	727	782	703	1.5	1.6	1.5
Rhode Island	54	48	47	1.4	1.4	1.5
South Carolina	409	418	412	1.7	1.8	1.8
South Dakota	13	11	11	0.4	0.3	0.3
Tennessee	188	195	219	1.3	1.3	1.5
Texas	2,450	2,414	2,394	1.8	1.7	1.7
Utah	36	38	35	0.7	0.7	0.6
Vermont	14	17	3	1.0	1.1	0.2
Virginia	433	433	306	1.4	1.5	1.0
Washington	79	78	75	0.5	0.5	0.4
West Virginia	25	19	25	0.5	0.4	0.5
Wisconsin	132	145	128	0.6	0.7	0.6
Wyoming	5	9	5	0.4	0.6	0.3
Northeast	5,484	5,051	4,787	3.2%	3.0%	2.9%
Midwest	1,814	1,869	1,658	0.8%	0.8%	0.7%
South	10,627	10,357	10,244	2.0%	2.0%	2.0%
West	2,148	2,013	1,826	0.7%	0.7%	0.6%

—Not reported.
[a]Counts published in previous reports may have been revised.
[b]Excludes data from Alaska due to incomplete reporting.
[c]Excludes inmates in jurisdictions that did not report data.
[d]The number of HIV/AIDS cases in Oregon was based on a 3/9/09 count for 2008, a 7/20/2010 count for 2009, and a 6/28/11 count for 2010.
Note: Excludes inmates held in private facilities.

SOURCE: Laura M. Maruschak, Table 1. "Inmates in Custody of State and Federal Prison Authorities and Reported to Be HIV Positive or Have Confirmed AIDS, by Jurisdiction, Yearend 2008–2010," in *HIV in Prisons, 2001–2010*, Bureau of Justice Statistics, September 2012, http://www.bjs.gov/content/pub/pdf/hivp10.pdf (accessed July 22, 2013)

TABLE 4.8

AIDS-related deaths among state and federal prison inmates, 2008–10

Jurisdiction	Number			Rate per 100,000 inmates		
	2008	2009	2010	2008	2009	2010
U.S. total	102	101	79	7	7	5
Federal	13	7	7	6	3	3
State	89	94	72	7	7	5

Note: Includes deaths in private facilities.

SOURCE: Laura M. Maruschak, "Table 4. AIDS-Related Deaths among State Prison Inmates in Custody, 2008–2010," in *HIV in Prisons, 2001–2010*, Bureau of Justice Statistics, September 2012, http://www.bjs.gov/content/pub/pdf/hivp10.pdf (accessed July 22, 2013)

Weekly Report, vol. 61, no. 5, November 9, 2012), Hrishikesh Belani et al. assert that prevention services are vital in jails, prisons, and juvenile detention centers. The researchers recommend a comprehensive range of services that can be delivered in correctional settings to people who use illicit drugs, including routine HIV testing, access to sterile drug injection or clean preparation equipment, and referral to appropriate care upon release. (See Table 4.10.) Figure 4.5 shows Belani et al.'s recommendations for monitoring and evaluating services that are delivered to people who use drugs illicitly across all settings and underscores the importance of integrated prevention and treatment services to improve how IDUs fare in terms of their health.

The CDC recommends in "HIV in Correctional Settings" (June 2012, http://www.cdc.gov/hiv/resources/factsheets/pdf/correctional.pdf) that "HIV screening be provided upon entry into prison and before release and that voluntary HIV testing be offered periodically during incarceration." Operational, legal, and financial challenges have also hampered HIV testing in correctional settings. For example, the regular turnover of jail inmates has prompted many jurisdictions to use rapid HIV tests and to test within the first 24 hours of incarceration. Some jurisdictions do not provide HIV testing because it increases their laboratory and medical costs.

Just as state policies on HIV testing vary, so do policies regarding HIV-positive inmates. For example, in "Ruling Soon on Isolation of Inmates with H.I.V." (NYTimes.com, November 18, 2012), Robbie Brown reports that Alabama and South Carolina isolate HIV-infected inmates from other prisoners to halt the spread of HIV (which may occur through consensual sex, rape, injection drug use, or even when inmates apply tattoos) and to control medical care costs. These policies are being scrutinized because inmates have testified that isolation is harmful and that they have been bullied and ridiculed because they are HIV infected. Medical experts feel isolation is unnecessary and observe that most states treat HIV-infected inmates with ART.

SEX WORKERS

In "Sex Workers and HIV/AIDS" (2013, http://www.avert.org/hiv-and-sex-work.htm), AVERT, an international HIV/AIDS charity, defines sex workers as "people who sell sex, and who work in a variety of environments. They include women, men and transgender people and people who may work either full time or part time, in brothels, or bars, on the street or from home." It suggests that because they have a high number of sexual partners, they are at risk of being infected with HIV and can potentially transmit the virus to many clients. The clients of sex workers serve as a so-called bridge population for the transmission of HIV—they convey the virus from this high-risk population to the general population.

Melissa Hope Ditmore and Dan Allman observe in "An Analysis of the Implementation of PEPFAR's Antiprostitution Pledge and Its Implications for Successful HIV Prevention among Organizations Working with Sex Workers" (*Journal of the International AIDS Society*, vol. 16, March 28, 2013) that U.S. government funding to address the HIV/AIDS epidemic has been subject to an antiprostitution clause—funded organizations must have a written policy that opposes prostitution. Interpretation of this requirement varies and some organizations mistakenly believe they must stop providing services to sex workers, thereby further limiting sex workers' access to prevention, treatment, care, and support. Ditmore and Allman assert that despite sex workers' description of the toll these actions have taken on their health, they remain stigmatized and are often denied services.

HEMOPHILIACS

Hemophilia is a group of genetic disorders in which defects in a number of genes located on the X chromosome disrupt the proper clotting of blood. The most common type of hemophilia—hemophilia A—is a deficiency of a clotting substance designated Factor VIII. Varying severities of hemophilia can occur, depending on the level of Factor VIII present in the patient's plasma. Treatment of hemophilia involves close attention to injury prevention and periodic intravenous administration of Factor VIII concentrates, commonly known as clotting factors.

Because screening for HIV antibodies was not available until 1985, many hemophiliacs were exposed to HIV-contaminated blood and clotting factors. The national distribution of clotting factor concentrates before 1985 led to a high prevalence of HIV infections among hemophiliacs. The prevalence of HIV infection differs by the type and severity of the coagulation (clotting) disorder.

According to the Hemophilia Foundation of America (NHF), in "Hemophilia Awareness Month" (2013, http://www.hemophiliafed.org/programs/meetings-events/hemophilia-awareness-month/#.Ue3KOxYSz7o), during the

TABLE 4.9

Inmates infected with HIV or diagnosed with AIDS, by sex, yearend 2009 and 2010

	Male				Female			
	Number		Percent		Number		Percent	
Jurisdiction	2009	2010	2009	2010	2009	2010	2009	2010
U.S. total*	19,027	18,337	1.5%	1.4%	1,853	1,756	1.9%	1.9%
Federal	1,495	1,498	0.9%	0.9%	95	80	0.8%	0.7%
State	17,532	16,839	1.6%	1.5%	1,758	1,676	2.1%	2.0%
Alabama	260	236	1.1%	1.0%	15	16	0.9%	1.0%
Alaska	20	—	0.6	—	8	—	1.5	—
Arizona	135	154	0.5	0.5	19	10	0.5	0.3
Arkansas	101	121	0.8	0.9	11	7	1.1	0.6
California	1,146	1,023	0.7	0.7	89	75	0.8	0.8
Colorado	160	159	1.0	1.0	25	22	1.3	1.1
Connecticut	268	261	1.6	1.6	52	40	4.8	3.9
Delaware	63	65	1.0	1.1	8	8	1.7	1.8
Florida	2,749	2,636	3.2	3.1	333	284	6.3	5.3
Georgia	864	832	1.7	1.8	87	80	2.3	2.1
Hawaii	18	14	0.7	0.5	6	4	1.2	0.7
Idaho	19	16	0.4	0.4	4	4	0.6	0.5
Illinois	411	439	1.0	1.0	49	48	1.9	1.6
Indiana	—	—	—	—	—	—	—	—
Iowa	27	31	0.3	0.4	1	5	0.1	0.6
Kansas	48	29	0.6	0.3	5	4	0.9	0.6
Kentucky	81	78	0.7	0.7	9	9	1.0	0.7
Louisiana	488	599	2.6	3.3	85	66	7.7	6.1
Maine	8	15	0.4	0.8	0	0	0.0	0.0
Maryland	533	658	2.5	3.0	32	64	3.1	6.6
Massachusetts	230	192	2.2	1.8	17	14	2.4	1.8
Michigan	385	231	0.9	0.5	19	2	1.1	0.1
Minnesota	45	43	0.5	0.5	3	4	0.5	0.7
Mississippi	196	221	1.9	2.2	26	33	1.8	2.6
Missouri	309	259	1.1	0.9	4	14	0.2	0.6
Montana	7	7	0.5	0.5	0	0	0.0	0.0
Nebraska	19	19	0.5	0.5	2	1	0.5	0.2
Nevada	111	118	1.0	1.0	21	15	2.2	1.6
New Hampshire	12	12	0.4	0.5	0	0	0.0	0.0
New Jersey	385	389	1.9	1.9	32	31	3.6	3.7
New Mexico	33	27	0.6	0.4	1	0	0.2	0.0
New York	2,930	2,820	5.2	5.2	270	260	10.8	11.7
North Carolina	716	650	1.9	1.7	75	70	2.6	2.5
North Dakota	7	9	0.6	0.7	0	0	0.0	0.0
Ohio	350	355	0.8	0.8	29	26	0.7	0.7
Oklahoma	136	146	0.9	0.9	10	9	0.4	0.4
Oregon	61	59	0.5	0.5	5	4	0.5	0.4
Pennsylvania	720	629	1.5	1.4	62	74	2.4	2.9
Rhode Island	40	40	1.2	1.3	8	7	4.3	3.9
South Carolina	391	388	1.8	1.8	27	24	1.8	1.6
South Dakota	11	9	0.4	0.3	0	2	0.0	0.5
Tennessee	181	199	1.3	1.4	14	20	1.2	1.7
Texas	2,182	2,153	1.7	1.6	232	241	2.3	2.3
Utah	32	30	0.7	0.6	6	5	1.1	0.9
Vermont	17	3	1.2	0.2	0	0	0.0	0.0
Virginia	398	275	1.5	1.0	35	31	1.5	1.3
Washington	72	70	0.5	0.4	6	5	0.5	0.4
West Virginia	18	23	0.4	0.5	1	2	0.2	0.4
Wisconsin	131	93	0.6	0.4	14	35	1.1	2.8
Wyoming	8	4	0.6	0.2	1	1	0.5	0.5
Northeast	4,610	4,361	2.9%	2.8%	441	426	5.2%	5.3%
Midwest	1,743	1,517	0.8%	0.7%	126	141	0.8%	0.9%
South	9,357	9,280	1.9%	1.9%	1,000	964	2.7%	2.5%
West	1,822	1,681	0.7%	0.6%	191	145	0.8%	0.7%

—Not reported.
*Excludes inmates in jurisdictions that did not report HIV/AIDS infection by sex.
Note: Excludes inmates held in private facilities.

SOURCE: Laura M. Maruschak, "Table 2. Inmates in Custody of State and Federal Prison Authorities and Reported to Be HIV Positive or Have Confirmed AIDS, by Jurisdiction Yearend 2009 and 2010," in *HIV in Prisons, 2001–2010*, Bureau of Justice Statistics, September 2012, http://www.bjs.gov/content/pub/pdf/hivp10.pdf (accessed July 22, 2013).

TABLE 4.10

Recommended prevention services for inmates who use illicit drugs, 2012

Correctional institution
Examples of integrated prevention services

Routine HIV testing, TB screening, and vaccination for viral hepatitis A and B
Screening of young women in jails and juvenile detention centers for gonorrhea and chlamydia
HCV testing conducted
HIV-infected inmates referred to HIV clinical services during and after incarceration, and progress tracked
Access to sterile drug injection or clean preparation equipment and condoms
Education on prevention of overdose
Persons addicted to opiates offered medication-assisted therapy while incarcerated or via referral at discharge
Comprehensive health risk assessment services for TB, HIV, STDs, and viral hepatitis as well as counseling for reproductive health, drug use, alcohol misuse, and mental health disorders
Case management for housing/drug/alcohol/mental health services and discharge planning to inmates for appropriate follow-up care in the community
Routine screening for syphilis, chlamydia, and gonorrhea
% of inmates screened for infection with HIV, TB, and viral hepatitis
No. of inmates diagnosed with syphilis, chlamydia, or gonorrhea
% of inmates receiving HAV/HBV vaccination
% of tested inmates who test positive for HIV, TB, or viral hepatitis
% of inmates with diagnosed HIV infection, syphilis, chlamydia, gonorrhea, TB, or viral hepatitis who receive comprehensive discharge planning and continued care

HAV = Hepatitis A Virus.
HBV = Hepatitis B Virus.
HIV = Human Immunodeficiency Virus.
STD = Sexually Transmitted Disease.
TB = Tuberculosis.

SOURCE: Adapted from Hrishikesh Belani et al., "Table. Examples of Integrated Prevention Services That Can Be Delivered in Different Settings to Persons Who Use Drugs Illicitly and Examples of Monitoring and Evaluation Indicators," in "Integrated Prevention Services for HIV Infection, Viral Hepatitis, Sexually Transmitted Diseases, and Tuberculosis for Persons Who Use Drugs Illicitly: Summary Guidance from CDC and the U.S. Department of Health and Human Services," *MMWR*, vol. 61, no. 5, November 9, 2012, http://www.cdc.gov/mmwr/pdf/rr/rr6105.pdf (accessed July 22, 2013)

early 1970s and 1980s about half of all people with hemophilia became infected with HIV through blood products. As a result, 70% of Americans with hemophilia were infected with HIV, and more than half of those infected died.

Thomas Tencer et al. explain in "Medical Costs and Resource Utilization for Hemophilia Patients with and without HIV or HCV Infection" (*Journal of Managed Care Pharmacy*, vol. 13, no. 9, November–December 2007) that although the possibility of contracting HIV or the hepatitis C virus has been virtually eliminated in the United States, at the close of 2007 about one-third of hemophiliacs were believed to be HIV infected or infected with both HIV and hepatitis C. Coinfected people have been found to have higher rates of illness, death, and utilization of clotting factor.

A Slow Reaction

Concentrated clotting factor, which is derived from human blood obtained from as many as 2,000 donors,

became available during the mid-1970s. Its success at stopping bleeding was so dramatic that hemophilia changed from a disease that produced intense pain, disability, and the possibility of premature death to one that allowed sufferers to lead nearly normal lives. Hemophiliacs could infuse clotting factors into their own blood if they felt bleeding was about to start. Patients were advised by their physicians to "infuse early and often."

During the late 1970s and early 1980s some clotting factor concentrates were inadvertently infected with HIV. Even after the first cases of HIV/AIDS appeared in people with hemophilia and the CDC, along with the NHF, identified this new disease as being bloodborne, physicians did not advise their patients to alter their clotting factor treatments. Hemophiliacs were encouraged to continue using their clotting factor because researchers and physicians were not sure there would be a major epidemic.

Anecdotal comments from hemophiliacs indicate that when many of them became infected, primary care doctors were slow to respond and supplied little information. There was no warning to practice safe sex to prevent the spread of HIV. Some hemophiliacs reported receiving more information from gay men's organizations than from their own hematologists (physicians who specialize in diseases and disorders of the blood).

In "The Aging Patient with Hemophilia: Complications, Comorbidities, and Management Issues" (*Hematology*, December 2010), Claire Philipp of the University of Medicine and Dentistry of New Jersey–Robert Wood Johnson Medical School explains that although clotting factor concentrates free of HIV contamination have been available since 1985, many older hemophiliacs are infected. However, since the advent of ART, the survival rate of HIV-infected hemophiliacs has improved, with 27% to 39% surviving 20 to 25 years.

ANGER AND COMPENSATION. Many hemophiliacs feel they are entitled to compensation or, at the very least, assistance in paying the overwhelming medical expenses they incurred as a result of HIV infection and AIDS treatment. They maintain that the companies that produced the clotting factors were slow to warn the public about HIV and slow to use heat treatment to eliminate the live virus from the clotting factors (although this procedure has not gained widespread acceptance among scientists as an adequate method to inactivate HIV).

Hemophilia foundations in some countries have convinced government pharmaceutical or insurance companies to compensate HIV-infected hemophiliacs. Peter D. Weinberg et al. report in "Legal, Financial, and Public Health Consequences of HIV Contamination of Blood and Blood Products in the 1980s and 1990s" (*Annals of Internal Medicine*, vol. 136, no. 4, February 19, 2002) that Armour Pharmaceuticals agreed to pay six

FIGURE 4.5

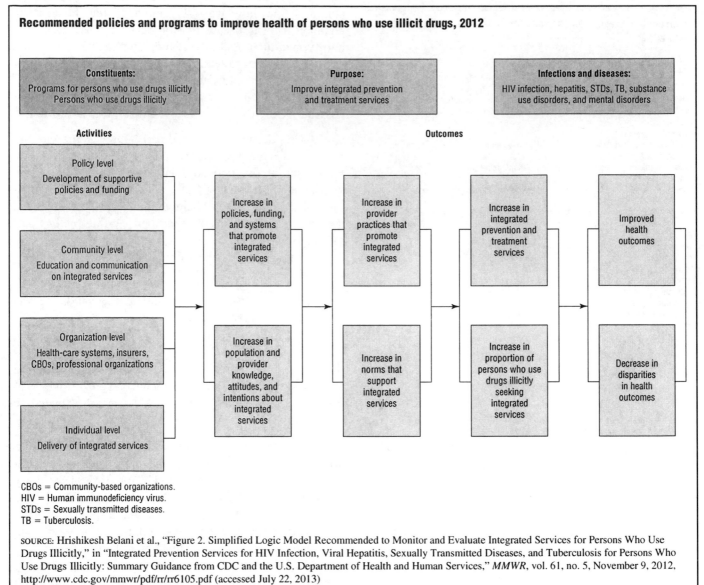

Recommended policies and programs to improve health of persons who use illicit drugs, 2012

Constituents:	Purpose:	Infections and diseases:
Programs for persons who use drugs illicitly Persons who use drugs illicitly	Improve integrated prevention and treatment services	HIV infection, hepatitis, STDs, TB, substance use disorders, and mental disorders

Activities

Policy level
Development of supportive policies and funding

Community level
Education and communication on integrated services

Organization level
Health-care systems, insurers, CBOs, professional organizations

Individual level
Delivery of integrated services

Outcomes

Increase in policies, funding, and systems that promote integrated services

Increase in population and provider knowledge, attitudes, and intentions about integrated services

Increase in provider practices that promote integrated services

Increase in norms that support integrated services

Increase in integrated prevention and treatment services

Increase in proportion of persons who use drugs illicitly seeking integrated services

Improved health outcomes

Decrease in disparities in health outcomes

CBOs = Community-based organizations.
HIV = Human immunodeficiency virus.
STDs = Sexually transmitted diseases.
TB = Tuberculosis.

SOURCE: Hrishikesh Belani et al., "Figure 2. Simplified Logic Model Recommended to Monitor and Evaluate Integrated Services for Persons Who Use Drugs Illicitly," in "Integrated Prevention Services for HIV Infection, Viral Hepatitis, Sexually Transmitted Diseases, and Tuberculosis for Persons Who Use Drugs Illicitly: Summary Guidance from CDC and the U.S. Department of Health and Human Services," *MMWR*, vol. 61, no. 5, November 9, 2012, http://www.cdc.gov/mmwr/pdf/rr/rr6105.pdf (accessed July 22, 2013)

Canadians $1.5 million each; Germany offered people infected with HIV and those who became ill with AIDS annual compensation; and Switzerland extended annual compensation of $12,216 to people with AIDS. France gave one-time compensation of $87,735 to hemophiliacs at the time they were diagnosed with AIDS due to tainted blood products. During the first decade of the 21st century, more than 20 developed countries acted to compensate HIV-infected hemophiliacs. In contrast, developing countries continued to grapple with blood-supply safety issues.

In 1995 the U.S. Supreme Court refused to hear a class action suit brought by hemophiliacs against a pharmaceutical company and other blood-product manufacturers (*Barton v. American Red Cross*, 826 F. Supp. 412 and 826 F. Supp. 407, append 43 F. 3rd 678, certiorari denied 116 S. Ct. 84). Regardless, some companies have

reached out-of-court settlements with affected people. For example, according to the article "4 Drug Companies Ordered to Pay Hemophiliacs" (NYTimes.com, May 8, 1997), in 1997 four manufacturers of blood clotting products were ordered by a federal judge to pay approximately $670 million to settle cases on behalf of more than 6,000 hemophiliacs who were infected in the United States during the early 1980s. The settlement compensated each infected hemophiliac with an estimated $100,000 payment.

The NHF explains in "Ricky Ray Program Office Set to Close" (September 29, 2005, http://www.hemophilia.org/NHFWeb/MainPgs/MainNHF.aspx?menuid=117&contentid=360) that the international catastrophe of HIV/AIDS in the hemophilia community was recognized by the U.S. federal government in 1998 with passage of the

Ricky Ray Hemophilia Relief Fund Act, named for a boy with hemophilia who died from AIDS. According to the NHF, the act provided "payments of $100,000 to individuals with hemophilia who were treated with HIV-contaminated clotting factor products between July 1, 1982, and December 31, 1987. Spouses and children who contracted HIV from these individuals, as well as specified family survivors were also eligible for compassionate payment." When the program closed in October 2005, it had paid over $559 million to more than 7,171 eligible individuals and survivors.

CHAPTER 5
CHILDREN, ADOLESCENTS, AND HIV/AIDS

HIV/AIDS IN CHILDREN: DIFFERENT FROM HIV/AIDS IN ADULTS

HIV can cause AIDS in adults and children. The virus attacks and damages the immune and central nervous systems of all infected people. However, the development and course of the disease in children differs considerably from its progression in adults.

Before the use of highly active antiretroviral therapy (HAART) and early intervention strategies, there were two patterns of HIV progression among children. The first pattern, which is called severe immunodeficiency, is apparent as recurring serious infections or encephalopathy (any of various diseases of the brain). The National Institute of Allergy and Infectious Diseases (NIAID) reports in the fact sheet "HIV Infection in Infants and Children" (September 10, 2008, http://www.niaid.nih.gov/topics/hivaids/understanding/population%20specific%20information/Pages/children.aspx) that severe immunodeficiency develops in 20% of infected infants during their first year of life. The second pattern, which occurs in the other 80% of infected children, is more gradual and is similar to the development and progression of the disease that is observed in adults.

HIV nucleic acid detection tests can detect the presence of HIV in nearly all infants aged one month and older. Before the development of these tests, detecting HIV infection, especially in babies, was difficult. This is because the earlier tests involved the detection of antibodies formed by the infant in response to HIV. However, infants have often not developed the full capacity to produce antibodies at the time of testing. Furthermore, HIV-infected mothers may transmit antibodies alone, without the virus, to their babies. In the latter instance, infants with positive results from antibody tests at birth may later test negative, indicating that the mother transmitted the HIV antibodies to the baby, but not the virus itself.

Among infants and children, the disease is characterized by wasting syndrome, the failure to thrive, and unusually severe bacterial infections. Except for *Pneumocystis carinii* pneumonia, children with symptomatic HIV infection rarely develop the same opportunistic infections that adults contract. Although adults and children with HIV may both suffer from chronic or recurrent diarrhea, its dehydrating effect may be particularly debilitating and life-threatening to children. Children infected with HIV may suffer recurrent bacterial infections such as severe forms of conjunctivitis (pink eye), ear infections, tonsillitis, and persistent or recurrent oral thrush (an infection of the mouth or throat that is caused by the fungus *Candida albicans*). They may also suffer from enlarged lymph nodes, chronic pneumonia, developmental delays, and neurological abnormalities. Simply stated, the immune system of HIV-infected children is destroyed even as it matures.

Whether HIV positive or not, babies born to HIV-infected mothers appear to be predisposed to a variety of heart problems. In the landmark study "Cardiovascular Status of Infants and Children of Women Infected with HIV-1 (P2C2 HIV): A Cohort Study" (*Lancet*, vol. 360, no. 9330, August 3, 2002), Steven E. Lipshultz et al. examined more than 500 infants born to HIV-positive women. They discovered that the babies suffered from significantly higher rates of abnormalities, such as defects in the heart wall and valve and reduced pumping action. These defects occurred in less than 1% of healthy children whose mothers were not infected with HIV. Lipshultz et al. recognize that HIV alone did not necessarily cause these anomalies. They observe that a mother's alcohol, drug, or nutrition problems can also interfere with fetal heart development.

Hamisu M. Salihu et al. analyzed over 1.6 million birth records in Florida. In "Maternal HIV/AIDS Status and Neurological Outcomes in Neonates: A Population-Based

Study" (*Maternal and Child Health Journal*, April 20, 2011), the researchers report that babies born to HIV-infected mothers are at higher risk of having feeding difficulties and seizures (sudden loss of consciousness).

A CASE DEFINITION FOR CHILDREN

Because data were limited during the first few years of HIV's acknowledged presence in the United States, the Centers for Disease Control and Prevention's (CDC) definition of AIDS did not differentiate between adults and children until 1987, when the classification system was revised. The CDC Division of HIV/AIDS Prevention, National Center for HIV/AIDS, Viral Hepatitis, STD, and TB Prevention updated the pediatric definition in 1994, 1999, and 2008 as more information about HIV and AIDS became available. The 2008 revision, which takes into account new testing technologies, is intended for public health surveillance purposes and not as a guide for clinical diagnosis.

Changes to the case definitions were published by Eileen Schneider et al. of the CDC in "Revised Surveillance Case Definitions for HIV Infection among Adults, Adolescents, and Children Aged <18 Months and for HIV Infection and AIDS among Children Aged 18 Months to <13 Years—United States, 2008" (*Morbidity and Mortality Weekly Report*, vol. 57, no. RR-10, December 5, 2008). No changes were made to the 27 AIDS-defining conditions listed in Table 2.2 in Chapter 2. However, the 2008 criteria stipulate that:

- Because of the greater uncertainty that is associated with diagnostic testing for HIV in this population (maternal antibodies from the HIV-infected mother might exist in the infant after birth, possibly affecting HIV diagnostic testing of the infant that occurs soon after birth), children whose illness meets clinical criteria for the AIDS case definition but does not meet laboratory criteria for definitive or presumptive HIV infection are still categorized as HIV infected when the mother has laboratory-confirmed HIV infection.

- For children aged 18 months to less than 13 years, laboratory-confirmed evidence of HIV infection is required to meet the surveillance case definition for HIV infection and AIDS.

- Diagnostic confirmation of an AIDS-defining condition alone, without laboratory-confirmed evidence of HIV infection, is no longer sufficient to classify a child as HIV infected for surveillance purposes.

Table 5.1 presents the criteria for HIV infection in children. These include laboratory criteria such as the results of the screening test for HIV antibodies or detection of HIV using a virologic (nonantibody) test. HIV infection based on confirmed laboratory test results and documented in a medical record also meets the criteria

TABLE 5.1

Surveillance case definitions for HIV infection in children aged 18 months to 12 years, 2008

These 2008 surveillance case definitions of HIV infection and AIDS supersede those published in 1987 and 1999 and apply to all variants of HIV (e.g., HIV-1 or HIV-2). They are intended for public health surveillance only and are not a guide for clinical diagnosis.

The 2008 laboratory criteria for reportable HIV infection among persons aged 18 months to <13 years exclude confirmation of HIV infection through the diagnosis of AIDS-defining conditions alone. Laboratory-confirmed evidence of HIV infection is now required for all reported cases of HIV infection among children aged 18 months to <13 years.

Criteria for HIV infection

Children aged 18 months to <13 years are categorized as HIV infected for surveillance purposes if at least one of laboratory criteria or the other criterion is met.

Laboratory criteria

Positive result from a screening test for HIV antibody (e.g., reactive EIA), confirmed by a positive result from a supplemental test for HIV antibody (e.g., Western blot or indirect immunofluorescence assay).

or

Positive result or a detectable quantity by any of the following HIV virologic (non-antibody) tests:—HIV nucleic acid (DNA or RNA) detection (e.g., PCR)—HIV p24 antigen test, including neutralization assay—HIV isolation (viral culture)

Other criterion (for cases that do not meet laboratory criteria)

HIV infection diagnosed by a physician or qualified medical-care provider based on the laboratory criteria and documented in a medical record. Oral reports of prior laboratory test results are not acceptable.

EIA = enzyme immunoassay. PCR = polymerase chain reaction.

SOURCE: Eileen Schneider et al., "2008 Surveillance Case Definitions for HIV Infection and AIDS among Children Aged 18 Months to <13 Years," in "Revised Surveillance Case Definitions for HIV Infection among Adults, Adolescents, and Children Aged <18 Months and for HIV Infection and AIDS among Children Aged 18 Months to <13 Years—United States, 2008," *MMWR*, vol. 57, no. RR-10, December 5, 2008, http://www.cdc.gov/mmwr/PDF/rr/rr5710.pdf (accessed July 23, 2013)

for HIV infection. Children aged 18 months to less than 13 years are categorized for surveillance purposes as having AIDS if the criteria for HIV infection are met and at least one of the AIDS-defining conditions listed in Table 2.2 in Chapter 2 has been documented.

There are three categories of HIV-infected children: those younger than 18 months who were perinatally exposed (acquired the virus from their mother), children older than 18 months with perinatal infection, and infants and children of all ages who acquired the virus through other types of exposure.

Children Younger Than 18 Months

The screening and confirmatory blood tests that accurately diagnose HIV in adults are not reliable for detecting HIV in children younger than 18 months old due to the presence of passively acquired maternal antibodies. Early recognition of HIV infection in infants younger than 18 months is accomplished using polymerase chain reaction (PCR). PCR amplifies the amounts of viral genetic material to detectable levels by the direct isolation of the HIV virus using viral culture techniques or by the detection of the p24 viral antigen. According to the NIAID, in "HIV Infection in Infants and Children," these tests can identify about 33% of infected babies at birth and 95% at three months of age. Those who are HIV-antibody positive and asymptomatic (without symptoms) without immune abnormalities have an HIV-infection status that cannot be determined unless a virus culture or other antigen-detection test is positive. As with any diagnostic test, the accuracy of detection is not absolute. The test does not detect 100% of people who are HIV positive because low levels of virus may escape detection. This possibility of a "false negative" result means that a negative culture does not necessarily rule out an infection. A small percentage of people who are infected with HIV can produce a negative result during testing.

The U.S. Public Health Service recommends that all HIV-infected expectant mothers be given antiretroviral therapy (ART) and that HIV-infected mothers be warned about the risks of transmission through breastfeeding. Infants with negative HIV tests at birth should be retested periodically during the first 18 months of life.

The 2008 criteria for indeterminate HIV infection stipulate that a child less than 18 months of age born to an HIV-infected mother is categorized as having perinatal exposure with an indeterminate HIV infection status if the criteria for infected with HIV and uninfected with HIV are not met. The CDC advises monitoring children with perinatal HIV exposure for potential complications of exposure to ART during the perinatal period and confirming the absence of HIV infection with repeat clinical and laboratory evaluations.

Classification

The 2008 changes in diagnostic criteria did not alter the existing classification system that was developed in 1994 for HIV infection in children less than 18 months or children aged 18 months to less than 13 years old. Table 5.2 shows the three categories of HIV infection that correspond to no evidence of immunological suppression, moderate immunosuppression, and severe suppression as defined by CD4+ T-lymphocyte counts and the percent of total lymphocytes for children less than one year old, one to five years old, and six to 12 years old.

PERINATAL INFECTION

According to the CDC, in *HIV Surveillance Report: Diagnoses of HIV Infection and AIDS in the United States and Dependent Areas, 2011* (February 2013, http://www.cdc.gov/hiv/pdf/statistics_2011_HIV_Surveillance _Report_vol_23.pdf), the overwhelming majority (88%) of the cumulative total number of children under the age of 13 years who were reported to have HIV infection through 2010 were infected perinatally. A number of factors are associated with an increased risk of an HIV-positive mother passing the infection to her baby. They include a low CD4+ T cell count, a high viral load (the concentration of the virus in the blood), advanced HIV progression, the presence of a particular HIV protein (p24) in serum, and placental membrane inflammation. Intrapartum (at the time of birth) events that result in increased exposure of the baby to maternal blood—breastfeeding, low vitamin A levels, premature rupture of membranes, prenatal use of illicit drugs, and premature delivery—also increase the risk of mother-to-child transmission. The risk of perinatal transmission also increases when the mother does not know she is infected until late in the course of the illness.

Despite these potential routes of transmission, the number of HIV-infected infants has been declining as a result of the more widespread use of HAART to prevent pregnant women from passing HIV infection to their offspring. Planned cesarean section delivery (the surgical delivery of a baby), the presence of neutralizing antibodies in the mother, and timely ART further reduce the chances of mother-to-infant HIV transmission. The CDC notes that survival is greatest among children with infection that is attributed to perinatal transmission.

TABLE 5.2

Pediatric HIV classification

Immunologic category	Age of child					
	<12 mos		1–5 yrs		6–12 yrs	
	µL	(%)	µL	(%)	µL	(%)
1: No evidence of suppression	≥1,500	(≥25)	≥1,000	(≥25)	≥500	(≥25)
2: Evidence of moderate suppression	750–1,499	(15–24)	500–999	(15–24)	200–499	(15–24)
3: Severe suppression	<750	(<15)	<500	(<15)	<200	(<15)

µL = microliter.

SOURCE: M. Blake Caldwell et al., "Table 2. Immunologic Categories Based on Age-Specific CD4+ T-Lymphocyte Counts and Percent of Total Lymphocytes," in "1994 Revised Classification System for Human Immunodeficiency Virus Infection in Children Less Than 13 Years of Age," *MMWR*, vol. 43, no. RR-12, September 30, 1994, http://www.cdc.gov/mmwr/preview/mmwrhtml/00032890.htm (accessed July 23, 2013)

FIGURE 5.1

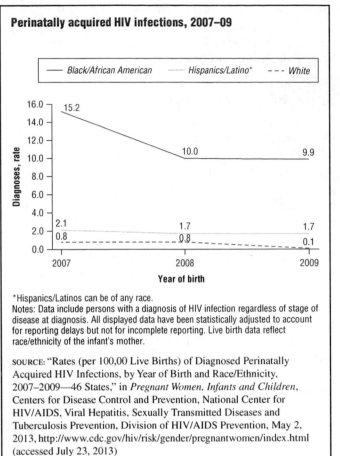

Perinatally acquired HIV infections, 2007–09

Legend: —— Black/African American ········ Hispanics/Latino* – – – White

(Y-axis: Diagnoses, rate; X-axis: Year of birth)

Black/African American: 15.2 (2007), 10.0 (2008), 9.9 (2009)
Hispanics/Latino: 2.1 (2007), 1.7 (2008), 1.7 (2009)
White: 0.8 (2007), 0.8 (2008), 0.1 (2009)

*Hispanics/Latinos can be of any race.
Notes: Data include persons with a diagnosis of HIV infection regardless of stage of disease at diagnosis. All displayed data have been statistically adjusted to account for reporting delays but not for incomplete reporting. Live birth data reflect race/ethnicity of the infant's mother.

SOURCE: "Rates (per 100,00 Live Births) of Diagnosed Perinatally Acquired HIV Infections, by Year of Birth and Race/Ethnicity, 2007–2009—46 States," in *Pregnant Women, Infants and Children*, Centers for Disease Control and Prevention, National Center for HIV/AIDS, Viral Hepatitis, Sexually Transmitted Diseases and Tuberculosis Prevention, Division of HIV/AIDS Prevention, May 2, 2013, http://www.cdc.gov/hiv/risk/gender/pregnantwomen/index.html (accessed July 23, 2013)

Antiretroviral Therapy

The use of ART to prevent mother-to-child transmission (PMTCT) has substantially decreased this route of HIV transmission. The CDC observes in "Pregnant Women, Infants, and Children" (May 2, 2013, http:// www.cdc.gov/hiv/risk/gender/pregnantwomen/index.html) that ART combined with timely, appropriate prenatal care can reduce the risk of transmission to less than 1%. In the United States the estimated numbers of perinatally acquired AIDS cases have dropped dramatically as a result of voluntary HIV testing of pregnant women, the use of ART for pregnant women and newborn infants, and the treatment of HIV infections that slow progression to AIDS. Although African Americans had the highest HIV rate per 100,000 live births each year, their rate decreased from 15.2 in 2007 to 9.9 in 2009. (See Figure 5.1.) The rates for Hispanic and white children were relatively unchanged during the same period.

According to the World Health Organization (WHO), in *Mother-to-child transmission of HIV data and statistics* (2013, http://www.who.int/hiv/topics/mtct/data/en/ index3.html), global efforts to reduce the rate of mother-to-child transmission have seen the most significant gains. In 2007 only 33% of HIV-positive pregnant women were getting drugs to prevent transmission, but as of 2011, 57% were receiving treatment. Likewise, the percentage of HIV-exposed infants receiving ART rose from 20% in 2007 to 41% in 2011.

Changing Thinking about How to Prevent Mother-to-Child Transmission

Worldwide, advising HIV-infected mothers to forgo breastfeeding has had mixed results in terms of its feasibility—specifically, the availability of infant formula and safe, uncontaminated water—and the overall health of infants. Hoosen M. Coovadia et al. find in "Mother-to-Child Transmission of HIV-1 Infection during Exclusive Breastfeeding in the First 6 Months of Life: An Intervention Cohort Study" (*Lancet*, vol. 369, no. 9567, March 31, 2007) that in areas where HIV-infected mothers chose to use formula and breastfeed or to feed their babies formula and soft foods exclusively, there were actually higher rates of mother-to-infant transmission of HIV.

Coovadia et al. indicate that exclusive breastfeeding reduced the risk of HIV transmission by nearly half compared with when formula was given with breast milk, and by more than 10 times compared with when solid foods were also part of the infants' diet. These findings are somewhat surprising. One might expect that the more breast milk the infants consumed, the greater the viral exposure and rate of infection. Coovadia et al. posit several ideas about how exclusive breastfeeding might protect against infection, including:

- Exclusive breastfeeding protects the integrity of the lining of the gastrointestinal tract (the mouth, esophagus, stomach, and intestines), and an intact gastrointestinal tract may prevent the HIV from entering to the blood.

- The consumption of foreign proteins such as cows' milk protein as in formula milk might stimulate the large numbers of immune receptors that ordinarily line the gastrointestinal tract and enable the virus to better adhere to the lining of the gastrointestinal tract and enter into the underlying tissues.

- Exclusive breastfeeding is also associated with a lower amount of HIV virus in the milk, compared with when the mother combines breastfeeding and formula feeding. When mothers supplement their infants' diet with formula, the breast is not entirely emptied and the remaining milk contains higher levels of the virus.

- Breast milk naturally contains several substances that can inhibit virus growth. Although more breast milk will present more virus, the effects may be countered because the infant also ingests more of the substances that inhibit virus growth.

In "Infant Feeding and HIV: Avoiding Transmission Is Not Enough" (*British Medical Journal*, vol. 334, no. 7592, March 10, 2007), Nigel C. Rollins of the Nelson R. Mandela School of Medicine in South Africa states that, in view of the results of this research, the WHO changed its recommendations in 2007. The new recommendations suggest that decision making be based on individual circumstances and acknowledge that infant survival, as opposed to simply preventing HIV transmission, should be the goal of infant feeding practices.

The WHO has revised its recommendations several times in response to new research findings. In *Guidelines on HIV and Infant Feeding 2010: Principles and Recommendations for Infant Feeding in the Context of HIV and a Summary of Evidence* (2010, http://whqlibdoc.who.int/publications/2010/9789241599535_eng.pdf), the WHO notes that HIV-infected women are recommended to breastfeed exclusively while taking ART to reduce transmission or to avoid breastfeeding altogether. In countries where ART is available, the WHO advises breastfeeding until infants are 12 months old.

Louise Kuhn et al. find in "HIV-1 Concentrations in Human Breast Milk before and after Weaning" (*Science Translational Medicine*, vol. 5, no. 181, April 2013) that HIV-infected mothers are less likely to transmit the virus to their newborns if they breastfeed their child exclusively for more than four months. Because even slight changes in breastfeeding patterns appear to increase HIV in the mother's breast milk, mothers are discouraged from supplementing their infants' diets with formula. Kuhn et al. also observe that when HIV-infected mothers adhere to ART during breastfeeding, the risk of transmission is very low.

TREATMENTS FOR CHILDREN

Prescribing drug therapy for children is often more difficult than prescribing for adults because children respond to drugs differently at different ages and because oral medication must have an acceptable taste to ensure that children will take it as prescribed.

In "Approved Antiretroviral Drugs for Pediatric Treatment of HIV Infection" (May 20, 2009, http://www.fda.gov/ForConsumers/ByAudience/ForPatientAdvocates/HIVandAIDSActivities/ucm118951.htm), the U.S. Food and Drug Administration (FDA) lists 28 drugs that are used to treat pediatric HIV patients. Nine of these, called protease inhibitors (PIs; used alone or in combination with other drugs to combat viral infection), were available for children two to 13 years old. PI compounds act by preventing the reproduction of HIV that is already in the host cells. However, safety and effectiveness had not been established for four of the PIs: tipranavir, saquinavir mesylate, darunavir, and atazanavir sulfate. The PIs approved for use and deemed safe and effective by the FDA are:

- Amprenavir
- Lopinavir/ritonavir
- Fosamprenavir calcium
- Ritonavir
- Nelfinavir mesylate

Another group of drugs approved for pediatric use are known as nucleoside reverse transcriptase inhibitors (NRTIs). NRTIs, which are structurally similar to a nucleoside constituent of deoxyribonucleic acid (DNA), limit HIV replication by incorporating themselves into a strand of DNA, which causes the chain to end. The NRTIs approved for pediatric use are:

- Lamivudine
- Emtricitabine
- Abacavir
- Zalcitabine and dideoxycytidine
- Zidovudine
- Tenofovir disoproxil fumarate
- Enteric-coated didanosine
- Didanosine and dideoxyinosine
- Tenofovir disoproxil/emtricitabine
- Stavudine

Another group of antiretroviral drugs are known as nonnucleoside reverse transcriptase inhibitors (NNRTIs). NNRTIs slow down the functioning of the enzyme that allows the virus to become a part of the infected cell's nucleus. Three NNRTIs are presently approved for pediatric use:

- Delavirdine
- Efavirenz
- Nevirapine

In March 1996 the Antiviral Drugs Advisory Committee of the FDA approved the use of the compound didanosine for pediatric use. The approval was based on the results of two separate U.S. AIDS Clinical Trials Group pediatric studies and an Australian study, all of which found that didanosine delayed the progression of AIDS and was superior to azidothymidine (ZDV) alone. ZDV, which is given to children and adults, had been the only drug widely recognized to help delay the progress of HIV infection and to reduce the risk of perinatal infection.

The study results generated high expectations for the performance of didanosine in both children and adults.

As promising as these early reports seemed, the effectiveness of didanosine alone or in combination with ZDV was short-lived because HIV susceptibility to the drugs decreased over time. Thus, although didanosine is still used, it has not proven to be a major breakthrough in HIV infections as was hoped.

In 1999 a study conducted jointly by the United States and Uganda demonstrated that the perinatal transmission of HIV from mother to child could be reduced by the drug nevirapine. The drug is given to the mother in labor and to the child within three days of birth. Initial study results showed the drug to be safe for both mother and child and relatively inexpensive ($4 per mother/child dose). In 2000 the Elizabeth Glaser Pediatric AIDS Foundation, a nonprofit organization that is dedicated to promoting and funding worldwide pediatric AIDS research, secured funds to implement this treatment in developing countries that lack health care resources and infrastructure.

By 2003 the administration of nevirapine to hundreds of thousands of pregnant women in Africa demonstrated the therapeutic potential of the drug in slowing the progression of pediatric AIDS. The WHO, governments throughout sub-Saharan Africa, and the National Institutes of Health have all recommended that nevirapine use be continued to prevent HIV transmission from mothers to infants.

Also in 2003 the drug enfuvirtide was approved for use by children over the age of six years. This drug is the first of the fusion inhibitor class of antiretroviral drugs. It acts by inhibiting the fusion of HIV to the host cell membrane.

In late 2007 two additional drugs—maraviroc and raltegravir—joined the FDA-approved list. Maraviroc is an entry inhibitor, meaning that it acts to block a receptor, CCR5, that HIV uses to enter white blood cells. Raltegravir is an HIV integrase strand transfer inhibitor, which means it targets integrase, an HIV enzyme that integrates the viral genetic material into human chromosomes.

Option B+ Reduces HIV Transmission

There are several ways to achieve PMTCT. Option A uses a single drug, zidovudine, during pregnancy and additional antiretroviral medications during labor, delivery, and the period following birth. Option B involves triple-drug ART during pregnancy and breastfeeding. Both options include additional ART for infants. In countries with limited resources, eligibility for ART is based on CD4 cell counts.

Frank Chimbwandira et al. report in "Impact of an Innovative Approach to Prevent Mother-to-Child Transmission of HIV—Malawi, July 2011–September 2012"

(*Morbidity and Mortality Weekly Report*, vol. 62, no. 8, March 1, 2013) that PMTCT is a challenge in countries with limited laboratory capacity. As a result, the key laboratory test used to determine when to begin ART, the CD4 count, is not performed and people, including pregnant and breastfeeding women, do not receive ART. To overcome this obstacle, Malawi, Rwanda, Uganda, and Haiti instituted a program called Option B+, which makes all HIV-infected pregnant and breastfeeding women eligible for lifelong ART regardless of their CD4 counts. In Malawi there was a sevenfold increase in the number of pregnant and breastfeeding women started on ART per quarter during the first year of Option B+. The program benefits women, their partners, and their children. It reduces the mother-to-child transmission of HIV to less than 5%, maintains the mother's health, and reduces HIV transmission to uninfected sexual partners.

CHILDREN ARE AT HIGHER RISK OF DRUG RESISTANCE

In "Risk of Triple-Class Virological Failure in Children with HIV: A Retrospective Cohort Study" (*Lancet*, vol. 377, no. 9777, May 7, 2011), the project team for the Collaboration of Observational HIV Epidemiological Research Europe looked at more than 1,000 children who had been infected with HIV perinatally and became resistant to the three major classes of drugs that are used to treat HIV: NRTIs, NNRTIs, and PIs. The team aimed to estimate the number of children who will need new classes of drugs as they age. It finds that 12% of the children developed resistance to all three drugs within five years of starting ART. The team also notes that the children who started ART at older ages were more likely to suffer drug resistance.

HOW MANY CHILDREN ARE INFECTED?

In 2011 an estimated 192 children under the age of 13 years were diagnosed with HIV infection in the United States. (See Table 3.2 in Chapter 3.) Of the estimated 32,052 AIDS diagnoses reported in 2011, just 15 were diagnosed in children under the age of 13 years. (See Table 5.3.)

The CDC indicates in *Pediatric HIV Surveillance* (June 2013, http://www.cdc.gov/hiv/pdf/statistics_surveillance _Pediatric.pdf) that of the 192 pediatric HIV cases reported in 2011 in the United States and dependent areas, 66% of the total were in African American children, even though they accounted for just 14% of the total number of children in the United States.

Geographic Distribution

According to the CDC, in *Pediatric HIV/AIDS Surveillance*, an estimated 5,134 people were living with

TABLE 5.3

AIDS diagnoses in children under age 13, 2008–11 and cumulative

Race/ethnicity	2008 No.	2008 Estimated[a] No.	2008 Estimated[a] Rate	2009 No.	2009 Estimated[a] No.	2009 Estimated[a] Rate	2010 No.	2010 Estimated[a] No.	2010 Estimated[a] Rate	2011 No.	2011 Estimated[a] No.	2011 Estimated[a] Rate	Cumulative[b] No.	Cumulative[b] Est. No.[a]
American Indian/Alaska Native	0	0	0.0	0	0	0.0	0	0	0.0	0	0	0.0	31	31
Asian[c]	1	1	0.0	1	1	0.1	1	1	0.0	0	0	0.0	47	47
Black/African American	23	24	0.3	7	7	0.1	13	14	0.2	9	12	0.2	5,737	5,761
Hispanic/Latino[d]	2	2	0.0	4	4	0.0	4	5	0.0	2	2	0.0	1,923	1,932
Native Hawaiian/other Pacific Islander	0	0	0.0	0	0	0.0	0	0	0.0	0	0	0.0	7	7
White	6	6	0.0	1	1	0.0	4	5	0.0	1	1	0.0	1,592	1,596
Multiple races	4	4	0.3	0	0	0.0	0	0	0.0	0	0	0.0	145	146
Total[e]	**36**	**37**	**0.1**	**13**	**14**	**0.0**	**22**	**24**	**0.0**	**12**	**15**	**0.0**	**9,483[f]**	**9,521**

[a]Estimated numbers resulted from statistical adjustment that accounted for reporting delays, but not for incomplete reporting. Rates are per 100,000 population.
[b]From the beginning of the epidemic through 2011.
[c]Includes Asian/Pacific Islander legacy cases.
[d]Hispanics/Latinos can be of any race.
[e]Because column totals for estimated numbers were calculated independently of the values for the subpopulations, the values in each column may not sum to the column total.
[f]Includes children of unknown race/ethnicity.
Note: Reported numbers less than 12, as well as estimated numbers (and accompanying rates and trends) based on these numbers, should be interpreted with caution because the numbers have underlying relative standard errors greater than 30% and are considered unreliable.

SOURCE: "Table 6a. Stage 3 (AIDS) among Children Aged <13 Years, by Race/Ethnicity, 2008–2011 and Cumulative—United States," in *HIV Surveillance Report: Diagnoses of HIV Infection in the United States and Dependent Areas, 2011*, vol. 23, Centers for Disease Control and Prevention, National Center for HIV/AIDS, Viral Hepatitis, STD, and TB Prevention, Division of HIV/AIDS Prevention, February 2013, http://www.cdc.gov/hiv/pdf/statistics_2011_HIV_Surveillance_Report_vol_23.pdf (accessed July 7, 2013)

perinatally acquired AIDS at year-end 2010. (See Figure 5.2.) New York (1,339) and Florida (842) reported the highest numbers of cases.

Global Outlook

In "Seven African Countries Cut Child HIV Infections by Half" (Reuters.com, June 25, 2013), Kate Kelland reports that seven countries in sub-Saharan Africa— Botswana, Ethiopia, Ghana, Malawi, Namibia, South Africa, and Zambia—reduced the numbers of new HIV infections in children by 50% between 2009 and 2012. This dramatic reduction was largely attributable to successful efforts to reduce mother-to-child transmission. Rates of ART for HIV-infected pregnant women exceeded 75% in many countries.

Kelland observes that some countries still have high numbers of new infections and mother-to-child transmission. In 2012 nearly 60,000 new HIV infections were reported in Nigeria. Furthermore, South Africa and Botswana made little progress in PMTCT, reducing their rates by less than 5%.

Gene Mutation in Some Babies May Help

A gene mutation that slows the progress of HIV in adults was shown during the late 1990s to help HIV-infected newborns avoid serious AIDS-associated illnesses longer than those who do not have the mutation. Michael Fischereder et al. report in "CC Chemokine Receptor 5 and Renal-Transplant Survival" (*Lancet*, vol. 357, no. 9270, June 2, 2001) that the gene CC chemokine receptor 5 (CCR5) is present in 10% to 15% of whites but is not found in Asian Americans or African Americans.

The gene codes for a protein called CCR5. This protein and another one called CXCR4 are located on the surface of a number of human cells. In "Analysis of the Mechanism by Which the Small-Molecule CCR5 Antagonists SCH-351125 and SCH-350581 Inhibit Human Immunodeficiency Virus Type 1 Entry" (*Journal of Virology*, vol. 77, no. 9, May 2003), Fotini Tsamis et al. demonstrate that CCR5 and CXCR4 can be used as receptors by HIV-1 to enter and infect CD4+ T cells, dendritic cells, and macrophages. Furthermore, CCR5 has been shown to be essential for viral transmission and replication during the early phase of the disease, even before symptoms of infection appear. Researchers expect that further investigation of the CCR5 gene will eventually help them develop drugs to prevent or destroy HIV in newborns.

Some researchers, such as Michael Marmor et al., in "Resistance to HIV Infection" (*Journal of Urban Health*, vol. 83, no. 1, January 2006), speculate that because several of the same genetic mutations have been found in both exposed uninfected populations and in long-term nonprogressor populations (people who become infected but do not develop AIDS), a single theory may explain both phenomena—that the genetic traits prevent or hinder HIV-1 entry into cells, which reduces the likelihood of infection and, should infection occur, slows or entirely eliminates the development of serious disease.

FIGURE 5.2

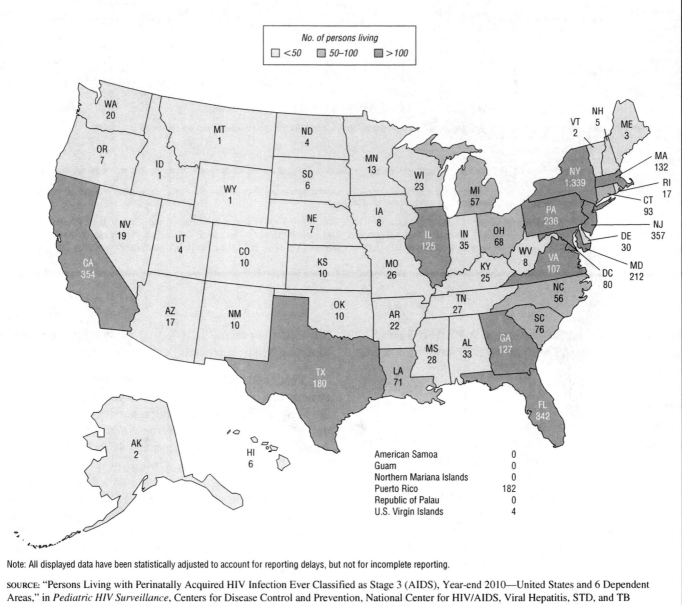

Persons living with perinatally acquired AIDS, yearend 2010

[United States and 6 dependent areas. Population = 5,134.]

No. of persons living
☐ <50   ▨ 50–100   ▪ >100

American Samoa	0
Guam	0
Northern Mariana Islands	0
Puerto Rico	182
Republic of Palau	0
U.S. Virgin Islands	4

Note: All displayed data have been statistically adjusted to account for reporting delays, but not for incomplete reporting.

SOURCE: "Persons Living with Perinatally Acquired HIV Infection Ever Classified as Stage 3 (AIDS), Year-end 2010—United States and 6 Dependent Areas," in *Pediatric HIV Surveillance*, Centers for Disease Control and Prevention, National Center for HIV/AIDS, Viral Hepatitis, STD, and TB Prevention, Division of HIV/AIDS Prevention, June 2013, http://www.cdc.gov/hiv/pdf/statistics_surveillance_Pediatric.pdf (accessed July 23, 2013)

ALL PREGNANT WOMEN SHOULD BE TESTED FOR HIV

When HIV-infected pregnant women know their HIV infection status, they are better able to make informed decisions about ART to reduce perinatal transmission of HIV to their infants. The U.S. Preventive Services Task Force recommends that all pregnant women be offered HIV counseling and voluntary HIV tests.

In September 2008 the American College of Obstetrics and Gynecology's (ACOG) Committee on Obstetric Practice expanded its recommendations about prenatal and perinatal HIV testing in "ACOG Committee Opinion No. 418: Prenatal and Perinatal Human Immunodeficiency Virus Testing: Expanded Recommendations" (*Obstetrics and Gynecology*, vol. 112, no. 3). The committee recommended that all pregnant women be screened for HIV infection as early as possible during each pregnancy and informed that they will receive an HIV test as part of routine prenatal testing unless they decline or opt-out of HIV screening. Repeat conventional or rapid HIV testing during the third trimester of pregnancy is recommended for:

- Women living in areas with high HIV prevalence rates

- Women known to be at high risk for acquiring HIV

- Women who declined testing earlier in the pregnancy

The CDC recommends treatment during three key periods—during pregnancy, during labor and delivery, and after birth—but not all mothers and infants receive treatment at each stage. Table 5.4 shows that between 2008 and 2011 ART was given to about 50% of mother-infant pairs during pregnancy, labor and delivery, and after birth.

SURVIVING INTO THEIR TEENS

The CDC indicates in *HIV Surveillance Report* that survival is greatest among children who are infected perinatally. Although many HIV-infected children die as infants and toddlers, most infected from birth now survive beyond age five, and it is not uncommon for others to reach their teens.

In "HIV Infection in Infants and Children," the NIAID distinguishes three distinct patterns of disease progression among HIV-infected children. The first group consists of those who display symptoms within their first 18 months following infection. Even with treatment, progression to AIDS in this group is rapid and most children die by age four. Children in the second group experience a less aggressive progression and often have milder or less prolonged symptomatic periods. These children tend to live longer. The third group is a recently emerging group of survivors. These children have grown up with few, if any, symptoms. Researchers are eager to determine precisely why and how these children remain asymptomatic in spite of their infection.

The CDC reports in "Ten Great Public Health Achievements—Worldwide, 2001–2010" (*Morbidity and Mortality Weekly Report*, vol. 60, no. 24, June 24, 2011) that more than two-thirds (68%) of deaths among children under the age of five years are attributable to infectious diseases, which includes AIDS. In "Forum on Women and HIV" (TheBody.com, 2013), Sharon Lee explains that with treatment, HIV-infected children may live for many years. Other experts assert in "Life Expectancy for Children Born with HIV" (2013, http://positive lyorphaned.org/2011/03/28/life-expectancy/) that medical professionals cannot accurately forecast life expectancy. During the early days of the epidemic life expectancy among those who were HIV infected or diagnosed with AIDS was extremely limited because many of them died from complications. However, some children who were born with HIV infection were, as of 2013, in their 30s and it is not yet known whether they will have normal life spans. Furthermore, because of ART, children who are born with HIV in the 21st century are living longer, healthier lives.

Research indicates that some of the difference in response to HIV is attributable to polymorphisms (common genetic variations). Kumud K. Singh and Stephen Spector find in "Host Genetic Determinants of HIV Infection and Disease Progression in Children" (*Pediatric Research*, vol. 65, May 2009) that HIV-infected children with a specific polymorphism called CCR5-delta32 had half the rate of disease progression compared with children with normal CCR5. They also observe that the most rapid progression of HIV symptoms occurred in children with normal CCR5 plus a polymorphism called 59029-A/A. This particular polymorphism was identified in about 25% of the HIV-infected children studied, representing the genotype that most often accelerated the

TABLE 5.4

Time of antiretroviral (ARV) treatment in HIV-infected women and infants, 2008–11

[United States]

| | Year of birth | | | | | | | |
| | 2008 | | 2009 | | 2010 | | 2011 | |
Time of ARV treatment	No.	%	No.	%	No.	%	No.	%
During pregnancy (DP) only	29	1.0	18	0.6	16	0.6	3	0.1
During labor and delivery (L&D) only	36	1.2	58	2.0	42	1.6	14	0.7
Infant received ARV after birth (Infant ARV) only	275	9.2	239	8.2	250	9.5	164	7.6
DP and L&D	66	2.2	62	2.1	41	1.6	34	1.6
DP and infant ARV	137	4.6	129	4.4	109	4.1	81	3.8
L&D and infant ARV	673	22.5	704	24.1	734	27.9	615	28.7
DP and L&D and infant ARV	1,467	49.1	1,520	52.0	1,258	47.8	1,049	48.9
No known treatment	303	10.1	195	6.7	181	6.9	186	8.7
Total	**2,986**	**100**	**2,925**	**100**	**2,631**	**100**	**2,146**	**100**

Note: Exposure data from 43 areas.

SOURCE: "Time of Antiretroviral (ARV) Treatment in HIV-Infected Pregnant Women or Perinatally Exposed Infants Birth Years 2008–2011—United States," in *Pediatric HIV Surveillance*, Centers for Disease Control and Prevention, National Center for HIV/AIDS, Viral Hepatitis, STD, and TB Prevention, Division of HIV/AIDS Prevention, June 2013, http://www.cdc.gov/hiv/pdf/statistics_surveillance_Pediatric.pdf (accessed July 23, 3013) rate of disease progression in children with normal CCR5. Furthermore, Singh and Spector find that there were some polymorphisms that had an impact in adults but not in children and some that seemed to have an important impact in children but only a modest impact in adults.

In "Host and Viral Genetic Correlates of Clinical Definitions of HIV-1 Disease Progression" (*PLoS One*, vol. 5, no. 6, June 11, 2010), Concepción Casado et al. describe patterns of HIV disease progression that are based on host genetic markers and viral factors. The researchers attempt to better define long-term nonprogressor elite controllers (HIV-infected people who show no signs of disease progression for over 12 years and remain asymptomatic), viremic controllers (HIV-infected people who progress to AIDS very slowly, after a long period, or in some instances do not progress to AIDS), viremic noncontrollers (HIV-infected people who have high levels of viral load), chronic progressors (HIV-infected people who progress to AIDS within 10 years of diagnosis), and rapid progressors (HIV-infected people who progress to AIDS within four years of diagnosis).

Dealing with Physical and Emotional Problems

When HIV-infected children died during the early years of the HIV/AIDS epidemic, they were generally unaware of what was happening to them. In the 21st century, at the Children's Evaluation and Rehabilitation Center of the Albert Einstein College of Medicine of Yeshiva University, school-aged children meet with social workers in a support group to handle the physical and emotional ordeals of growing up with HIV/AIDS. These children are part of the increasing number born with HIV who have survived long enough to realize what it means. They must learn to cope with the physical, psychological, and emotional consequences of HIV/AIDS.

Claude A. Mellins and Kathleen M. Malee review in "Understanding the Mental Health of Youth Living with Perinatal HIV Infection: Lessons Learned and Current Challenges" (*Journal of the International AIDS Society*, vol. 16, June 18, 2013) studies that examine the mental health problems of children aged 10 years and older living with perinatal HIV infection. The researchers find that although many of these youth fare well in terms of mental health, a substantial proportion experience emotional and behavioral problems, including psychiatric disorders, at higher than expected rates. Adolescents coping with lifelong HIV infection must contend with medical treatment, hospitalizations, and physical pain as well as the psychosocial impact of HIV, a stigmatized and sexually transmittable illness that may make their teen years especially challenging. Mellins and Malee cite building resilience—positive development despite exposure to significant adversity—as a preventive measure that can be used to promote mental health and emotional well-being.

Lisa Henry-Reid, Lori Wiener, and Ana Garcia observe in "Caring for Youth with HIV" (*Achieve*, Winter 2009) that adolescents with HIV require significant psychological and emotional support because they face unique challenges, including:

- Experiencing stigma and fear of rejection
- Dealing with the side effects of HIV drugs
- Coping with a potentially life-threatening illness and an uncertain life span
- Dealing with disclosure and transmission
- Enduring the impact of loss
- Navigating the health care system

Henry-Reid, Wiener, and Garcia report that adolescents who share their HIV diagnosis with others fare better psychologically and socially than those who do not disclose their HIV status. They assert that HIV-infected adolescents must deal with the normal challenges of adolescence and illness as well as with additional stressors such as poverty, barriers to care and social services, violence, racism, homophobia, broken families, homelessness, and child abuse.

Global HIV Infection in Young People

In *UNAIDS World AIDS Day Report, 2012* (November 2012, http://www.unaids.org/en/media/unaids/content assets/documents/epidemiology/2012/gr2012/JC2434_World AIDSday_results_en.pdf), the Joint United Nations Programme on HIV/AIDS (UNAIDS) notes that most parts of the world have seen a reduction in new HIV infections among young people. In 2011 there were 2.5 million new HIV infections, 1.7 million AIDS-related deaths, 14.8 million people eligible for HIV treatment, and 8 million receiving treatment.

According to UNAIDS, in 2011, 40% of all new adult HIV infections were in young people. It also indicates that between 2003 and 2011 HIV infections in children dropped 43%. Between 2009 and 2011 alone, new HIV infections in children decreased 24%. Two-thirds of this decrease was attributable to PMTCT.

Nearly none of the children who acquired HIV in 2011 lived in high-income countries and more than 90% lived in sub-Saharan Africa. Regardless, the situation is improving in sub-Saharan Africa—new infections in children decreased 24% during the first decade of the 21st century. Globally, new HIV infections in youth aged 15 to 24 years dropped 27%, and in Burundi, Kenya, Namibia, South Africa, Togo, and Zambia the number of newly infected children fell by between 40% and 59%

from 2009 to 2011. In 16 other countries declines of between 20% and 39% occurred during the same period.

The number of children becoming HIV infected has decreased significantly in the Caribbean (32%) and Oceania (36%) and modestly in Asia (12%). Likewise, new infections dropped in both Latin America (24%) and eastern Europe and Central Asia (13%). The Middle East and North Africa was the only region that did not report a decrease in the number of newly infected children.

WHO WILL CARE FOR THEM?

The HIV/AIDS epidemic has created many tragedies, including millions of orphans. The United Nations Children's Fund estimates in "Orphan Estimates" (April 2013, http://www.childinfo.org/hiv_aids_orphanestimates.php) that in 2011 there were 17.3 million orphans due to AIDS worldwide. According to UNAIDS, in *Global Report: UNAIDS Report on the Global Aids Epidemic, 2010* (November 2010, http://www.childinfo.org/files/20101123_GlobalReport_em.pdf), nearly 90% of these orphaned children live in sub-Saharan Africa.

It is not always possible to find someone to care for an orphan of parents who died of AIDS, particularly if the child also has HIV or AIDS. Some family members may be hesitant to take in the child for fear he or she may spread the infection. In a growing number of cases, however, grandparents (in most cases, grandmothers) are taking these orphans into their home. This may be a burden on older people who have lost their own children and may feel too old, tired, or impoverished to rear another family. They may also fear that they will die before their grandchildren do, leaving no one to care for them. It is no less difficult for the children who have lost their parents and fear they will probably miss the advantages they would have had with younger parents, such as being able to play more active childhood games.

Older orphans struggle with the rage, shame, and isolation of losing a parent to AIDS. Observers are finding that the HIV/AIDS epidemic is creating a class of particularly troubled youth. All children who lose a parent suffer to some degree, but for those whose parents die from AIDS, embarrassment and secrecy often compound the trauma. Teens whose parents became infected as a result of injecting drugs or practicing unsafe sex are often torn between feeling sorry for their parents and blaming them for their illness.

ADOLESCENTS, YOUNG ADULTS, AND HIV/AIDS
Patterns of Infection

The transmission and course of AIDS among adolescents aged 13 to 19 years and young adults aged 20 to 24 years follow similar patterns to those over the age of 25 years. The CDC reports in *HIV Surveillance in Men Who*

FIGURE 5.3

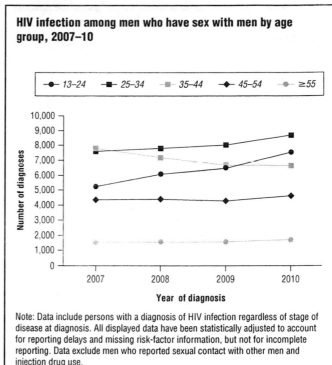

HIV infection among men who have sex with men by age group, 2007–10

Note: Data include persons with a diagnosis of HIV infection regardless of stage of disease at diagnosis. All displayed data have been statistically adjusted to account for reporting delays and missing risk-factor information, but not for incomplete reporting. Data exclude men who reported sexual contact with other men and injection drug use.

SOURCE: "Diagnosis of HIV Infection among Men Who Have Sex with Men, by Age Group, 2007–2010—46 States and 5 U.S. Dependent Areas," in *HIV Surveillance in Men Who Have Sex with Men (MSM)*, Centers for Disease Control and Prevention, National Center for HIV/AIDS, Viral Hepatitis, STD, and TB Prevention, Division of HIV/AIDS Prevention, May 2012, http://www.cdc.gov/hiv/topics/surveillance/resources/slides/msm/slides/MSM_2010.pdf (accessed July 23, 2013)

Have Sex with Men (MSM) (May 15, 2012, http://www.cdc.gov/hiv/topics/surveillance/resources/slides/msm/slides/MSM_2010.pdf) that between 2007 and 2010 HIV infections in males aged 13 to 24 years attributed to men who had sex with men increased 44%. (See Figure 5.3.) By contrast, female adolescents and young adults aged 13 to 19 years became infected through heterosexual contact (92.7%) or injection drug use (7%). (See Table 4.3 in Chapter 4.)

The characteristics of adolescence—a time of development, uncertainty, and a misleading sense of bravado and immortality, often combined with pushing the boundaries of good sense—create the potential for some young people to become particularly vulnerable to HIV infection. For many, this is a time of experimentation and risk-taking, often in terms of sexual behavior or use of alcohol and illicit drugs.

Many Adolescents Are Sexually Active

More than one-third of adolescents are sexually active. In "The Youth Risk Behavior Surveillance—United States, 2011" (*Morbidity and Mortality Weekly Report*, vol. 61, no. 4, June 8, 2012), Danice K. Eaton et al. indicate that in

TABLE 5.5

TABLE 5.6

Percent of high school students that used a condom during last sexual intercourse[a], 2011

| | Condom use | | |
| | Female | Male | Total |
Category	%	%	%
Race/ethnicity			
White[b]	53.4	66.3	59.5
Black[b]	53.8	75.4	65.3
Hispanic	53.0	63.4	58.4
Grade			
9	56.3	67.0	62.2
10	56.7	69.9	63.3
11	55.5	67.0	61.1
12	48.9	64.7	56.3
Total	**53.6**	**67.0**	**60.2**

[a]Among the 33.7% of students nationwide who were currently sexually active.
[b]Non-Hispanic.

SOURCE: Adapted from Danice K. Eaton et al., "Table 67. Percentage of High School Students Who Used a Condom during Last Sexual Intercourse and Who Used Birth Control Pills before Last Sexual Intercourse, by Sex, Race/Ethnicity, and Grade—United States, Youth Risk Behavior Survey, 2011," in "The Youth Risk Behavior Surveillance–United States, 2011," *MMWR*, vol. 61, no. 4, June 8, 2012, http://www.cdc.gov/mmwr/pdf/ss/ss6104.pdf (accessed July 23, 2013)

Percentage of high school students taught in school about HIV/AIDS by sex, 2011

| | Were taught in school about AIDS or HIV infection | | |
| | Female | Male | Total |
Site	%	%	%
State surveys			
Alabama	87.6	84.3	86.0
Alaska	81.0	83.4	82.2
Arizona	—*	—	—
Arkansas	85.5	79.6	82.5
Colorado	82.6	77.8	80.2
Connecticut	92.0	90.8	91.4
Delaware	87.1	84.4	85.7
Florida	85.3	83.7	84.5
Georgia	89.0	86.8	87.6
Hawaii	83.7	83.4	83.6
Idaho	80.9	82.7	81.9
Illinois	87.4	84.9	86.1
Indiana	90.3	89.0	89.6
Iowa	84.9	83.0	84.0
Kansas	85.5	80.4	82.7
Kentucky	86.8	81.3	83.9
Louisiana	79.3	70.2	74.9
Maine	89.4	88.3	88.6
Maryland	85.4	81.9	83.5
Massachusetts	83.5	84.7	84.0
Michigan	88.3	88.7	88.5
Mississippi	78.0	75.6	76.9
Montana	85.2	85.6	85.4
Nebraska	77.6	79.4	78.5
New Hampshire	88.1	85.5	86.7
New Jersey	—	—	—
New Mexico	81.8	80.3	81.1
New York	—	—	—
North Carolina	—	—	—
North Dakota	—	—	—
Ohio	—	—	—
Oklahoma	83.7	83.0	83.3
Rhode Island	83.3	83.4	83.3
South Carolina	82.0	80.6	81.1
South Dakota	79.5	80.0	79.7
Tennessee	81.9	79.6	80.6
Texas	81.1	81.1	81.0
Utah	86.0	86.8	86.3
Vermont	—	—	—
Virginia	87.8	85.5	86.6
West Virginia	89.8	86.2	88.0
Wisconsin	89.5	88.6	89.1
Wyoming	82.1	83.1	82.6
Median	*85.2*	*83.4*	*83.7*
Range	*77.6–92.0*	*70.2–90.8*	*74.9–91.4*
Large urban school district surveys			
Boston, MA	73.4	73.2	73.3
Broward County, FL	88.1	86.7	87.3
Charlotte-Mecklenburg, NC	85.9	82.9	84.3
Chicago, IL	75.0	71.0	72.9
Dallas, TX	82.2	79.7	80.9
Detroit, MI	82.7	79.0	80.8
District of Columbia	85.6	82.6	83.8
Duval County, FL	82.4	80.3	81.3
Houston, TX	75.9	73.2	74.6
Los Angeles, CA	84.2	79.9	82.0
Memphis, TN	78.6	75.7	77.2
Miami-Dade County, FL	79.3	76.3	77.9
Milwaukee, WI	83.8	79.9	81.7
New York City, NY	—	—	—
Orange County, FL	88.3	85.1	86.6
Palm Beach County, FL	87.5	83.8	85.5
Philadelphia, PA	83.0	80.5	81.8

2011 nearly half (47.4%) of high school students said they had had sexual intercourse and about six out of 10 (60.2%) said they had used a condom during their last sexual intercourse. (See Table 5.5.)

In 2011 the overwhelming majority (83.7%) of teens said they had been taught in school about HIV/AIDS. (See Table 5.6.) Just 12.9% of high school students received HIV testing in 2011, and more females and African Americans were tested. (See Table 5.7.)

SEXUALLY TRANSMITTED INFECTIONS. Teenagers engaging in sexual activity before becoming sufficiently mature, with inadequate regard for contraceptive methods or safe sex practices, have led to record high rates of sexually transmitted infections (STIs) among adolescents and young adults. According to the CDC, in the fact sheet "STD Trends in the United States: 2011 National Data for Chlamydia, Gonorrhea, and Syphilis" (March 2013, http://www.cdc.gov/std/stats11/trends-2011.pdf), approximately 20 million new STIs occur every year, and most chlamydia and gonorrhea infections occur among young people aged 15 to 24 years. (See Figure 5.4.)

Although overall rates of infection for some STIs, such as gonorrhea, declined during the 1990s and leveled off during the first decade of the 21st century, syphilis and chlamydia infections among adolescents are increasing. The CDC notes in "STDs in Adolescents and Young Adults" (December 13, 2012, http://www.cdc.gov/std/stats11/adol.htm) that young people aged 15 to 24 years

TABLE 5.6

Percentage of high school students taught in school about HIV/AIDS by sex, 2011 [CONTINUED]

Site	Were taught in school about AIDS or HIV infection		
	Female	Male	Total
	%	%	%
San Bernardino, CA	80.5	79.1	79.8
San Diego, CA	87.0	85.4	86.1
San Francisco, CA	84.4	78.0	81.1
Seattle, WA	87.5	85.3	86.2
Median	*83.4*	*79.9*	*81.5*
Range	*73.4–88.3*	*71.0–86.7*	*72.9–87.3*

*Not available.
Note: Among students who were currently sexually active.

SOURCE: Adapted from Danice K. Eaton et al., "Table 74. Percentage of High School Students Who Drank Alcohol or Used Drugs before Last Sexual Intercourse and Who Were Ever Taught in School about Acquired Immunodeficiency Syndrome (AIDS) or Human Immunodeficiency Virus (HIV) Infection, by Sex—Selected U.S. Sites, Youth Risk Behavior Survey, 2011," in "The Youth Risk Behavior Surveillance–United States, 2011," *MMWR*, vol. 61, no. 4, June 8, 2012, http://www.cdc.gov/mmwr/pdf/ss/ss6104.pdf (accessed July 23, 2013).

TABLE 5.7

Percentage of high school students tested for HIV by sex and race/ethnicity, 2011

Category	Female	Male	Total
	%	%	%
Race/ethnicity			
White*	12.6	8.7	10.6
Black*	24.2	23.7	24.0
Hispanic	14.0	11.0	12.5
Grade			
9	10.2	10.3	10.3
10	13.1	9.7	11.3
11	16.9	10.3	13.5
12	19.1	14.6	16.9
Total	**14.6**	**11.2**	**12.9**

*Non-Hispanic.
Note: Does not include tests conducted when donating blood.

SOURCE: Danice K. Eaton et al., "Table 75. Percentage of High School Students Who Were Tested for Human Immunodeficiency Virus (HIV), by Sex, Race/Ethnicity, and Grade—United States, Youth Risk Behavior Survey, 2011," in "The Youth Risk Behavior Surveillance–United States, 2011," *MMWR*, vol. 61, no. 4, June 8, 2012, http://www.cdc.gov/mmwr/pdf/ss/ss6104.pdf (accessed July 23, 2013).

acquire nearly half of all new STIs. Between 2010 and 2011 gonorrhea rates for people aged 15 to 19 years were relatively unchanged, but among people aged 20 to 24 years they increased 5.8%. Chlamydia rates for young people aged 15 to 19 years and 20 to 24 years rose 4% and 11%, respectively.

The rates of syphilis infection are different. The rates among 15- to 19-year-old females decreased from 2.9 cases per 100,000 population in 2010 to 2.4 cases in 2011. (See Figure 5.5.) Among women aged 20 to 24 years there were 3.8 cases in 2011. Among 15- to 19-year-old males the rate rose from 1.3 cases in 2009 to 5.4 cases in 2011. Men aged 20 to 24 years had the highest rates of any age group—23.4 cases in 2011. Figure 5.6 shows increasing rates of syphilis among men aged 15 to 44 years.

LEADING THE WAY: YOUNG PEOPLE AS AIDS ACTIVISTS AND ORGANIZATIONS THAT HELP YOUNG PATIENTS

Almost since the beginning of the HIV/AIDS epidemic, children and teenagers have been among the activists campaigning for HIV/AIDS reforms and awareness of the disease. Their role has been a profoundly personal one. For example, until his death from AIDS in April 1990, Ryan White—an Indiana teenager—generated worldwide attention to the disease and, in particular, to the stigmas and misconceptions surrounding it. White, who contracted the virus during treatment for his hemophilia, was a white, middle-class, heterosexual boy, which ran counter to the public's perception of AIDS at the time as a disease of gay men.

Being expelled from school because of the supposed health risk to other students galvanized White to educate others on the nature of HIV/AIDS. His legacy includes the Ryan White Comprehensive AIDS Resources Emergency Act, the multibillion-dollar program that funds programs to help provide primary health care and support to those living with HIV/AIDS.

The National Association of People with AIDS, founded in 1983, advocates for people, including children, who live with HIV/AIDS. The nonprofit organization—the oldest national AIDS organization in the United States—is a strong advocate for HIV/AIDS social programs and research funding.

The AIDS Alliance for Children, Youth, and Families was established in 1994 to publicize the concerns of women, children, young people, and families who are affected by HIV/AIDS. The nonprofit organization is also a clearinghouse for relevant information and advocates for public policy changes in the areas of HIV/AIDS social welfare and disease prevention.

Metro TeenAIDS focuses on prevention, education, and treatment needs of teenagers. Through its website (http://www.metroteenaids.org/) and in-person contact at schools, nightclubs, youth centers, shelters, and on the street, Metro TeenAIDS connects with teenagers in a language that is relevant to them. The intent is to help teenagers protect themselves from the risks of HIV exposure and contamination and in securing medical care for HIV infection and AIDS.

FIGURE 5.4

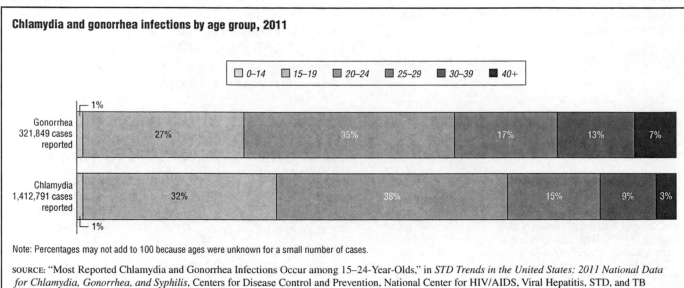

Chlamydia and gonorrhea infections by age group, 2011

☐ *0–14*   ☐ *15–19*   ☐ *20–24*   ☐ *25–29*   ☐ *30–39*   ■ *40+*

Gonorrhea
321,849 cases
reported

┌ 1%
27%   35%   17%   13%   7%

Chlamydia
1,412,791 cases
reported

32%   38%   15%   9%   3%
└ 1%

Note: Percentages may not add to 100 because ages were unknown for a small number of cases.

SOURCE: "Most Reported Chlamydia and Gonorrhea Infections Occur among 15–24-Year-Olds," in *STD Trends in the United States: 2011 National Data for Chlamydia, Gonorrhea, and Syphilis*, Centers for Disease Control and Prevention, National Center for HIV/AIDS, Viral Hepatitis, STD, and TB Prevention, Division of HIV/AIDS Prevention, March 2013, http://www.cdc.gov/std/stats11/trends-2011.pdf (accessed July 25, 2013)

FIGURE 5.5

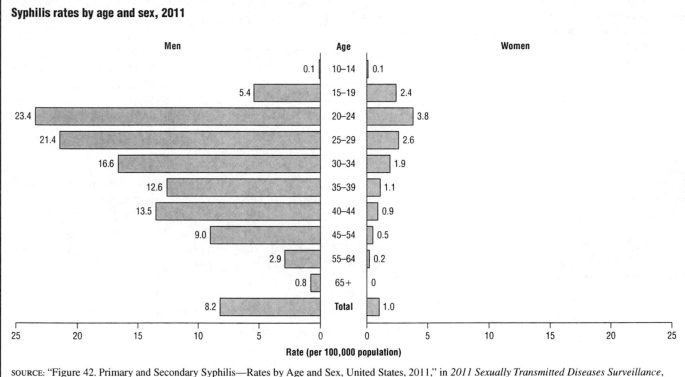

Syphilis rates by age and sex, 2011

Men	Age	Women
0.1	10–14	0.1
5.4	15–19	2.4
23.4	20–24	3.8
21.4	25–29	2.6
16.6	30–34	1.9
12.6	35–39	1.1
13.5	40–44	0.9
9.0	45–54	0.5
2.9	55–64	0.2
0.8	65+	0
8.2	Total	1.0

Rate (per 100,000 population)

SOURCE: "Figure 42. Primary and Secondary Syphilis—Rates by Age and Sex, United States, 2011," in *2011 Sexually Transmitted Diseases Surveillance*, Centers for Disease Control and Prevention, National Center for HIV/AIDS, Viral Hepatitis, STD, and TB Prevention, Division of HIV/AIDS Prevention, December 13, 2012, http://www.cdc.gov/std/stats11/figures/42.htm (accessed July 25, 2013)

Metro TeenAIDS has been working in conjunction with other youth and AIDS activist groups since 1994 to host annual conferences around the country that focus on educating young people about HIV/AIDS. In 1995 the conference became known as the Ryan White National Youth Conference on HIV and AIDS (RWNYC). In 2001

the first Positive Youth Institute—a one-day gathering specifically focusing on the needs of HIV-positive young people—was held before and in conjunction with the RWNYC. Each year several hundred young people, health care workers, and AIDS activists attend the conference.

FIGURE 5.6

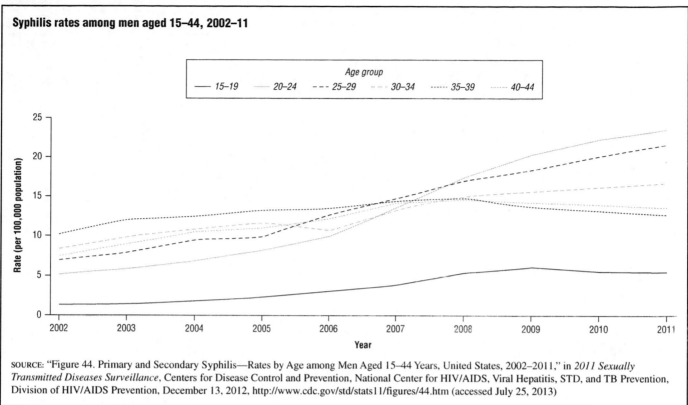

Syphilis rates among men aged 15–44, 2002–11

SOURCE: "Figure 44. Primary and Secondary Syphilis—Rates by Age among Men Aged 15–44 Years, United States, 2002–2011," in *2011 Sexually Transmitted Diseases Surveillance*, Centers for Disease Control and Prevention, National Center for HIV/AIDS, Viral Hepatitis, STD, and TB Prevention, Division of HIV/AIDS Prevention, December 13, 2012, http://www.cdc.gov/std/stats11/figures/44.htm (accessed July 25, 2013)

Many other organizations work to provide HIV/AIDS prevention, treatment, and support programs, including:

- Save the Children (2013, http://www.savethechildren .org/), which supports children and youth at risk for, and affected by, HIV. Save the Children focuses on orphans and others who are at risk and supports PMTCT efforts.

- Keep a Child Alive (http://keepachildalive.org/) supports innovative, community-based initiatives to

improve access to HIV treatment and care and support for children and families living with and affected by HIV in Kenya, Rwanda, South Africa, Uganda, and India.

- The Elizabeth Glaser Pediatric AIDS Foundation (http://www.pedaids.org/) is dedicated to preventing pediatric HIV infection and eliminating HIV/AIDS in children through research, advocacy, and prevention. It operates care and treatment programs in 15 countries around the world.

CHAPTER 6
HIV/AIDS COSTS AND TREATMENT

FINANCING HEALTH CARE DELIVERY

Care for HIV/AIDS patients is expensive. Drug treatments, most prominently highly active antiretroviral therapy (HAART), have high per-unit costs. Nonetheless, their introduction in 1996 reduced total health care spending on AIDS by decreasing the rate of hospitalization and outpatient care. According to Samuel A. Bozzette et al., in "Expenditures for the Care of HIV-Infected Patients in the Era of Highly Active Antiretroviral Therapy" (*New England Journal of Medicine*, vol. 344, no. 11, March 15, 2001), the average HIV patient incurred costs of approximately $1,410 per month in 1998. Extended over the full year, a patient's drug treatment for HIV could cost as much as $18,300. People with AIDS could spend up to $77,000 per year on treatment. By the second decade of the 21st century, the costs of treating AIDS increased more than sixfold. Jessica Camille Aguirre reports in "Cost of Treatment Still a Challenge for HIV Patients in U.S." (NPR.org, July 27, 2012) that in 2012 the average drug treatment cost was between $2,000 and $5,000 per month, and the lifetime cost was estimated at more than $500,000.

Longer survival following infection with HIV leads to even greater costs for care and treatment. The lifetime costs of care for HIV-infected people depend on the disease stage at which people are diagnosed and when antiretroviral therapy (ART) is started. For example, Paul G. Farnham et al. note in "Updates of Lifetime Costs of Care and Quality-of-Life Estimates for HIV-Infected Persons in the United States: Late versus Early Diagnosis and Entry into Care" (*Journal of Acquired Immune Deficiency Syndromes*, vol. 64, no. 2, October 1, 2013) that average lifetime costs vary from $253,000 to $402,000 (in 2011 dollars). HIV-infected patients who enter care early incur greater lifetime costs, improved quality of life, and reduced transmissions compared with patients who enter care late. Farnham et al. conclude that early

ART initiation and early entry into care increases the costs of care, in large part because it extends patients' years of life and treatment.

This finding prompted the World Health Organization (WHO) to issue new HIV treatment guidelines calling for earlier ART. In the press release "WHO Issues New HIV Recommendations Calling for Earlier Treatment" (June 30, 2013, http://www.who.int/), the WHO asserts that earlier ART has the potential to prevent an additional 3 million deaths and 3.5 million new HIV infections between 2013 and 2025.

Some HIV/AIDS patients rely on health insurance to help pay these costs. Many patients, however, are not insured. Also, until enactment of the Patient Protection and Affordable Care Act of 2010, which beginning in 2014 prohibits preexisting condition exclusions and lifetime limits, many policies excluded or denied coverage to people with preexisting conditions, and, as a result, many HIV-positive people were denied private health insurance.

According to AIDS.com, in "The Affordable Care Act and HIV/AIDS" (March 29, 2013, http://aids.gov/federal-resources/policies/health-care-reform/), 17% of people living with HIV/AIDS have private insurance and nearly 30% do not have any coverage. Many people living with HIV/AIDS in the United States have the costs of their treatment paid for by Medicaid and Medicare. Medicaid is an entitlement program that is run by the federal and state governments to provide health care insurance to patients under the age of 65 years who cannot afford to pay for private health insurance. Medicare is the federal health insurance program for adults aged 65 years and older and younger adults with permanent disabilities. Medicaid eligibility requirements vary from state to state. Generally, however, Medicaid covers people with very little income who cannot support themselves financially due to a physical or mental impairment—an impairment that is expected to last at least one year or result in death. The operation of Medicaid programs also varies widely by jurisdiction. Many states supplement federal funding with their own funds, and each state determines its eligibility criteria and benefits—the number and type of treatments that are provided through the program. The Ryan White HIV/AIDS Program is another key source of funding for health and social services for this population.

The toll of HIV/AIDS on Medicaid and Medicare is huge. The Kaiser Family Foundation estimates in the fact sheet "U.S. Federal Funding for HIV/AIDS: The President's FY 2014 Budget Request" (May 23, 2013, http://kff.org/hivaids/fact-sheet/u-s-federal-funding-for-hivaids-the-presidents-fy-2014-budget-request/) that the federal contribution to Medicaid for HIV/AIDS care rose from $4.7 billion in fiscal year (FY) 2010 to $5.9 billion in FY 2014. Medicare accounts for approximately a quarter of federal spending on HIV/AIDS care in the United States. The Kaiser Family Foundation projects that Medicare spending for HIV/AIDS will grow from $5.1 billion in FY 2010 to $6.6 billion in FY 2014.

AIDS Drug Assistance Programs

During the late 1980s state-administered programs were established to help AIDS patients pay for zidovudine, the most effective drug at the time. The AIDS drug assistance programs (ADAPs) provide free drugs to low-income AIDS patients who are not poor enough to qualify for Medicaid coverage but who do not have private health insurance coverage or who have used up their prescription drug coverage. The federal government provides two-thirds of the funding for the state programs, and the balance comes mostly from the states. These programs financed most of the cost of medication for low-income patients until 2006, when the Medicare prescription drug benefit Part D took effect. People eligible for both Medicaid and Medicare have the cost of their drugs covered by Part D.

During the late 1990s, however, the development of new and more effective antiretroviral drugs prompted more patients to take advantage of the ADAPs. This growing demand has put a financial strain on the ADAPs, and many states have to ration HIV/AIDS drugs or turn patients away to remain solvent. Some states are making it harder for people to qualify for the programs, and a few are beginning to charge small co-payments (a percentage of the total cost that the patient is responsible for paying) to offset the cost of the drugs. Others are attempting to obtain larger price discounts or rebates on HIV/AIDS drugs in an effort to reduce their costs so they can continue to provide the drugs to an expanding population of patients.

The National Alliance of State and Territorial AIDS Directors (NASTAD) reports in *National ADAP Monitoring Project Annual Report Module One* (January 2013, http://nastad.org/docs/NASTAD-National-ADAP-Monitoring-Project-Report-Module-1-2013-1.pdf) that as of June 2012 the ADAPs provided medications to 143,941 clients, an increase of 5% from June 2011. Most clients were low income and uninsured and more than half were African American (32%) or Hispanic (23%). ADAP spending on prescription drugs totaled over $139 million, and 10 states accounted for 74% of all drug spending. In 2012 the average per client expenditure was $12,648.

According to the NASTAD, drug spending increased more than ninefold between 1996 and 2012, almost three times the rate of client growth during this same period. Congress has increased the ADAP budget to accommodate rising drug costs—in 2012 the U.S. Department of Health and Human Services (HHS) transferred $75 million in "emergency funding" to the ADAPs to meet the needs of their growing waiting lists. In 2013 legislation was passed that capped spending for the ADAPs at about $900 million.

Changes to the Health Care System

Since the 1960s U.S. government spending on health services has consistently increased. The Centers for Medicare and Medicaid Services' Office of the Actuary reports in *National Health Expenditure Projections 2011–2021* (June 2012, http://www.cms.gov/) that health care spending will grow at an average annual rate of 5.7% between 2011 and 2021. By 2021 government spending for health care is projected to reach nearly 50% of total national health expenditures, with the federal government accounting for about two-thirds.

Along with Medicaid and Medicare, managed-care plans (also known as managed-care organizations [MCOs]), which control the use of and reimbursement for services in an effort to contain costs, rely heavily on primary care practitioners (general and family physicians). These plans have become the health care providers for increasing numbers of HIV/AIDS patients. Since 2000 many HIV-infected people have enrolled in managed-care plans. This is partly because more companies are only offering employees managed-care plans and partly because government insurance programs are directing Medicaid recipients to such programs.

A MANAGED-CARE PLAN FOR HIV/AIDS PATIENTS: THE TENNESSEE "CENTERS OF EXCELLENCE" PROGRAM. On January 1, 1994, Tennessee withdrew from the federal Medicaid program and began implementing a state health care reform plan called Tennessee Medicaid (TennCare). In May 1998 TennCare introduced a voluntary managed-care plan for its members with HIV or AIDS. The model plan features "Centers of Excellence" providers—practitioners with expertise in the care of HIV/AIDS patients. The providers must agree to adopt and adhere to a clinical protocol (practice and care guidelines) developed by a committee composed of providers, consumers, MCOs, and public health officials. The committee meets up to twice a month to evaluate and recommend new drug therapies as they become available and to inform participating providers about new treatments.

Providers may be individual practitioners with access to needed services or full-service clinics composed of a group of practitioners. There are no financial incentives to participate in the program. However, providers who meet the Centers of Excellence criteria do not have to obtain prior authorization when they prescribe drugs or treatments that fall under the clinical protocols.

The Centers of Excellence program frees MCOs from the clinical and administrative responsibility of keeping close tabs on HIV/AIDS care. It also allows MCOs to remain confident that providers are capable and have access to a wide range of services needed by members. MCO members know that participating providers meet high standards of HIV/AIDS clinical care. Other managed-care plans are developing comparable programs to meet the unique health and social service needs of people living with HIV/AIDS.

With an annual budget of more than $9 billion, TennCare (2013, http://www.tennessee.gov/tenncare/) provides health care to 1.2 million people per year. Darin Gordon, Wendy Long, and Casey Dungan report in *Health Care Finance and Administration FY 2014 Budget Presentation* (March 2013, http://www.tn.gov/tenncare/forms/HCFAbudgetFY14.pdf) that in 2012 TennCare exceeded its goal of achieving member satisfaction above 90% for the fourth consecutive year. It also received the Mercy Award for "outstanding dedication to provide health care services to the underserved in Tennessee," and was recognized by the AARP as "one of the top Medicaid managed care [long-term services and support] programs in the nation."

CHALLENGES FOR THE DELIVERY SYSTEM

HIV/AIDS poses a major challenge to health care institutions, health care professionals, and others who provide direct health care services. Since its emergence and identification, HIV infection has undergone a dramatic transformation—it has gone from being an infectious disease that was an almost certain death sentence to a chronic disease that for many can be managed for decades. Furthermore, unlike most chronic diseases that afflict older Americans, HIV/AIDS affects people of all ages, and young adults are disproportionately affected. The health care system cares for more than a million people in the United States suffering from a disease that is still only partly understood. The system must also plan to deliver services to the tens of thousands of people in the United States who are HIV positive and will require specialized health care services during the coming years, even though only a small proportion will need intensive medical care at any one time.

The number of indigent people in need of HIV/AIDS care, particularly those who bring the added complications of drug addiction, homelessness, and other socioeconomic problems, has strained public hospitals in particular. Patients in public hospitals are often different from those in private hospitals. They generally seek care later in the course of the disease's progression and are, therefore, sicker. The scarcity of resources—trained personnel, hospital beds, and support services—in the community, combined with inadequate funding and reimbursement for HIV/AIDS care, are significant obstacles to effective health care delivery for poor HIV/AIDS patients.

Health Care Reform Legislation Promises to Improve Access to Care

In March 2010 President Barack Obama (1961–) signed the Patient Protection and Affordable Care Act (PPACA) into law. The PPACA is considered to be the most comprehensive and important health care reform legislation since the 1965 passage of Medicaid and Medicare. The provisions of the legislation that aim to improve access to care for people with HIV/AIDS include:

- Eliminating the Medicaid disability requirement (people with HIV no longer must wait for an AIDS diagnosis to be eligible for Medicaid coverage) and extending access to Medicaid to people with an income 133% of the federal poverty line in 2014

- Closing the Medicare Part D donut hole (a gap in Medicare that stops paying for prescriptions and the beneficiary must pay the entire cost) by 2020, and allowing the ADAP to be used to meet the Medicare Part D True Out of Pocket Spending Limit

- Requiring pharmaceutical companies to offer a 50% discount on brand-name drugs in the donut hole

- Increasing access to private health insurance in 2014 by prohibiting discrimination or higher premiums based on health status or gender and banning preexisting condition exclusions and lifetime limits on coverage

- Expanding the scope of coverage in 2014 by mandating benefits that include prescription drugs, mental health and substance abuse treatment, preventive care, and chronic disease management

- Increasing affordability of insurance coverage by providing subsidies for people with incomes up to 400% of the federal poverty line

Preventing HIV Is Cost-Effective

Although HIV treatment increases health care costs, prevention efforts are cost-effective. In "The Cost and

Impact of Scaling up Pre-exposure Prophylaxis for HIV Prevention: A Systematic Review of Cost-Effectiveness Modelling Studies" (*PLoS Medicine*, vol. 10, no. 3, March 2013), Gabriela B. Gomez et al. evaluate the anticipated health gains and costs of HIV pre-exposure prevention efforts—giving people at high risk for HIV exposure ART to reduce their risk of becoming infected. The researchers find that pre-exposure prophylaxis has "the potential to be a cost-effective addition to HIV prevention programmes in some settings."

Hospital Care

The American Hospital Association reports in "Fast Facts on US Hospitals" (January 3, 2013, http://www.aha.org/research/rc/stat-studies/fast-facts.shtml) that in 2011 there were 5,724 hospitals. These hospitals are also feeling the pinch of Medicare rate limits, reduced payments from MCOs, and intense competition from other providers, such as ambulatory surgical centers and hospices. Many are struggling to remain profitable. During the 1970s and 1980s the steady growth of for-profit hospitals lured many privately insured, middle-class patients away from community hospitals, leaving most of the uninsured, sicker patients to seek care from inner-city public hospitals.

Most HIV/AIDS patients are cared for in inner-city public hospitals that are already overburdened with inadequate revenues, staff shortages, lack of referral facilities, and emergency departments that are used by many poor neighborhood residents as sources of primary medical care. Many health care professionals praise a model of hospital care that was pioneered in San Francisco, California. The city was hit hard during the early days of the HIV/AIDS epidemic and developed a range of innovative, effective programs in response to acute need. This model of care relies on extensive outpatient services and volunteer social support services that are provided by the well-established and well-organized gay and lesbian community.

Changes in Health Care Delivery

Although fewer people are acquiring HIV/AIDS, the evolution of HIV care is altering the ways in which health care is delivered. In the late stages of AIDS, most patients require intermittent hospitalization and home health care. Those who are not as severely affected and have symptoms or conditions that once required intravenous therapy (which had to be administered in a hospital or by home health professionals) are now able to self-medicate at home. Many drugs are now available for oral administration in pill or liquid form. These home care and community-based measures lessen the burden on the health care delivery system and make it easier for HIV/AIDS patients to care for themselves.

People with AIDS (PWAs) who receive informal home health care (such as care from friends and family) often use fewer hospital services, perhaps reflecting a greater desire to remain at home. PWAs who have strong social support systems and who prefer to remain at home may also be less likely to demand an aggressive approach to treating their illness. Those who receive formal home health care (visits from physicians, nurses, therapists, social workers, case managers, and other paid caregivers) often use more hospital services. This may reflect a greater use of all types of health services by PWAs with weaker social support systems and/or an aggressive approach to treatment by medical professionals.

An AIDS Care Alternative

In an effort to offer uninsured AIDS patients in Atlanta, Georgia, treatment equal to that available to patients with private insurance, Grady Memorial Hospital (2013, http://www.gradyhealth.org/specialty/ponce-de-leon-center.html/) opened in 1986 the Ponce De Leon Center, one of the largest centers that is dedicated to the treatment of advanced HIV/AIDS. The center provides internal medicine and infectious disease care, mental health counseling, social and support services, HIV research and education, and case management. It also works closely with many local AIDS service organizations, some housed on-site, to meet the complex needs of people living with HIV/AIDS. The Ponce De Leon Center is the largest publicly funded program of its kind in the eastern United States and is consistently named as one of the top-three HIV/AIDS outpatient clinics in the country.

Hospice Care

The AIDS epidemic has had a significant impact on hospices. According to the National Center for Health Statistics, in *Health, United States, 2012* (May 2013, http://www.cdc.gov/nchs/data/hus/hus12.pdf), the number of certified hospice care agencies grew from 164 in 1985 to 3,509 in 2010. Hospice care, both in the home and in specialized centers, offers care that is aimed at comfort rather than cure. This includes expert pain relief, along with emotional, psychological, and spiritual support for patients, their families, and friends. Most hospice patients are older adults who suffer from terminal diseases such as cancer and face imminent death.

At the beginning of the AIDS epidemic, patients did not fit well into the hospices of the day. AIDS patients were younger than traditional hospice patients, and the progression of their disease was less predictable than many cancers. However, during the first decade of the 21st century home-based hospice programs were designed to meet the needs of AIDS patients, their partners, and families and gained acceptance in the medical community as well as among HIV-infected people and the voluntary social service agencies that are organized to support them.

HEALTH CARE PROVIDERS
Physicians

There are physicians from many medical specialties— primary care physicians such as family practitioners, internists, and specialists in infectious diseases, pulmonary medicine, and cancer medicine—who care for people infected with HIV or those suffering from AIDS. Physicians who treat AIDS patients often perform a wide variety of services. Many are also AIDS activists and may be involved in developing policies, planning for care needs, and dealing with the media.

One challenge in the training of physicians to treat AIDS patients is that AIDS care requires skills and training in the multitude of conditions that are known to be part of HIV/AIDS. However, the amount of experience— rather than the kind of training—may be a better predictor of the quality of care the physician is able to deliver.

Maria Zolfo et al. describe in "A Telemedicine Service for HIV/AIDS Physicians Working in Developing Countries" (*Journal of Telemedicine and Telecare*, vol. 17, no. 2, March 2011) an Internet-based service to assist physicians and other health care workers in countries where medical resources are limited. Between April 2003 (when it began) and December 2009 the service had fielded 1,058 queries from more than 40 countries. Most of the questions were posed in a web-based telemedicine discussion forum and some were submitted via e-mail. About half of the questions were about the use of antiretroviral drugs. A survey of users of the service revealed that it helped them manage specific cases and influenced their future patient management.

In parts of the world such as sub-Saharan Africa a shortage of health care workers has impeded the provision of HIV treatment. Connor A. Emdin, Nicholas J. Chong, and Peggy E. Millson analyze in "Non-physician Clinician Provided HIV Treatment Results in Equivalent Outcomes as Physician-Provided Care: A Meta-analysis" (*Journal of International AIDS Society*, vol. 16, July 3, 2013) the results of nine studies that examined how patients with HIV infection fare when treated by non-physicians (nurses and others). The researchers find that nonphysician-provided care produced comparable outcomes to physician-provided treatment and also decreased the number of patients who did not return for follow-up care.

Nurses

Nurses often have different viewpoints than some physicians about their professional obligations to patients with HIV/AIDS. As hospital employees, nurses seldom have the option of choosing whether to treat a particular patient (nor do patients have much choice of nurses). Nurses, however, report that caring for HIV/AIDS patients can take an enormous emotional toll because they are often the primary source of continuous physical and emotional care for these patients, who generally require more intensive care and services than other patients.

Nurses face a wide range of emotional issues when caring for these patients, from feelings of failure when treatment is unsuccessful to grief when witnessing the untimely deaths of patients. In "How Caring for Persons with HIV/AIDS Affects Rural Nurses" (*Issues in Mental Health Nursing*, vol. 30, no. 5, May 2009), Iris L. Mullins of New Mexico State University explains that caring for patients with HIV/AIDS affects nurses in three distinct areas of their personal and professional lives: their personal sense of self as a nurse in practice; their interactions with their family members, friends, and colleagues; and their interactions with patients with HIV/AIDS. Nurses caring for HIV/AIDS patients in rural areas expressed additional concerns including the need for ongoing continued education about the care of people with HIV/AIDS.

Irish Patrick Williams and Lorona Searcy examine in "Study: Is Bedside Nursing Still Affected by HIV Stigma?" (*HIV Clinician*, vol. 24, no. 4, Fall 2012) nurses' feelings about HIV/AIDS and whether stigma associated with the disease influences the care nurses deliver. The researchers find that some nurses remain reluctant to care for patients with HIV/AIDS because of fear of contracting the disease and that stigmatization continues to challenge efforts to optimize treatment of this vulnerable patient population. Williams and Searcy assert that improved HIV/AIDS education for nursing students and professional development for nurses is needed.

Centers for Disease Control and Prevention Guidelines

In response to an incident in which five patients acquired HIV from David J. Acer (1949–1990), a Florida dentist, the Centers for Disease Control and Prevention (CDC) addressed occupational exposure to bloodborne pathogens in "Recommendations for Preventing Transmission of Human Immunodeficiency Virus and Hepatitis B Virus to Patients during Exposure-Prone Invasive Procedures" (*Morbidity and Mortality Weekly Report*, vol. 40, no. RR-8, July 12, 1991). The updated guidelines were intended to prevent the accidental spread of the infection from health care providers to patients and from patients to health care workers. The recommendations stressed the careful and consistent use, with all patients, of standard infection control procedures for bloodborne agents—the so-called universal precautions—that were published by the CDC in 1987.

The CDC guidelines also recommended that HIV-infected health care workers stop performing exposure-prone invasive procedures and that professional medical and dental groups draw up lists of exposure-prone procedures for their disciplines. The CDC recommended that HIV-infected health care workers consult with a panel of experts to determine which, if any, limits should be placed on their medical practices and further advised practitioners to inform patients of their HIV-infection status before performing medical procedures.

The CDC guidelines resulted in some unforeseen consequences. Professional groups, hospital attorneys, state courts, legislatures, and Congress reacted with alarm to a perception of dangers to patients posed by HIV-infected health care professionals totally out of proportion to the largely theoretical risk. Adelisa L. Panlilio et al. of the CDC note in "Updated U.S. Public Health Service Guidelines for the Management of Occupational Exposures to HIV and Recommendations for Postexposure Prophylaxis" (*Morbidity and Mortality Weekly Report*, vol. 54, no. RR-9, September 30, 2005) that the average risk of HIV infection after skin contact with HIV-infected blood is estimated to be about 0.3%, and the risk for transmission is even lower from contact with bodily fluids or tissues other than blood. In "Surveillance of Occupationally Acquired HIV/AIDS in Healthcare Personnel, as of December 2010" (May 2011, http://www.cdc.gov/HAI/organisms/hiv/Surveillance-Occupationally-Acquired-HIV-AIDS.html), the CDC indicates that 57 documented cases had been reported between 1981 and 2010 (although no documented cases were reported between 2000 and 2010), and it was possible that 143 additional cases of HIV infection were linked to occupational exposures.

According to Panlilio et al., the CDC recommends that the following procedures and philosophies would best serve patients and health care workers:

- The universal and meticulous use of well-understood infection-control procedures, particularly those developed from the study of hepatitis B (another blood-borne infection that is 100 times more infectious and 10 times more common in health professionals), should be applied in all health care settings, whether hospital, office, or home based.

- Operative or other invasive procedures, in which injury to health care professionals occurs with any frequency, should be discontinued or modified to the greatest extent possible. This involves developing new instruments and investigating new operative techniques.

- All health care professionals should consider being tested for HIV. However, an HIV-positive result should not justify restricting the practice of health care professionals.

HEALTH CARE WORKERS AND INFECTION
Health Care Workers with HIV and AIDS

In "Surveillance of Occupationally Acquired HIV/AIDS in Healthcare Personnel, as of December 2010," the CDC indicates that as of May 2011 it was aware of only 57 documented cases of health care workers other than surgeons in the United States who had become infected with HIV as a result of occupational exposures. The breakdown of those who were infected was as follows:

- Nurses (24)
- Clinical laboratory workers (16)
- Nonsurgical physicians (6)
- Nonclinical laboratory technicians (3)
- Housekeeper/maintenance workers (2)
- Surgical technicians (2)
- Dialysis technician (1)
- Embalmer/morgue technician (1)
- Health aide/attendant (1)
- Respiratory therapist (1)

The CDC was also aware of 143 cases of HIV infection or AIDS that were possibly linked to occupational exposure among health care workers. These workers had not reported other risk factors for HIV infection. They reported a history of occupational exposure to blood, bodily fluids, or HIV-infected laboratory material, but they did not document infection after a specific exposure.

The known and possible cases of occupational acquisition of HIV undoubtedly represent an underestimate. There are likely unknown numbers of people who acquired their infection through occupational exposures, although, even in 2013, this is purely conjecture.

According to the National Institute for Occupational Safety and Health, in "Overview of State Needle Safety Legislation" (December 29, 2011, http://www.cdc.gov/niosh/topics/bbp/ndl-law.html), as of June 2002, 21 states had enacted needle-safety legislation to safeguard health care workers from bloodborne pathogen (agents that cause disease) exposures. State laws aim to supplement and strengthen the federal standards mandated by the Occupational Safety and Health Administration. Many of the state laws require the creation of a written exposure plan that is periodically reviewed and updated; protocols for safety device identification and selection; logs to document and report injuries with sharp instruments; and strict requirements and training for workers on how to use safety devices.

In "Updated U.S. Public Health Service Guidelines for the Management of Occupational Exposures to HBV, HCV, and HIV and Recommendations for Postexposure

Prophylaxis" (*Morbidity and Mortality Weekly Report*, vol. 50, no. RR-11, June 29, 2001), the U.S. Public Health Service updated the guidelines for treatment to prevent health care workers with occupational exposure to HIV from becoming infected with the virus. Known as postexposure prophylaxis (PEP), the recommendation was that affected workers be given a four-week regimen of two antiretroviral drugs such as zidovudine and lamivudine, with the addition of a third drug for HIV exposures that pose an increased risk of transmission. Another update was issued by Panlilio et al. in September 2005 because since publication of the 2001 update the U.S. Food and Drug Administration (FDA) had approved new antiretroviral agents and additional information had become available about the use and safety of PEP. Although the best strategy to protect health care workers is to avoid exposure to HIV and other bloodborne pathogens, PEP has, as of 2013, proven generally effective in preventing HIV infection in workers who have been exposed.

Risks to Patients

Health care officials are not the only ones worried about HIV transmission in the health care setting. Patients also fear that infected health care workers can transmit the virus to them. In the landmark study "HIV Transmission from Health Care Worker to Patient: What Is the Risk?" (*Annals of Internal Medicine*, vol. 116, no. 10, May 15, 1992), Mary E. Chamberland and David M. Bell of the CDC develop a model of the risk of HIV transmission to patients and estimate that the risk of a patient becoming infected by an HIV-positive surgeon during a single operation is anywhere from 1 out of 42,000 to 1 out of 420,000. This risk is considerably less than the risks that are associated with many other medical procedures.

The CDC indicates in "HIV and Its Transmission" (July 1999, http://www.hivlawandpolicy.org/sites/www .hivlawandpolicy.org/files/CDC%2C%20HIV%20and%20 its%20transmission.pdf) that of more than 22,000 patients of 63 HIV-infected health care workers, no documented evidence has been found that links HIV infection to medical or dental care, except for the five patients of Acer in 1990. Medical researchers have tried without success to determine how Acer infected his patients and whether the exposure was accidental or deliberate. One theory is that he did not properly sterilize his dental tools; another is that he accidentally cut his finger or jabbed himself with a hypodermic needle, did not notice it, and bled into the patients' mouths. Before his death in 1990, Acer denied intentionally exposing his patients.

Although HIV transmission through transplanted organs occurs very rarely, in November 2007 the first known cases in 20 years of HIV transmission from a high-risk donor were reported by the national media. The most likely explanation for this transmission is that the donor, who was deceased when the organs were harvested, had tested HIV negative because the infection was recent and antibodies had not yet formed to the virus. In "Provider Response to a Rare but Highly Publicized Transmission of HIV through Solid Organ Transplantation" (*Archives of Surgery*, vol. 146, no. 1, January 2011), Lauren M. Kucirka et al. examine how transplant surgeons' practices changed following the cases of HIV transmission. The researchers determine that nearly one-third (31.6%) of transplant surgeons said their practices changed following this exceedingly rare event. Over four out of 10 (41.7%) decreased use of high-risk donors, 34.5% intensified efforts to obtain patients' informed consent, and 16.7% increased their use of nucleic acid amplification testing, which is a more difficult and time-consuming test, but it does detect viral infection earlier than traditional antibody tests.

As described in Chapter 2, another instance of HIV transmission from a kidney transplant—the first documented case of this kind—was reported in March 2011.

WHAT DOES IT COST TO TREAT HIV/AIDS PATIENTS?

The Kaiser Family Foundation notes in "U.S. Federal Funding for HIV/AIDS: The President's FY 2014 Budget Request" that in FY 2012 federal government spending for domestic and global HIV-related activities totaled $27.8 billion. President Obama's federal budget request for FY 2014 included an estimated $29.7 billion—$23.2 billion for domestic programs and $6.5 billion for global initiatives and activities. Federal funding has increased significantly throughout the course of the epidemic, and the FY 2014 federal budget for domestic programs and research represented a 7% increase over FY 2012. Much of the federal funding for HIV/AIDS care, as opposed to other assistance such as housing, was for Medicaid and Medicare, which were budgeted for 11.3% and 13.8% increases, respectively, in funding.

HIV/AIDS-related costs are expected to increase in response to the rising costs of hospitalization, home care, insurance premiums and co-payments, physician services, and pharmaceutical drugs. Growing concern about rising drug prices led to a self-imposed price freeze by some pharmaceutical companies in 2002. However, price increases were eventually instituted. For example, in "Gilead under Pressure to Produce Stand-Alone Version of New HIV Drug" (Nature.com, July 3, 2013), Liz Devitt reports that Gilead Sciences plans to sell its antiretroviral drug, tenofovir alafenamide, only in combination with the drugs elvitegravir, cobicistat, and emtricitabine, rather than as a stand-alone drug. This decision makes the drug prohibitively expensive for health programs in poorer countries.

Regardless, some HIV/AIDS care-related expenses have actually been reduced by relocating services from the hospital to outpatient settings. Examples of cost-saving services include outpatient transfusions and outpatient treatment for opportunistic infections such as *Pneumocystis carinii* pneumonia and cryptococcal meningitis. Increased volunteer-based social service programs that enable patients to be cared for at home can also prevent expensive hospital stays.

The Ryan White Comprehensive AIDS Resources Emergency Act

As of 2013, the Ryan White Comprehensive AIDS Resources Emergency (CARE) Act was the only federal program that exclusively funded medical and supportive services for people with HIV/AIDS. The act was named after Ryan White, who died of AIDS in 1990. White was an Indiana teenager with hemophilia who was infected through a blood transfusion. Shunned by his community because many people feared becoming infected through any kind of contact with him, White fought to attend school and attain rights for those infected with HIV/AIDS. White's efforts helped change the way the world treated those with the disease.

The Ryan White HIV/AIDS Program meets the needs of people living with HIV/AIDS who are not covered by other resources or payers and serves as payer of last resort. According to the HHS, in *FY 2014 Congressional Justification for the Health Resources and Services Administration* (April 2013, http://www.hrsa.gov/about/budget/budgetjustification2014.pdf), every year the program serves over 500,000 low-income people with HIV/AIDS. More than one-quarter (27.6%) are uninsured and an additional 54% are underinsured. The CARE Act was

signed in 1990 and reauthorized in 1996, 2000, 2006, and 2009. Funding priority is given to urban areas with the highest number of people living with AIDS, while helping eligible metropolitan areas (EMAs) and midsized cities with emerging needs, which are called transitional grant areas.

The 2009 reauthorization, called the Ryan White HIV/AIDS Treatment Extension Act of 2009, required planning councils to characterize not only the demographics of people with HIV/AIDS but also the population of people unaware of their HIV status. The councils had to develop plans to identify people with HIV/AIDS who do not know their status and to assist these people in obtaining health care services. The councils also had to work to eliminate "barriers to routine testing and disparities in access to services for minorities and underserved communities."

The funds from the Ryan White HIV/AIDS Treatment Extension Act are appropriated using five formulas. Part A funds eligible EMAs that are disproportionately affected by HIV/AIDS and transitional grant areas. Part B funds states to improve the quality, availability, and organization of HIV/AIDS health care and support services. Part C funds early intervention services and ambulatory care. Part D funds do not have to be used for primary care; instead, they may be used to help improve access to clinical trials and research. Part F funds encompass Special Projects of National Significance, which support the demonstration and evaluation of innovative models of HIV/AIDS care delivery for hard-to-reach populations as well as for AIDS Education and Training Centers, dental programs, and the Minority AIDS Initiative.

To qualify for Part A funds, EMAs must have more than 2,000 cumulative AIDS cases reported during the preceding five years and a population of at least 500,000. (The population provision does not apply to any EMA that was named and funded before FY 1997.) Table 6.1 is

TABLE 6.1

Ryan White Act, fiscal years 2012–14

	Fiscal year 2012 enacted	Fiscal year 2013 annualized CR	Fiscal year 2014 president's budget	Fiscal year 2014 +/− fiscal year 2012
Budget authorization	$2,367,178,000	$2,336,479,000	$2,387,178,000	+$20,000,000
ADAP (non add)	933,299,000	903,797,000	943,299,000	+10,000,000
MAI (non add)	160,722,000	169,077,000	161,026,000	+304,000
SPNS	25,000,000	25,000,000	25,000,000	—
Total funding	**$2,392,178,000**	**$2,361,479,000**	**$2,412,178,000**	**+$20,000,000**
FTE	141	141	141	—

ADAP = AIDS Drug Assistance Program. CR = Continuing resolution. FTE = Full-time equivalent. FY = Fiscal year. MAI = Minority AIDS Initiative. SPNS = Special Projects of National Significance.
Note: The amounts include funding for SPNS funded from Department Public Health Service Act evaluation set-asides in fiscal year 2012 and fiscal year 2013 proposed for fiscal year 2014.

SOURCE: "Ryan White HIV/AIDS Treatment Extension Act of 2009 Overview," in *FY 2014 Congressional Justification for the Health Resources and Services Administration (HRSA)*, Health Resources and Services Administration, 2013, http://www.hrsa.gov/about/budget/budgetjustification2014.pdf (accessed July 25, 2013) an overview of funding by the Ryan White HIV/AIDS Treatment Extension Act for FYs 2012, 2013, and 2014.

THE PPACA AND THE RYAN WHITE HIV/AIDS PROGRAM. As the provisions of the PPACA take effect in 2014, it is anticipated that uninsured people living with HIV/AIDS will enroll in private health insurance or be covered under expanded Medicaid. This should reduce the number of people in need of services funded by the "payer of last resort." As a result, grantees will be able to use a greater percentage of their grants to support services not covered by public or private insurance but that are crucial to getting people living with HIV/AIDS into treatment to suppress the virus and help prevent the spread of the epidemic.

The actual scope of coverage for Ryan White HIV/AIDS services under the expanded Medicaid program will be determined by the states. It is anticipated that in many states coverage for the Ryan White service categories will be included in the benefits package in each state's Medicaid program and in the health plans offered through the exchanges. For example, it is likely that the Ryan White program will no longer have to pay full costs for ambulatory health services, prescription drugs, mental health services, substance abuse services, rehabilitation services, and some early intervention services. Regardless, Medicaid and other insurance coverage are unlikely to be sufficient for people living with HIV/AIDS because of limitations in the scope of coverage. This prediction is supported by the fact that nearly three-quarters of current Ryan White clients have private insurance, Medicaid, and/or Medicare. Services that may not be covered by Medicaid or plans offered by the exchanges include oral health care, medical case management, counseling, and psychosocial support services.

Private Insurance and Medicaid

The financing of HIV/AIDS care has increasingly become the responsibility of Medicaid. The greater reliance on Medicaid funding is due in large part to the increase in the number of HIV/AIDS cases among injection drug users and poor people who are unlikely to be covered by private health insurance. In addition, patients who once had private insurance through their workplace lost their coverage when the illness made them too sick to work, or they lost their job and job-related health benefits during the so-called Great Recession (which lasted from late 2007 to mid-2009), forcing them to turn to Medicaid and other public programs.

Added to this list are those whose employment or economic status would normally ensure them insurance coverage, but who became virtually ineligible for private health insurance coverage once they tested positive for HIV. Others need assistance because some insurance companies consider HIV infection to be a preexisting condition, making it ineligible for payment of claims. Even insurance companies that do cover HIV treatment often impose caps, limiting coverage to relatively small dollar amounts.

The National Association of Health Underwriters explains in "Consumer Guide to Individual Health Insurance" (2013, http://www.nahu.org/consumer/individual insurance.cfm) that in 2013 a person with HIV could be turned down for individual coverage by private insurers in most states. However, many states provide uninsurable people with access to individual health insurance coverage through high-risk pools. The PPACA resolves this problem. In 2014 private health insurance companies are prohibited from discriminating against or denying people coverage because they have preexisting conditions.

Death Benefits

Since 1988 an industry has developed that offers dying AIDS patients the opportunity to collect a portion of their life insurance benefits before they die, either to pay for their treatment or to spend as they wish during their remaining time. These viatical (money for necessities given to a person dying or in danger of death) settlements are reached when an insured person sells his or her life insurance policy to an independent insurance company at a reduced or discounted price. This enables the patient to have some cash from the policy while he or she is still alive. After the patient dies, the company that bought the policy is paid the full death benefits. Regulators with the U.S. Securities and Exchange Commission are scrutinizing some practices they believe may victimize AIDS patients.

Some larger companies, such as Prudential, offer policyholders more than 90% of their policy payouts, but only with a physician's certification that they have less than six months to live. Smaller companies usually pay 50% to 80% of the benefit payable at death, although they will pay benefits to people who still have up to five years to live. The longer the policyholders are expected to live, the less the cash disbursement they receive.

Most insurers will not write new life insurance policies for people known to have AIDS. Those that do offer life insurance policies to people infected with HIV or people with AIDS often have stringent requirements and limited benefits. For example, some policies for AIDS patients stipulate that should death occur due to illness during the first two or three years of coverage, then the benefits paid are simply a return of premiums paid plus an annual interest rate. Others offer an initial two- or three-year incremental period; after that initial period full benefits are paid whether death occurs due to accident or to illness.

TABLE 6.2

Office of AIDS Research budget allocation by activity, fiscal years 2010–14

[Dollars in thousands]

Area of emphasis	Fiscal year 2010 actual	Fiscal year 2011 actual	Fiscal year 2012 actual	Fiscal year 2013 CR	Fiscal year 2014 president's budget	Fiscal year 2014 +/− fiscal year 2012
HIV microbicides	$143,162	$120,982	$129,919	$134,627	$133,800	$3,881
Vaccines	534,972	548,834	556,613	560,962	574,966	18,353
Behavioral and social science	429,313	412,163	420,084	421,684	430,209	10,125
Etiology and pathogenesis	744,649	730,978	668,244	674,697	693,851	25,607
Therapeutics						
Therapeutics as prevention	67,734	65,064	56,561	58,126	66,026	9,465
Drug discovery, development, and treatment	617,257	615,475	650,059	659,261	651,168	1,109
Total, therapeutics	**684,991**	**680,539**	**706,620**	**717,387**	**717,194**	**10,574**
Natural history and epidemiology	275,098	278,998	257,973	253,342	247,385	(10,588)
Training, infrastructure, and capacity building	216,329	232,624	280,775	281,474	272,062	(8,713)
Information dissemination	56,832	54,159	54,567	50,708	52,249	(2,318)
Total	**$3,085,346**	**$3,059,277**	**$3,074,795**	**$3,094,881**	**$3,121,716**	**$46,921**

Note: CR = Continuing resolution.

SOURCE: "National Institutes of Health Office of AIDS Research Budget Authority by Activity," in *Office of AIDS Research Trans-NIH AIDS Research Budget*, U.S. Department of Health and Human Services, National Institutes of Health, 2013, http://www.oar.nih.gov/budget/pdf/2014_OAR_CJ_Trans-NIH.pdf (accessed July 29, 2013)

TREATMENT RESEARCH

Medical and pharmaceutical research to develop and conduct clinical trials of antiretroviral drugs is expensive. According to the National Institutes of Health (NIH), nearly $3.1 billion was allocated for AIDS research in FY 2012 and over $3.1 billion was budgeted for FY 2014. Table 6.2 shows budget allocations by the type of activity funded between FYs 2010 and 2014.

Decisions about how much is spent to research a particular disease are not based solely on how many people develop the disease or die from it. Rightly or wrongly, economists base the societal value of an individual on his or her earning potential and productivity (the ability to contribute to society as a worker). The bulk of the people who die from heart disease, stroke, and cancer are older adults. Many have retired from the workforce and their potential economic productivity is often minimal. This economic measure of present and future financial productivity should not be misinterpreted as a casting-off of older adults; instead, it is simply an economic measure of present and future financial productivity.

In contrast, AIDS patients are usually much younger and, until recently, often died young—in their 20s, 30s, and 40s. Until they develop AIDS, the potential productivity of these people, measured in economic terms, is high. The number of work years lost when they die is considerable. Using this economic equation to determine how disease research should be funded, it may be considered economically wise to invest more money to research AIDS because the losses, measured in potential work years rather than in lives, are so much greater.

The primary goals of HIV/AIDS therapy are to prolong life and improve its quality. Even though during the early days of AIDS research a cure for the disease was envisioned, few researchers at the turn of the 21st century realistically expected any one drug to cure HIV infection in all people. The bottom-line objective became making the virus less deadly by foiling its efforts to reproduce within the body.

A major obstacle to the discovery of such treatments is the cost of drug research and development. Pharmaceutical manufacturers spend millions of dollars researching and developing new medicines. According to the Pharmaceutical Research and Manufacturers of America (PhRMA), since 1992 U.S. pharmaceutical companies have consistently spent more money each year on research and development (R&D) activities than the NIH has spent on its annual budget. For example, PhRMA reports in *2013 Profile Bioharmaceutical Industry* (July 2013, http://phrma.org/sites/default/files/pdf/PhRMA%20Profile%202013.pdf) that in 2012 the estimated total pharmaceutical R&D budget was $48.5 billion. By contrast, the HHS states in *Fiscal Year 2013 Budget in Brief: Strengthening Health and Opportunity for All Americans* (February 2012, http://www.hhs.gov/budget/budget-brief-fy2013.pdf) that the NIH budget for research was $31.6 billion in 2012. Furthermore, private-sector spending has been outpacing government spending since 1995.

PhRMA explains that pharmaceutical manufacturers must cover the cost not only of R&D for the approximately two out of 10 drugs that succeed but also for many of the drugs—eight out of 10—that fail to make it to the marketplace. Because of this cost, once a new drug receives FDA approval, its manufacturer ordinarily holds a patent or gains exclusivity rights, which guarantee that it will be the sole marketer for a specified time (usually from three to 20 years) to recoup its investment. During this time the drug is priced much higher than if other manufacturers were allowed to compete by producing generic versions of the same drug. In contrast to the original manufacturer, the generic manufacturer does not have to pay for the successes and failures that occurred in the drug development pathway or pursue the complicated, time-consuming process of seeking FDA approval. The producer of generic drugs has the formula and must simply manufacture the drugs properly. Because of the lower cost of the generic drug after the original patent or exclusivity period has expired, competition among pharmaceutical manufacturers generally lowers the price. HIV/AIDS drugs are granted seven years of exclusivity under legislation that is aimed at encouraging research and promoting development of new treatments.

The issue of patent protection for HIV/AIDS drugs is understandably contentious. Pharmaceutical manufacturers and others argue that patent protection is necessary to allow for the financial investments necessary to breed innovation. However, to those directly affected by HIV/AIDS and those governments or health care systems that provide care, the enormous costs can be infuriating, especially with the knowledge that generic drugs carrying a lower price tag are possible. The need for less expensive HIV/AIDS drugs is especially urgent in the developing world.

In light of this need, the Medicines Patent Pool (2013, http://www.medicinespatentpool.org), a United Nations–backed organization, was established in 2010 with the intent to foster generic competition by reducing the price of drugs and stimulating development of new formulations. It negotiates for licenses from key HIV medicines patent holders (pharmaceutical companies, research institutes, governments, and universities) and then makes sublicenses available to generic companies, enabling them to produce low-cost HIV drugs for use in developing countries before the patent terms expire.

FDA-APPROVED DRUGS

The first drug thought to delay symptoms was zidovudine. Although initially promising, zidovudine's effects were found to be temporary at best. Several other drugs worked using the same mechanism of action as zidovudine—exclusion of HIV from the host chromosome. A newer class of drugs called protease inhibitors (PIs) prevents HIV already in the host cells from reproducing. PIs block the ability of HIV to mature and infect new cells by suppressing a protein enzyme of the virus, called protease, which is crucial to the progression of HIV. Roy M. Gulick et al. indicate in the landmark study

"Treatment with Indinavir, Zidovudine, and Lamivudine in Adults with Human Immunodeficiency Virus Infection and Prior Antiretroviral Therapy" (*New England Journal of Medicine*, vol. 337, no. 11, September 11, 1997) that a combination of indinavir, zidovudine, and lamivudine reduces the viral load and CD4 cell count. In the researchers' study, reduction in the viral load and the CD4 cell count lasted for as long as 52 weeks and the drugs were generally well tolerated.

Even if the effectiveness of PIs proves to be transient, they improve patients' prospects simply by creating more roadblocks for HIV, which mutates so rapidly that it becomes resistant to most drugs when the drugs are used alone. These drugs, when used in various combinations, have helped transform HIV infection from a certain death sentence to a chronic but manageable disease, much like diabetes.

Types of Antiretroviral Agents

The FDA notes in "Antiretroviral Drugs Used in the Treatment of HIV Infection" (August 20, 2013, http://www.fda.gov/ForConsumers/byAudience/ForPatientAdvocates/HIVandAIDSActivities/ucm118915.htm) that it approves seven classes of antiretroviral agents for the treatment of HIV/AIDS.

PROTEASE INHIBITORS. As of August 2013, the FDA had approved the following PIs:

- Amprenavir (no longer marketed)
- Tipranavir
- Indinavir
- Saquinavir (no longer marketed)
- Saquinavir mesylate
- Lopinavir and ritonavir
- Fosamprenavir calcium
- Ritonavir
- Darunavir
- Atazanavir sulfate
- Nelfinavir mesylate

NUCLEOSIDE REVERSE TRANSCRIPTASE INHIBITORS. Nucleoside reverse transcriptase inhibitors (NRTIs) were among the first compounds shown to be effective against viral infections. Research during the 1970s led to the development of the drug acyclovir, which is still being used to treat herpes infections. The first four anti-HIV drugs to be approved—zidovudine, didanosine, dideoxycytosine, and stavudine—were nucleoside analogs.

As their name implies, NRTIs exert their action based on their three-dimensional structure, which mimics the structure of the nucleoside building blocks of deoxyribonucleic acid (DNA). By becoming incorporated into the DNA as the molecule is replicated, the analogs can preserve the structure of DNA but make it impossible for the HIV to use its reverse transcriptase to hijack the host replication machinery to make new viral copies.

As of August 2013, the following NRTIs had received FDA approval for use with HIV/AIDS:

- Lamivudine and zidovudine
- Emtricitabine
- Lamivudine
- Abacavir and lamivudine
- Zalcitabine and dideoxycytidine (no longer marketed)
- Zidovudine and azidothymidine
- Abacavir, zidovudine, and lamivudine
- Tenofovir disoproxil fumarate and emtricitabine
- Enteric coated didanosine
- Didanosine and dideoxyinosine
- Tenofovir disoproxil fumarate
- Stavudine
- Abacavir sulfate

NONNUCLEOSIDE REVERSE TRANSCRIPTASE INHIBITORS. Another class of antiretroviral drugs that were approved during the late 1990s is nonnucleoside reverse transcriptase inhibitors (NNRTIs). NNRTI compounds slow down the process of the reverse transcriptase enzyme that allows the virus to become part of the infected cell's nucleus. The compounds accomplish this by binding to the viral enzyme, which blocks the ability of the enzyme to function.

As of August 2013, there were six NNRTIs approved for use by the FDA:

- Rilpivirine
- Etravirine
- Delavirdine
- Efavirenz
- Nevirapine (immediate release)
- Nevirapine (extended release)

MULTICLASS COMBINATION PRODUCTS. The FDA approves another class of HIV medications that consist of combinations of specific drugs. As of August 2013, there were three combinations approved for use:

- Efavirenz, emtricitabine, and tenofovir disoproxil fumarate
- Emtricitabine, rilpivirine, and tenofovir disoproxil fumarate
- Elvitegravir, cobicistat, emtricitabine, tenofovir disoproxil fumarate

OTHER APPROVED DRUGS. As of August 2013, the FDA also approved the fusion inhibitor drug enfuvirtide, which interferes with the fusion of HIV with the host cell membrane; the entry inhibitor drug maraviroc, which binds CCR5, an essential co-receptor for most HIV strains, and blocks them from entering T cells; and the HIV integrase strand inhibitor drugs raltegravir, which acts against an enzyme that HIV uses to integrate its viral material into the host's chromosomes, and dolutegravir, which is a once-daily integrase inhibitor that prevents HIV replication and reduces the amount of HIV in the blood.

Aggressive Treatment

With new drugs in the anti-HIV/AIDS arsenal, many people with HIV/AIDS who had given up hope of effective treatment returned to clinics and doctors' offices. Although treatment guidelines previously promoted early intervention with zidovudine, recommended treatment now combines PIs with other antiretroviral drugs. Treatment recommendations change rapidly in response to the development of new drugs and clinical trials indicating the effectiveness of different combinations of antiretroviral drugs. Because HIV mutates to resist any drug it faces, including all PIs, researchers find that varying the combination of drugs prescribed can "fool" the virus before it has time to mutate.

Patients undergoing therapy with new drugs or drug combinations must be highly disciplined. For example, indinavir must be taken on an empty stomach, every eight hours, not less than two hours before or after a meal, and with large amounts of water to prevent the development of kidney stones. Patients must also be careful to never skip doses of indinavir, otherwise the virus will quickly grow immune to the drug. (Indinavir has been found to generate cross-resistance, meaning it makes patients resistant to other PIs.) Saquinavir mesylate must be taken in large doses. Ritonavir must be carefully prescribed and administered because it interacts negatively with some antifungals and antibiotics used by AIDS patients. Because there are many minor and serious risks that are associated with use of these drugs, patients must be closely monitored.

When effective AIDS drugs were introduced, patients sometimes had to wake up during the middle of the night to take pills, and some treatment regimens consisted of as many as 50 or 60 pills administered several times a day. Even with intense pressure to simplify treatment regimens, pharmaceutical companies remained skeptical about an effective once-a-day pill despite the consensus opinion that it would help more people start, and stick with, treatment. Even as recently as 2005, many combined HIV/AIDS medication regimens were administered two to three times per day. Once-a-day regimens were not available until 2006.

Once-a-Day AIDS Treatment

In July 2006 the FDA approved the first once-a-day AIDS treatment, a combination of efavirenz, emtricitabine, and tenofovir disoproxil fumarate. Although this once-a-day drug combination reduces the number of pills a patient must take and as a result improves adherence to treatment, it is probably not the sole drug an AIDS patient needs. Many patients also require additional prescription medications to support their immune system and help them resist infection. In August 2010 the FDA approved a second once-a-day AIDS treatment, a combination of emtricitabine, rilpivirine, and tenofovir disoproxil fumarate. A third once-a-day treatment became available in August 2012, a combination of elvitegravir, cobicistat, emtricitabine, and tenofovir disoproxil fumarate.

THE DISCOVERY OF AN HIV-RESISTANT GENE

In August 1996 scientists working independently at the Aaron Diamond AIDS Research Center in New York City and the Free University of Brussels, Belgium, announced that some white (Caucasian) people have genes that may protect them from HIV, regardless of how many times they are exposed to the virus. The researchers hoped that their findings would lead to new HIV/AIDS therapies or to the development of drugs or vaccines to prevent HIV infection.

The researchers discovered that a gene called CCR5 is associated with HIV resistance. The gene codes for a protein called CC chemokine receptor 5 (CCR5) that is located on the surface of host cells including macrophages, monocytes, and T cells. HIV exploits this protein by using it as a receptor to bind to, and subsequently infect, cells such as T cells. The CCR5 mutation blocks the manufacture of CCR5. Thus, HIV loses its surface target and cannot invade the immune system.

Subsequent studies conducted in the United States found that one out of 100 people inherits two copies of this gene—one from each parent—and is completely immune to HIV infection. One out of five people with only one copy of the CCR5 gene can become infected, but will remain healthy two to three years longer than those without the altered gene. This may be because these people have half as many CCR5 receptors as normal, which limits or slows the spread of the virus.

According to Michael Fischereder et al., in "CC Chemokine Receptor 5 and Renal-Transplant Survival" (*Lancet*, vol. 357, no. 9270, June 2, 2001), the gene is most common in white Americans (10% to 15% of the population). It is rarely found in African Americans and almost never in Asian Americans, perhaps reflecting the origins of the mutation.

Certain populations appear to be resistant to HIV because they lack or have a mutated form of the CCR5 receptor. Most populations that carry the mutant CCR5 gene come from Europe, and there are indications that the mutation arose only about 700 years ago. For a mutation to be sustained in a population at a rate of 10%, there must be some benefit bestowed by the mutation. It is likely nothing to do with HIV, because HIV did not appear until the late 20th century.

The exact nature of the selective pressure that caused the appearance of the CCR5 mutation is the subject of considerable debate. The prevailing theory has been that the selective pressure was the bubonic plague; however, new research suggests that smallpox may have been the trigger. Which of these, if either, is true remains to be determined.

Research is also under way to learn more about other genes such as CCR2 that, when expressed dominantly, appears to slow the progression of AIDS. Vijay Kumar et al. confirm in "Genetic Basis of HIV-1 Resistance and Susceptibility: An Approach to Understand Correlation between Human Genes and HIV-1 Infection" (*Indian Journal of Experimental Biology*, vol. 44, no. 9, September 2006) that site-specific mutations in these genes determine the susceptibility or resistance to HIV-1 infection and AIDS. Researchers hope that the study of host genes in relation to HIV-1 infection may speed the development of drug therapies to prevent or cure HIV-1 infection effectively.

ENGINEERING AN HIV-RESISTANT GENE

In 2013 researchers announced that they had found a way to engineer key cells of the immune system so they remain resistant to HIV infection. In "Generation of an HIV Resistant T-cell Line by Targeted 'Stacking' of Restriction Factors" (*Molecular Therapy*, vol. 21, no. 4, April 2013), Richard A. Voit et al. describe the use of a kind of molecular scissors to insert a series of HIV-resistant genes into T cells. By inactivating a receptor gene and inserting additional anti-HIV genes, the virus was completely blocked from entering the cells, effectively preventing it from harming the immune system.

OTHER RESEARCH LOOKS FOR PROTECTION AGAINST HIV INFECTION
A Natural Barrier to HIV

Olivier Schwartz of the Pasteur Institute identifies in "Langerhans Cells Lap up HIV-1" (*Nature Medicine*, vol. 13, no. 3, March 2007) a protein that acts as a natural barrier to HIV infection. The protein is called langerin, because it is produced by Langerhans cells, which form a network in the skin and mucosa (the membrane lining the vagina) and were previously thought to promote the spread of HIV. Instead, the Langerhans cells contain a protein that eats viruses. Langerin scavenges for viruses in the surrounding environment and thereby helps prevent infection. Langerhans cells do not become infected by HIV-1 because they have langerin on their surfaces. It appears that HIV infection occurs when levels of invading HIV are high or if langerin activity is especially weak. In either of these instances, Langerhans cells can become overwhelmed by the virus and infected.

In "Elevated Elafin/Trappin-2 in the Female Genital Tract Is Associated with Protection against HIV Acquisition" (*AIDS*, vol. 23, no. 13, August 24, 2009), Shehzad M. Iqbal et al. identify the protein elafin/trappin-2 as a novel innate immune factor that is strongly associated with HIV resistance. This innate immune factor was found in the mucosal secretions from the genital tracts of HIV-resistant women who are sex workers. Discovery of this factor enhances understanding of natural immunity to HIV infection.

Researchers are also looking at so-called elite suppressors, a small fraction (0.5%) of people who are infected with HIV that appear able to control infection without antiretroviral drugs. Robert W. Buckheit, Robert F. Siliciano, and Joel N. Blankson of the Johns Hopkins University School of Medicine find in "Primary CD8+ T Cells from Elite Suppressors Effectively Eliminate Nonproductively HIV-1 Infected Resting and Activated CD4+ T Cells" (*Retrovirology*, vol. 10, July 2013) that elite suppressors have much lower levels of HIV integrated into their immune cells than do HIV-infected people treated with antiretroviral drugs. This finding is believed to reflect the fact that elite suppressors mount a more effective immune response to HIV—meaning that their T cells more effectively combat the virus. Elite suppressors are able to efficiently eliminate CD4+ T cells shortly after viral entry and before they produce infection. Buckheit, Siliciano, and Blankson note that elite suppressors are significantly more effective at eliminating these cells than are chronic progressors. The researchers posit that a vaccine that helps generate killer T cells comparable to those in active elite suppressors might help others to more effectively combat infection.

Morning-After Treatment

Some physicians prescribe drugs that are used to treat established infections as "morning-after" pills in an attempt to prevent the transmission of HIV after risky sexual encounters. As of 2013, there was no scientific consensus on the validity of this approach, and no medications were approved for this use. Because some forms of HIV are halted by prompt use of the drugs, some doctors believe it is a worthwhile approach. Taryn Young

et al. describe the results of a review of the medical literature on PEP in "Antiretroviral Post-exposure Prophylaxis (PEP) for Occupational HIV Exposure" (*Cochrane Database of Systematic Reviews*, vol. 1, January 24, 2007) and conclude that "there is no direct evidence to support the use of multi-drug antiretroviral regimens following occupational exposure to HIV. However, due to the success of combination therapies in treating HIV-infected individuals, a combination of antiretroviral drugs should be used for PEP."

This "off-label" use of potent PIs in an attempt to prevent the spread of HIV is controversial. All the drugs that are used in the treatment of HIV have side effects, some of which may be potentially life threatening. PIs may cause high blood sugar and diabetes, lipodytrophy (problems with fat metabolism that can result in dangerously high cholesterol levels), and liver problems. Furthermore, some researchers fear that if people believe morning-after treatment will prevent HIV infection, they may stop taking precautions, such as using condoms, to prevent exposure to HIV. Others feel that the treatment is not appropriate as a preventive measure for people who are exposed to ongoing risk, such as relationships where only one partner is infected, because the drugs are too toxic. Other methods, such as the continued use of condoms, are much safer.

Finally, postexposure treatment is expensive. The costs of two or three drugs taken for a month, plus laboratory tests and visits to the doctor, may cost more than $1,000. Of course, this is a fraction of the cost for lifetime treatment of HIV infection and certainly money well spent if it prevents a person from acquiring the virus.

In "Antiretroviral Therapy for Prevention of HIV Transmission in HIV-Discordant Couples" (*Cochrane Database of Systemic Review*, vol. 5, May 11, 2011), a meta-analysis of seven studies, Andrew Anglemyer et al. find that antiretroviral drugs may prevent the transmission of HIV from an infected person to an uninfected sexual partner by suppressing viral replication. In couples in which the infected partner was taking antiretroviral drugs, the uninfected partner had more than five times the lower risk of becoming infected than in couples where the infected partner was not receiving antiretroviral treatment.

Topical Drugs to Block HIV Infection

In recent years there have been many efforts to develop topical microbicides—preparations to prevent HIV infection. Anita B. Garg, Jeremy Nuttall, and Joseph Romano report in "The Future of HIV Microbicides: Challenges and Opportunities" (*Antiviral Chemistry and Chemotherapy*, vol. 19, no. 4, 2009) that ongoing clinical trials of "vaginal gels containing non-specific compounds" had met with some success. One of the potential drawbacks of these gels is that they must be applied close to the time of sexual intercourse to be optimally effective.

In 2013 researchers in India reported that extracts of banaba (Lagerstroemia speciosa L.) demonstrate anti-HIV activity. In "Ellagic Acid and Gallic Acid from Lagerstroemia speciosa L. Inhibit HIV-1 Infection through Inhibition of HIV-1 Protease and Reverse Transcriptase Activity" (*Indian Journal of Medical Research*, vol. 137, no. 3, March 2013), Satish Kumar Gupta et al. assert that gallic acid and ellagic acid, the active components responsible for anti-HIV activity, could be promising candidates for the development of topical anti-HIV agents.

THE PROMISE OF GENE THERAPY

In 2011 researchers reported progress using genetic engineering techniques to create HIV-resistant blood cells. This effort was inspired by the apparent cure of Timothy Rae Brown after he received a transplant of blood stem cells in 2007 to treat the leukemia (cancer of the blood cells) he had in addition to his AIDS diagnosis. Brown's physician, Gero Huetter, knew that the best chance of curing the leukemia was with a blood stem cell transplant, so he searched for a donor who was not only a tissue match for Brown but was also among the 1% of people with gene mutations that confer resistance to HIV. In preparation for the transplant, Brown was given chemotherapy and radiation treatment to destroy his immune system so that he would not reject the donor blood stem cells. Remarkably, four years after the procedure Brown was still disease free—there was no evidence of HIV in his body and he no longer required antiretroviral drug treatment. Although this treatment is not feasible for everyone with HIV/AIDS—because it is physically grueling, involves considerable risk, and is prohibitively expensive—it offers tantalizing clues about new approaches for HIV/AIDS treatment.

In 2013 two HIV-infected men who were taking ART prior to bone marrow transplants to treat cancer appeared to be cured of HIV as well. The mechanism of the apparent cure is different from the cure affected in Brown because neither of the two patients received bone marrow from donors with mutations that confer immunity to HIV infection. As of July 2013, researchers were cautiously optimistic that the cure would be a lasting one and that it would inform new avenues of treatment.

IN SEARCH OF A VACCINE

Some pharmaceutical companies claim that the high costs of R&D and the relatively low return on their investments (because the period of patent protection is limited to seven years) leave little financial incentive to develop new HIV/AIDS drugs. The development of such drugs is, for better or worse, an economically driven, rather than strictly humanitarian, enterprise. Similarly,

FIGURE 6.1

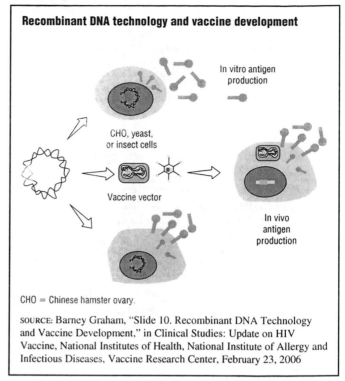

Recombinant DNA technology and vaccine development

In vitro antigen production

CHO, yeast, or insect cells

Vaccine vector

In vivo antigen production

CHO = Chinese hamster ovary.

SOURCE: Barney Graham, "Slide 10. Recombinant DNA Technology and Vaccine Development," in Clinical Studies: Update on HIV Vaccine, National Institutes of Health, National Institute of Allergy and Infectious Diseases, Vaccine Research Center, February 23, 2006

the companies allege that they have little economic motivation to research and develop HIV vaccines. In February 1996 Anthony S. Fauci (1940–), the head of the National Institute of Allergy and Infectious Diseases (NIAID), issued guidelines to promote cooperation between the government and private industry. The plan's goal was to overcome the alleged unfavorable market forces that have caused some companies to abandon research of potential HIV vaccines.

There are several vaccines under trial. Some vaccines use a weakened and medically safe version of viruses as a delivery vehicle to carry various HIV genes into the human participants. The hope is that antibody production of the HIV-critical proteins encoded by these genes will occur and that this production will offer protection from HIV infection. Other vaccines use a DNA plasmid to ferry HIV genes into the human participants; the aim again is to stimulate antibody production.

Unsurprisingly, there are experimental design challenges and ethical considerations involved in vaccine trials using human volunteers. Vaccines may be made using recombinant DNA technology—DNA that has been altered by joining genetic material from two different sources. Figure 6.1 shows how recombinant DNA is used to develop vaccines. Although some recombinant technology uses live attenuated viruses (viruses that are genetically altered so they are less virulent), this is not feasible with HIV because it would be unwise to create any risk of infection. The challenges are to elicit cell-mediated immune responses against HIV and the need for a balanced immune response consisting of not only cellular immunity but also a broad and strong antibody response that can prevent infection with HIV. Concerning ethical considerations, most volunteers for a vaccine have behaviors that put them at risk for contracting HIV. Some may mistakenly believe that participating in the clinical trial of an experimental vaccine—which may be a vaccine or a placebo (which contains no active drug)—protects them and, with a false sense of security, they may resume high-risk behaviors.

Despite optimistic projections during the early 1990s that a vaccine would be found in a few years, a considerable number of promising experimental HIV vaccines have proven ineffective against strains of HIV taken from infected people. Researchers reported developing antibodies that worked successfully against HIV grown in test tubes, but in every case they failed when used against HIV in human beings. The progress and setbacks in vaccine development as well as the results of recent clinical trials of vaccines are described in Chapter 1. As of October 2013, none of the candidate vaccines had shown sufficient promise in clinical trials to warrant approval, manufacture, and widespread use.

History of Human Vaccine Trials

In "F.D.A. Authorizes First Full Testing for H.I.V. Vaccine" (NYTimes.com, June 4, 1998), Lawrence K. Altman reports that in 1998 the FDA granted permission to VaxGen to conduct the first full-scale test of a vaccine to prevent HIV infection. The VaxGen vaccine—a genetically engineered molecule called AIDSvax—had been found "safe in tests involving 1,200 uninfected volunteers beginning in March 1992 and induced production of antibodies in more than 99 percent of the vaccinated participants." The 1998 test involved 5,000 volunteers in 40 clinics throughout the United States and Canada and 2,500 volunteers in 16 clinics in Thailand.

AIDSvax was made from part of HIV's outer coat, specifically a molecule called gp120, which functions in the attachment of the virus to host cells. The vaccine did not contain the intact virus, only the gp120 protein from two strains of HIV. The two strains of the vaccine that were tested in North America were made with strains common in North America. The vaccine used in Thailand contained strains common to that part of the world. Participants in the North American study were men who have sex with men and uninfected partners of HIV-positive people. In Thailand, volunteers were uninfected injection drug users. Two-thirds of the North American volunteers were given the vaccine, and the rest received a placebo. In Thailand, half the group received the vaccine and half were given a placebo. The four-year trial ended in 2002.

The trial results were reported in February 2003. David R. Baker explains in "Vaccine Has No Impact, AIDSVAX's Failure a Blow to Treatment" (SFGate.com,

November 13, 2003) that AIDSvax was determined to be a failure, as the comparison of those who received the vaccine versus those who received a placebo demonstrated a slight reduction in new HIV infections in the vaccine population. Surprisingly, Asian Americans and African Americans who received the vaccine displayed a lower rate of infection than their racial counterparts who received the placebo. Considerable debate has arisen concerning these latter observations. Was this a statistical fluke? Or did AIDSvax display demographically specific protection, and if so, why?

One potential problem with AIDSvax, and perhaps a partial explanation of the poor overall results, is that previous tests indicated that it boosted only one part of the immune system—the component of the immune system that is responsible for antibody production. It is generally believed that a truly effective anti-HIV vaccine must boost another part of the immune system: the killer T cells that destroy virus-infected cells. Some experts consider the vaccine a long shot, but others point out that a failed vaccine does not mean that the experiment failed. Negative results can teach researchers what not to do in the future.

In 2011 another vaccine trial reported disappointing results. According to Glenda E. Gray et al., in "Safety and Efficacy of the HVTN 503/Phambili Study of a Clade-B-Based HIV-1 Vaccine in South Africa: A Double-Blind, Randomised, Placebo-Controlled Test-of-Concept Phase 2b Study" (*Lancet Infectious Diseases*, vol. 11, no. 7, July 2011), researchers conducted a clinical trial in South Africa with a vaccine that was designed to elicit T cell–mediated immune responses capable of providing complete or partial protection from HIV-1 infection or a decrease in viral load after acquisition. When the researchers compiled the results following the completion of the trial, they determined that the vaccine failed to accomplish either of these objectives. Gray et al. opine that there are lessons to be learned from such trials, noting that "this is now the third study in human beings that has failed after initial successful data from studies in non-human primates, highlighting once again that human HIV-1 vaccines should not be based simply on non-human primate models. We should still strive for innovative strategies that prevent HIV, despite the success of antiretroviral drugs in those for whom they are available. It would not be surprising if further prophylactic studies yielded new mechanistic and therapeutic insights outside the remit of the initial endpoints, ultimately enabling the eradication of HIV."

As detailed in Chapter 1, two vaccine trials were halted in 2013 when it was found that HIV infections occurred as often among the vaccine recipients as they did in subjects who received the placebo vaccine and that the vaccine failed to reduce viral load among volunteers who acquired HIV infection.

Vaccine Research Center

In 2000 the Dale and Betty Bumpers Vaccine Research Center (VRC) opened on the NIH campus in Bethesda, Maryland. The facility brings together private companies and federal agencies to research, develop, and produce vaccines. The VRC is not exclusively devoted to HIV research and works to develop vaccines for other diseases.

Johannes F. Scheid et al. report in "Broad Diversity of Neutralizing Antibodies Isolated from Memory B Cells in HIV-Infected Individuals" (*Nature*, vol. 458, no. 7238, April 2, 2009) that they made progress in the development of an AIDS vaccine. The researchers looked at HIV patients who progress very slowly to AIDS because they have a range of neutralizing antibodies that identify and attack the virus. The researchers isolated 433 neutralizing antibodies from the blood of these slow-to-progress HIV patients and uncovered how the antibodies disarm the virus.

In 2011 a study that was directed by NIAID researchers uncovered another genetic mechanism of protection that may be helpful in the design of an HIV vaccine for humans. The researchers administered to monkeys a vaccine made from DNA that encodes immunodeficiency virus proteins, followed by a booster vaccine containing an inactivated cold virus (adenovirus) and immunodeficiency virus proteins to help protect monkeys from simian immunodeficiency virus (the monkey analog of HIV). Norman L. Letvin et al. find in "Immune and Genetic Correlates of Vaccine Protection against Mucosal Infection by SIV in Monkeys" (*Science Translational Medicine*, vol. 3, no. 81, May 4, 2011) that neutralizing antibodies are a key component of the immune response needed to prevent HIV infection. This finding may help future vaccine development efforts.

Most researchers are optimistic that an effective vaccine will be developed, but many believe that perfecting a vaccine will take years. VRC researchers believe that more than one vaccine formulation, or a vaccine that works two ways—by boosting immunity provided by T cells and producing antibodies to attach to HIV and mark it for destruction—may be necessary to provide complete protection.

In "Co-evolution of a Broadly Neutralizing HIV-1 Antibody and Founder Virus" (*Nature*, vol. 496, no. 7446, April 25, 2013), Hua-Xin Liao et al. report increased understanding of how HIV and a strong antibody response develop in an HIV-infected person who naturally develops antibodies to the virus after several years of infection. This understanding is helping researchers create a vaccine that mimics the virus and results in the body generating neutralizing HIV antibodies.

Arik Cooper et al. note in "HIV-1 Causes CD4 Cell Death through DNA-Dependent Protein Kinase during Viral Integration" (*Nature*, vol. 498, no. 7454, June 20, 2013) the discovery of how HIV triggers a signal that tells infected immune cells—the very cells that mobilize to fight the infection—to die. These findings suggest that treating HIV-infected individuals with drugs that block the first steps of viral replication can not only prevent viral replication but may also improve CD4+ T cell survival and immune function. This discovery may also help researchers figure out how to eliminate reservoirs of the resting virus.

Renewed Optimism

Reports of the stem-cell therapy cure of Timothy Rae Brown and the two patients with no detectable virus after receiving bone marrow transplants lead many to believe that a cure is close at hand. According to the article "Cure for Aids 'Possible' Says Nobel Prize–Winning Scientist Who Helped Discover HIV" (Telegraph.co.uk, March 5, 2013), Françoise Barré-Sinoussi (1947–), who along with Luc Montagnier (1932–) and Harald zur Hausen (1936–) was awarded the 2008 Nobel Prize in Physiology or Medicine for pinpointing the cause of AIDS, expresses optimism about the possibility of a cure. Barre-Sinoussi suggests, "We are now in a position that we have evidence suggesting a cure might be possible. We have to stimulate funding for research into cures. It's ongoing, and it will take time, but more and more data [are] indicating that we have to move forward and work on a cure."

Similarly, the article "HIV 'Cure' Looks 'Promising,' Danish Scientists Contend" (USNews.com, April 29, 2013) indicates that Danish scientists conducting a trial of a new HIV treatment in 15 patients are confident their strategy will result in a cure. Ole Sogaard describes a technique that "involves freeing the HIV virus from DNA cells, where it collects in 'reservoirs,' and bringing it to the surface of the cells" where "it can be permanently destroyed." Sogaard asserts, "I am almost certain that we will be successful in releasing the reservoirs of HIV."

CHAPTER 7
PEOPLE WITH HIV/AIDS

Large numbers of people are afflicted with HIV/AIDS in the United States. An increasing proportion of the population lives with HIV infection. In the second decade of the 21st century more Americans than ever before are likely to know someone who is affected by HIV or AIDS. Even people who live in remote geographic areas and do not believe they are personally at risk of acquiring HIV are aware of the epidemic from ongoing public health education campaigns, reports in the media, school health programs, and health and social service agencies, all of which are dedicated to improving community awareness of HIV/AIDS.

PUBLIC FIGURES WITH HIV/AIDS

Perhaps one of the most famous HIV-infected people in the world is Magic Johnson (1959–), an internationally known former basketball player for the Los Angeles Lakers. When Johnson announced his HIV infection in November 1991, the world was shocked. He had no idea he was infected until he received the results of a routine physical examination for life insurance. He freely admitted that before his marriage he had unprotected sexual contact with many women.

Following this announcement, Johnson became an HIV/AIDS spokesperson and began working in prevention programs. In 1991 he started the Magic Johnson Foundation, which seeks to fund and establish community-based education and social and health programs (including HIV/AIDS awareness) in inner-city communities, and briefly served on the President's Commission on AIDS. Although he officially retired from professional basketball in 1996, he continues to play on the Magic Johnson All-Stars Team and is an active spokesperson for HIV/AIDS.

In 1992 the former tennis star Arthur Ashe (1943–1993) announced that he had become infected with HIV from a blood transfusion in the mid-1980s during a heart bypass

operation. His was not a voluntary announcement, but one made necessary when the news media discovered his HIV infection and threatened to announce it before he did. Ashe was reluctant to make his condition public, fearing the effect on his five-year-old daughter. He maintained that because he did not have a public responsibility, he should have been allowed to maintain his privacy. He died of pneumonia, a complication of AIDS, in 1993.

The diver Greg Louganis (1960–), who competed in the 1976, 1984, and 1988 Olympic games, was diagnosed with HIV infection in 1988, before his competition in the 1988 games. During the games, Louganis hit his head on the diving board while competing. Although his injury was not serious, it did result in an open wound—making Louganis concerned that his blood might have entered the pool. However, Louganis did not reveal his HIV status at the time. The Olympic gold medalist announced that he had HIV in 1995. Louganis now competes in dog agility competitions with his dogs, is a published author of two books, and coaches athletes in diving. He advocates safe sexual practices, because he attributes his HIV infection to unsafe sexual behavior.

Other sports figures diagnosed with HIV infection include Rudy Galindo (1969–), an American figure skater who earned a bronze medal at the 1996 world championships, and Roy Simmons (1956–), an American athlete who played for the National Football League.

Another sports celebrity who succumbed to AIDS was the National Association for Stock Car Auto Racing (NASCAR) racecar driver Tim Richmond (1955–1989). During his heyday on the NASCAR race circuit in the 1980s, Richmond was one of the circuit's premier drivers. He was also well known for his expensive tastes and playboy lifestyle. Whether his lifestyle contributed to his illness is conjecture. Nonetheless, by the end of the 1986 racing season Richmond had become noticeably ill. He was diagnosed with AIDS that same year. He was able to race again in 1987, but soon thereafter his health deteriorated precipitously. During another attempted comeback in 1988, when his illness was still unpublicized, Richmond faced the hostility and innuendo of his fellow drivers, who, guessing the nature of the illness, speculated about his sexual orientation and the possibility of drug abuse. In response, Richmond filed a defamation of character lawsuit against NASCAR. He subsequently withdrew the lawsuit to avoid making his condition public. Richmond ultimately retired from competitive racing and lived in seclusion with his mother until his death. After his death, as news of his illness and the treatment he received from his fellow drivers and NASCAR became public, many people were outraged at the NASCAR organization, which as of October 2013 had not apologized.

Mary Fisher (1948–), a heterosexual and nondrug user who contracted HIV from her husband, stood before her peers during the 1992 Republican National Convention and announced that she was infected with HIV. A former television producer and assistant to President Gerald R. Ford (1913–2006), she said she considered her announcement part of her contribution to the fight against HIV/AIDS. The wealthy and well-educated Fisher was among the first women to publicly dispel the image that still comes to mind when many people think of HIV/AIDS: homosexual, poor, drug addicted, and lacking access to support systems or adequate medical care and housing.

Fisher established the Mary Fisher Clinical AIDS Research and Education Fund at the University of Alabama, Birmingham, in 2000. She is an accomplished artist, public speaker, and author of four books. In 2006 Peter Piot (1949–), the under secretary-general of the United Nations, appointed Fisher to a two-year term as a special representative of the Joint United Nations Programme on HIV/AIDS, which Piot directed.

The actor Anthony Perkins (1932–1992), who is best known for his role as Norman Bates in the classic Alfred Hitchcock (1899–1980) film *Psycho* (1960), also died of AIDS. Forever typecast by that performance, Perkins was in fact an accomplished film and stage actor. He was bisexual and had relationships with a number of men. Shortly before his death in 1992, Perkins commented in a press release about a *National Enquirer* article that revealed his AIDS-positive status by saying, "I have learned more about love, selflessness, and human understanding from the people I have met in this great adventure in the world of AIDS than I ever did in the cutthroat, competitive world in which I spent my life." Perkins's widow, Berry Berenson (1948–2001), was one of the passengers on American Airlines Flight 11, which was hijacked and crashed into the World Trade Center on September 11, 2001.

Another movie star who succumbed to AIDS was Rock Hudson (1925–1985). Indeed, Hudson was the first major U.S. celebrity known to have died from AIDS. His death was especially noteworthy, given his status during the 1950s as the quintessential rugged, all-American male. Despite his many movie roles as a leading man opposite many beautiful actresses, Hudson was homosexual, a fact that was covered up by movie studios. His 1955 marriage to the studio employee Phyllis Gates (1925–2006), which ended in divorce in 1958, is thought to have been a studio-orchestrated attempt to cover up his sexual orientation. Hudson died at the age of 59.

The African American rap star Eazy-E (c. 1963–1995) rose to fame as one of the members of the group N.W.A. (Niggaz with Attitude), based in Compton, California. Using money obtained from illegal drug sales, Eazy-E founded Ruthless Records. Soon after, he recruited Ice Cube (1969–), Dr. Dre (1965?–), MC Ren (1969–), DJ Yella (1967–), and Arabian Prince (1965–) to form N.W.A. Following the dissolution of N.W.A., Eazy-E went on to have a successful solo career. In 1995 he entered the hospital for treatment of what he thought was asthma. However, he was diagnosed with AIDS and died soon after. Eazy-E is now regarded as one of the influential founders of the style of music known as gangsta rap. Every year, the city of Compton celebrates his life by observing Eazy-E Day.

Another music icon who died of AIDS was Freddie Mercury (1946–1991), the lead vocalist of the British rock band Queen. His more than three-octave vocal range and operatic compositional approach to rock resulted in classic hits such as "Bohemian Rhapsody," "Somebody to Love," and "We Are the Champions." The video made for the 1975 release of "Bohemian Rhapsody" is considered by some music insiders to be one of the decisive influences that spurred the popularity of music videos. Mercury was well known for his extravagance and bisexuality. His diagnosis and deteriorating physical condition were kept private. Indeed, his eventual announcement that he had AIDS was made only one day before his death in 1991.

Rudolf Nureyev (1938–1993) was a Soviet-born dancer of ballet and modern dance who defected to the West in 1961. As one of the most celebrated dancers of the 20th century, Nureyev tested positive for HIV in 1984 and died of AIDS at the age of 54. The British actor and Oscar-winning director Tony Richardson (1928–1991), the former husband of Vanessa Redgrave (1937–), died of AIDS at the age of 63.

Elizabeth Glaser (1947–1994), the wife of the actor Paul Michael Glaser (1943–), was motivated to cofound the Pediatric AIDS Foundation in 1988 (now called the Elizabeth Glaser Pediatric AIDS Foundation), following the discovery that she and her children, Ariel (1981–1988) and Jake (1984–), were all infected with HIV. She originally contracted the virus from contaminated blood that was administered during pregnancy, but she was unaware of her illness until much later, already having passed it to her children. In the ensuing years she became a vocal AIDS activist. The foundation that is her legacy contributes more than $1 million annually to pediatric AIDS research. Ariel died at the age of seven, and Elizabeth died in 1994. Because Jake has a mutation of the CCR5 gene that delays onset by restricting the virus's ability to enter white blood cells, he remains symptom free and no longer takes HIV medication. He and Paul continue to raise money and AIDS awareness through Elizabeth's foundation.

Although he did not confirm his HIV status when he was alive, an autopsy performed on the flamboyant entertainer Liberace (1919–1987) confirmed that he was HIV infected. The award-winning playwright and lyricist Howard Ashman (1950–1991) also died of AIDS. Ashman wrote the lyrics for several Disney films, including *The Little Mermaid*, *Alladin*, and *Beauty and the Beast*, which was dedicated to him.

The artist and photographer Robert Mapplethorpe (1946–1989) was 42 when he died of AIDS complications. The artist Keith Haring (1958–1990), who was known for his striking murals and political themes, also died of AIDS-related complications.

Finally, in a list of examples that is by no means complete, the prolific and influential science-fiction author Isaac Asimov (1920–1992) contracted HIV from infected blood that was given to him in a transfusion during heart bypass surgery in 1983. He died in 1992 of heart and renal failure that were complications of AIDS.

OLDER PEOPLE WITH HIV/AIDS

In "AIDS among Persons Aged Greater Than or Equal to 50 Years—United States, 1991–1996" (*Morbidity and Mortality Weekly Report*, vol. 47, no. 2, January 23, 1998), the Centers for Disease Control and Prevention (CDC) reports that most older people infected with HIV early in the epidemic were typically infected through contaminated blood or blood products. Through 1989 only 1% of HIV/AIDS cases of people aged 13 to 49 years was due to contaminated blood. However, during this same period 6% of cases of people aged 50 to 59 years, 28% of cases of people aged 60 to 69 years, and 64% of cases of people aged 70 years and older resulted from contaminated blood or blood products.

Improved safety of the nation's blood supply, including routine screening of blood donations for HIV, sharply reduced the risk of contracting the virus from contaminated blood or blood products. Subsequently, the proportion of people aged 50 years and older who acquired HIV from other types of exposure increased. Although male-to-male

sexual contact and injection drug use remain the primary means by which HIV is transmitted among all age groups in the United States, heterosexual transmission of HIV is steadily increasing in people aged 50 years and older.

HIV/AIDS Cases among Older People

The CDC notes in *Diagnoses of HIV Infection among Adults Aged 50 Years and Older in the United States and Dependent Areas, 2007–2010* (February 2013, http://www.cdc.gov/hiv/pdf/statistics_2010_HIV_Surveillance_Report_vol_18_no_3.pdf) that in 2010 the largest percentage of HIV diagnoses (47%) were for adults aged 50 to 54 years, who had a prevalence rate of 17.8 per 100,000 population. The proportion of adults over the age of 50 years with HIV/AIDS is expected to increase as HIV-infected people of all ages live longer as a result of effective drug therapy and other advances in medical treatment.

Through 2011 an estimated 295,339 cases of AIDS in people over the age of 45 years had been reported. (See Table 3.1 in Chapter 3.) Of these reported cases, 133,612 (45% of the cumulative total) were among people aged 45 to 49 years, 77,843 (26%) were among people aged 50 to 54 years, 42,372 (14%) were among people aged 55 to 59 years, 22,369 (8%) were among people aged 60 to 64 years, and 19,143 (6%) were among people aged 65 years and older.

HIV Testing for Those over the Age of 50 Years

Many older adults do not seek routine screening for HIV infection because they do not believe they are at risk of acquiring HIV. Figure 7.1 shows that in 2012 the lowest rates of testing among adults over the age of 18 years were among people aged 65 years and older—just 12.7% of older adults had ever been tested for HIV, compared with 49.5% of those aged 25 to 34 years, 49% of those aged 35 to 44 years, and 34% of those aged 45 to 64 years. Among women over the age of 50 years, the absence of the risk of pregnancy may lead to a false sense of security and the mistaken belief that they are at less risk for sexually transmitted infections, including HIV. The failure to test or the late testing of older patients may be because:

- Physicians are less apt to look for HIV in people of this age group

- Some AIDS-related illnesses that occur in older people, such as encephalopathy (any of various diseases of the brain) and wasting disease, have similar symptoms to other diseases that are associated with aging, such as Alzheimer's disease (a progressive form of dementia that is characterized by impairment of memory and intellectual functions), depression, and malignancies

It is vitally important to overcome older adults' reluctance to seek testing and other delays to diagnosis

FIGURE 7.1

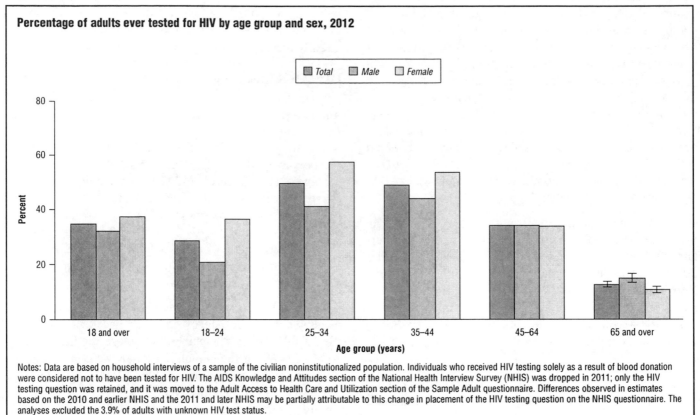

Percentage of adults ever tested for HIV by age group and sex, 2012

Notes: Data are based on household interviews of a sample of the civilian noninstitutionalized population. Individuals who received HIV testing solely as a result of blood donation were considered not to have been tested for HIV. The AIDS Knowledge and Attitudes section of the National Health Interview Survey (NHIS) was dropped in 2011; only the HIV testing question was retained, and it was moved to the Adult Access to Health Care and Utilization section of the Sample Adult questionnaire. Differences observed in estimates based on the 2010 and earlier NHIS and the 2011 and later NHIS may be partially attributable to this change in placement of the HIV testing question on the NHIS questionnaire. The analyses excluded the 3.9% of adults with unknown HIV test status.

SOURCE: "Figure 10.2. Percentage of Adults Aged 18 Years and over Who Had Ever Been Tested for Human Immunodeficiency Virus (HIV), by Age Group and Sex: United States, 2012," in *Early Release of Selected Estimates Based on Data from the 2012 National Health Interview Survey*, Centers for Disease Control and Prevention, June 2013, http://www.cdc.gov/nchs/data/nhis/earlyrelease/earlyrelease201306_10.pdf (accessed July 29, 2013)

because research shows that age speeds the progression of HIV to AIDS and blunts CD4 response to highly active antiretroviral therapy. Equally important is continuing the research to improve the treatment of HIV-infected older adults and the development of effective education programs to prevent infection in this population.

LIVING WITH HIV/AIDS

To gain a more complete view of the impact of HIV/AIDS, it is important to understand the psychosocial and emotional consequences of diagnosis with a potentially fatal disease.

A Worrisome Diagnosis

By the dawn of the 21st century, a diagnosis of HIV infection was no longer a certain death sentence, but it was still likely to elicit feelings of fear, confusion, depression, and anger. Researchers have identified another reason that people who are diagnosed with HIV infection require additional emotional support: there is an association between psychosocial stress and HIV disease progression. Yoichi Chida and Kavita Vedhara report in "Adverse Psychosocial Factors Predict Poorer Prognosis in HIV Disease: A Meta-analytic Review of Prospective

Investigations" (*Brain, Behavior, and Immunity*, vol. 23, no. 4, May 2009) the results of a review of 36 articles describing the association between psychosocial factors such as personality types, coping styles, psychological distress, and HIV disease progression. The researchers find a strong relationship between adverse psychosocial factors such as difficulty coping with stress and HIV disease progression.

The 2011 release of *Aging with HIV: A Gay Man's Guide* by James Masten and James Schmidtberger offers guidance to the growing numbers of men who are living with HIV/AIDS. Masten and Schmidtberger address many of the issues that are related to aging with HIV/AIDS. They outline strategies for maintaining physical and emotional health and well-being and approaches to help men break unhealthy habits. They also offer examples of coping strategies that have worked for men, many of whom are surprised to have lived to midlife and old age and never dreamed they would have to plan for a future.

Coping with Discrimination

Unlike people who are diagnosed with other terminal or catastrophic illnesses such as cancer or multiple sclerosis, people with HIV/AIDS often confront the social isolation and discrimination that accompany a stigmatized status. Many people continue to mistakenly characterize HIV/AIDS as exclusively a disease of homosexual men and drug users and condemn HIV-infected people for inflicting themselves with the condition. Some still believe that AIDS is divine retribution for an "immoral lifestyle." The fear of unfavorable judgment keeps many infected individuals from disclosing their HIV infection to others, even friends and family. Others simply do not want the pity that is often extended to people with potentially fatal conditions. Still others worry that friends and family, fearing infection, will abandon them.

Under the Americans with Disabilities Act (ADA) of 1990, people infected with HIV and those diagnosed with AIDS are considered disabled and as such are subject to the antidiscrimination provisions of this landmark legislation. As a result, employers may not ask job applicants if they are HIV infected or have AIDS, nor can they require an HIV test of prospective employees. The only exceptions to this provision are those employers who can demonstrate that such questions or testing are job-related and absolutely necessary for the employer to conduct business.

More important, the ADA requires employers to make "reasonable accommodations" for disabled employees. Reasonable accommodation is an adjustment to a job or modification of the responsibilities or work environment that will enable the worker with a disability to gain equal employment opportunity. Examples include flexible work schedules to allow for medical appointments, treatments, and counseling and the provision of additional unpaid leave.

PRESIDENT PROCLAIMS JUNE 2013 AS LESBIAN, GAY, BISEXUAL, AND TRANSGENDER PRIDE MONTH. On May 31, 2013, President Barack Obama (1961–; http://www .whitehouse.gov/the-press-office/2013/06/03/presidential-proclamation-lgbt-pride-month) issued a proclamation naming June 2013 as Lesbian, Gay, Bisexual, and Transgender (LGBT) Pride Month. President Obama stated that his administration lifted the HIV entry ban, eliminating the 20-year-old U.S. travel ban against people with HIV and developed the National HIV/AIDS Strategy, which "addresses the disparate impact of the HIV epidemic among certain LGBT sub-communities. We have a long way to go, but if we continue on this path together, I am confident that one day soon, from coast to coast, all of our young people will look to the future with the same sense of promise and possibility."

THE STIGMA OF AIDS. In "A Comparison of HIV Stigma and Discrimination in Five International Sites: The Influence of Care and Treatment Resources in High Prevalence Settings" (*Social Science and Medicine*, vol. 68, no. 12, June 2009), a study designed to examine HIV stigma and discrimination in five high prevalence settings, Suzanne Maman et al. observe that the factors that contribute to HIV stigma and discrimination include the fear

of transmission, the fear of suffering and death, and the burden of caring for people with AIDS.

According to Maman et al., the family, access to antiretroviral drugs, and other resources offered some protection against HIV stigma and discrimination. Variation in the availability of health and social services designed to lessen the impact of HIV/AIDS helps explain differences in HIV stigma and discrimination across the settings. The researchers opine that "increasing access to treatment and care resources may function to lower HIV stigma, however, providing services is not enough." They also assert that it is necessary to develop "effective strategies to reduce HIV stigma as treatment and care resources are scaled up in the settings that are most heavily impacted by the HIV epidemic."

Three decades after the first diagnosis of AIDS and widespread public health and community education efforts to inform people about HIV infection and prevent the spread of HIV, ignorance and misunderstanding of HIV/AIDS persist. Health educators and HIV/AIDS activists stress the importance of intensified, ongoing education to destigmatize people who are affected by HIV/ AIDS and prevent discrimination. Reducing the stigma that is associated with HIV/AIDS may also encourage individuals to get tested and, for those who are infected, begin treatment as soon as possible.

Because stigma, even among personnel who work with people with HIV/AIDS, persists, efforts to reduce it continue. The HIV/AIDS Stigma Program, which is funded by the Health Resources and Services Administration's HIV/AIDS Bureau, offers training programs that explore the stigma associated with HIV/AIDS. The programs, which are made available to staff employed by agencies and organizations funded by the Ryan White Comprehensive AIDS Resources Emergency Act of 1990, focus on:

- Defining stigma and its origins in society

- The impact of stigma on an individual's decision-making process and how it deters him or her from seeking HIV testing and counseling services

- How stigma affects access to care and disclosure of HIV-positive status

Dealing with Emotions

Not unexpectedly, anger and depression are natural and common reactions to discovering that one is infected with HIV. Experts stress the importance of recognizing and expressing anger and depression; however, if these feelings become all consuming, they can prevent health- and life-improving actions. Many people with HIV/AIDS admit that sharing feelings with friends and family members and participating in support groups ease anguish and help generate more positive attitudes and actions.

Many HIV/AIDS sufferers report that the most difficult thing they had to do after being diagnosed with HIV was to inform people in their present or recent past whom they might have exposed to the virus. If the patient is unable to do this, a physician or public health official can notify present or former sexual partners without revealing the infected person's name.

Early Medication Improves Outlook and Protects against Spread of HIV

The earlier people learn of their infection, the earlier they can begin medical treatment to suppress the virus's destructive growth, delay the onset of AIDS symptoms, and extend life. Along with antiretroviral drugs there are medications that fight the life-threatening opportunistic infections that eventually may afflict people who are HIV infected. Although these drugs do not eliminate HIV infection, they have been shown to keep HIV/AIDS patients healthy and symptom free for increasingly longer periods.

In 2011 the results of an international study definitively concluded that prompt treatment of HIV infection, before a person develops symptoms, dramatically reduces the risk that the person with HIV will transmit the virus to a sexual partner. According to the article "Early HIV Therapy Protects against Virus Spread" (Associated Press, May 12, 2011), the study followed 1,763 couples in which one partner was HIV infected and the other was not. The study participants were from Botswana, Brazil, India, Kenya, Malawi, South Africa, Thailand, the United States, and Zimbabwe. Half of the couples received early treatment of the infected partner and the other half waited until the infected partner's CD4 cell count fell below 250 per cubic millimeter of blood or until symptoms appeared. Among the untreated couples, 28 previously uninfected partners were infected. Among the treated couples, just one previously uninfected person became infected. Anthony S. Fauci (1940–), the head of the National Institute of Allergy and Infectious Diseases, said the study's finding "promises to change practice worldwide."

Practicing Good Health Habits

Experts advise HIV-infected people to exercise and maintain a balanced diet with sufficient lean protein. Not only does exercise improve overall fitness and generate a sense of well-being but also it releases endorphins, which are natural substances produced by the brain that boost immunity, reduce stress, and elevate mood. People with HIV/AIDS are advised to avoid smoking, excessive alcohol consumption, and using illegal drugs, all of which can act to depress the immune system.

HOUSING PROBLEMS

The difficulty of finding affordable and appropriate housing can be an acute crisis for people living with HIV/AIDS. HIV-infected people need more than just a safe shelter that provides protection and comfort; they may also require a base from which to receive services, care, and support. Adherence to complicated medical regimens is challenging for many HIV-infected people, but for some homeless people it is nearly impossible.

Some individuals are homeless when they acquire the HIV infection, whereas others lose their home when they are no longer able to hold jobs or cannot afford to pay for health care and housing costs. The National AIDS Housing Coalition (NAHC) indicates in the fact sheet "Breaking the Link between Homelessness and HIV" (February 2011, http://www.nationalaidshousing.org/PDF/Factsheets-Homelessness.pdf) that:

- Housing status is a key factor affecting access to care and health behaviors among people with HIV/AIDS—housing assistance reduces HIV health risk behaviors, improves health outcomes, and reduces use of costly emergency and inpatient hospital services

- Housing remains one of the greatest unmet needs of Americans with HIV/AIDS—at least half of all people with HIV/AIDS experience housing instability or homelessness

- Although about 500,000 households affected by HIV/AIDS will require some form of housing assistance during the course of their illness, the federal program Housing Opportunities for Persons with AIDS (HOPWA) serves less than 60,000 households per year

In the fact sheet "Housing Is HIV Prevention & Care" (2013, http://nationalaidshousing.org/PDF/Fact Sheet.pdf), the NAHC describes the relationship between HIV risk and housing instability and homelessness. More than 145,000 households living with HIV/AIDS have unmet housing needs and less than 60,000 are currently served by the HOPWA. The NAHC asserts, "Improved housing status also prevents new HIV infections by reducing HIV risk behaviors by as much as half and by facilitating effective [antiretroviral therapy] that lowers viral load to an undetectable level, virtually eliminating ongoing HIV transmission."

According to the NAHC, in the fact sheet "Housing Is Cost-Effective HIV Prevention and Care" (February 2011, http://nationalaidshousing.org/PDF/Factsheets-Cost%20 Effective.pdf), housing for people with HIV/AIDS not only saves lives but also saves money. The NAHC observes that housing assistance improves health outcomes, reduces utilization of emergency and other costly health services such as hospitalization by 57%, and reduces involvement with the criminal justice system. Each new HIV infection that is prevented saves an estimated $300,000 in lifetime health care costs.

SUICIDE

Depression is a common psychiatric problem among patients who are seriously ill with HIV/AIDS. Although this is a normal grief response, the combination of alienation, hopelessness, guilt, and lack of self-esteem can lead some to contemplate and plan for suicide in search of lost dignity and control. Others counter that the real dignity is in seeing the disease to the end. Those who encourage people with HIV/AIDS to "stick it out" often see the disease as becoming increasingly manageable with drugs and improved treatment techniques.

Several factors make HIV/AIDS patients more likely to commit suicide. They may feel they are certain to die sooner than they expected and worry that their death will be prolonged and emotionally and physically painful. They may also be despondent about the prospects of losing their job, their insurance, or their home. Furthermore, they may be ostracized from society. Researchers find that factors that have a considerable impact on the quality of life include security, family, love, pleasurable activity, and freedom from pain, suffering, and debilitating disease. AIDS patients may lose all of these, or they may be consumed by the fear of losing vital capacities and freedoms. For some, suicide seems like a reasonable alternative; it offers an end to pain and suffering, insecurity, self-pity, dependency, and hopelessness.

William Breitbart et al. examine in "Impact of Treatment for Depression on Desire for Hastened Death in Patients with Advanced AIDS" (*Psychosomatics*, vol. 51, no. 2, March 2010) the impact of treatment for depression on advanced AIDS patients who expressed a desire for hastened death. The researchers interviewed 372 patients shortly after they were admitted to a palliative care unit (palliative care focuses on symptom relief rather than on cure) and reinterviewed them monthly for two months. Patients who were identified as depressed were treated with antidepressant medication and reinterviewed weekly. Breitbart et al. find that the desire for death was highly associated with depression and that it decreased dramatically in patients who responded to antidepressant treatment. In contrast, patients whose depression did not improve with treatment had little or no change in their desire for hastened death. Although relief from symptoms of depression was not significantly associated with the use of antidepressant medication, patients receiving antidepressant drugs had the largest decreases in the desire for hastened death.

According to Pablo Aldaz et al., in "Mortality by Causes in HIV-Infected Adults: Comparison with the General Population" (*BMC Public Health*, May 11, 2011), people with HIV infection have higher mortality (deaths) than uninfected people of the same age and sex for many causes of death including suicide. The researchers analyzed deaths among HIV-infected people aged 20 to 59 years between 1999 and 2006 and compared mortality from the same causes in the general population. Aldaz et al. conclude that "in agreement with other studies, we found a high mortality from suicide among HIV-infected persons."

The Physician's Role

During the 1990s there were heated debates, voter initiatives, and court decisions about the legalization of physician-assisted suicide. As of October 2013, only four states—Oregon (in 1994), Washington (in 2008), and Vermont (in 2013) through legislation and Montana (in 2009) through court order—had legalized physician-assisted suicide. Voters in Oregon, Washington, and Vermont determined that the right to end one's own life is intensely personal and should not be forbidden by law. (Although attempts and acts of suicide are no longer subject to criminal prosecution in the United States, aiding a suicide is considered a criminal offense.)

Both the public and physicians themselves are divided about the issue of physician-assisted suicide. People who support the practice believe that doctors should make their skills available to patients to end anguish and suffering. Those who oppose physician-assisted suicide argue that better end-of-life care—effective pain management, emotional and spiritual support, and widespread education to reduce anxiety about dying—may reduce the frequency of requests for physician-assisted suicide. Opponents also fear that the legal right to assist suicide can be misused or abused and that such abuses might victimize already vulnerable populations.

In May 2013, the same month that Vermont legalized physician-assisted suicide, a Gallup survey found that 70% of Americans supported allowing physicians to end patients' lives by "some painless means." (See Table 7.1.) According to Lydia Saad of the Gallup Organization, in *U.S. Support for Euthanasia Hinges on How It's Described* (May 29, 2013, http://www.gallup.com/poll/162815/support-euthanasia-hinges-described.aspx), only 51% of Americans support the idea when it is described as physicians helping patients "commit suicide."

TABLE 7.1

Public opinion about the acceptability of physician-assisted suicide, 2013

(FORM A) WHEN A PERSON HAS A DISEASE THAT CANNOT BE CURED, DO YOU THINK DOCTORS SHOULD BE ALLOWED BY LAW TO END THE PATIENT'S LIFE BY SOME PAINLESS MEANS IF THE PATIENT AND HIS OR HER FAMILY REQUEST IT?

(FORM B) WHEN A PERSON HAS A DISEASE THAT CANNOT BE CURED AND IS LIVING IN SEVERE PAIN, DO YOU THINK DOCTORS SHOULD OR SHOULD NOT BE ALLOWED BY LAW TO ASSIST THE PATIENT TO COMMIT SUICIDE IF THE PATIENT REQUESTS IT?

	"End the patient's life by some painless means"	"Assist the patient to commit suicide"
	%	%
Should be allowed	70	51
Should not be allowed	27	45
No opinion	3	4

May 2–7, 2013

SOURCE: Lydia Saad, "Support for Physician-Assisted Suicide—Two Question Wordings," in *U.S. Support for Euthanasia Hinges on How It's Described*, The Gallup Organization, May 29, 2013, http://www.gallup.com/poll/162815/support-euthanasia-hinges-described.aspx (accessed July 29, 2013). Copyright © 2013 Gallup, Inc. All rights reserved. The content is used with permission; however, Gallup retains all rights of republication.

CHAPTER 8
TESTING, PREVENTION, AND EDUCATION

HIV TESTING

Voluntary, Not Mandatory

Few issues about the HIV/AIDS epidemic have prompted more controversy than the use of antibody tests to identify people who are infected with HIV. Soon after the enzyme-linked immunosorbent assay test was developed and licensed in 1985, many public health officials supported testing in an attempt to change "undesirable" behaviors that were determining the course of the epidemic (such as unsafe male-to-male sexual contact and injection drug use). Those who favored testing claimed that if a person knew he or she was HIV positive, the infected person would change his or her behavior. Others argued that aggressive public health education and thoughtful counseling would be more productive strategies to achieve the desired results, even if people did not know their HIV status.

During the early years of the epidemic, health care officials in the public and private sectors refrained from advocating mandatory testing; instead, they focused on HIV testing that would be performed by physicians for patients they considered to be at risk for infection. In 1990 the House of Delegates of the American Medical Association voted to declare HIV/AIDS a sexually transmitted disease (STD). This designation allowed physicians more freedom to decide the conditions under which HIV testing should take place.

During the late 1980s, when the research community announced that HIV-infected, symptom-free people could receive early intervention with azidothymidine (now called zidovudine) to slow the effects of the illness and delay the onset of *Pneumocystis carinii* pneumonia, the debate took another turn. Gay rights advocates, such as the Gay Men's Health Crisis in New York, began encouraging those who were at risk for HIV infection to get tested rather than discouraging testing, as they had previously done. In June 1997 the Gay Men's Health Crisis Center opened its own

testing facility. This service was still available in 2013 as part of the range of care and support services offered by the Michael Palm Center (http://www.gmhc.org/). The center also offered a 12-week "harm reduction program" that was designed to curb risky behaviors such as substance abuse and unprotected sex. The intent of the program was to encourage people to change their risky behavior in a supportive atmosphere of care.

Another controversy surrounding testing concerns reporting HIV-positive patients by name. Every state is required to report AIDS cases. Since 2011, all 50 states and six dependent areas (American Samoa, Guam, the Northern Mariana Islands, Palau, Puerto Rico, and the U.S. Virgin Islands) have implemented HIV case surveillance using the same confidential system for name-based case reporting for both HIV infection and AIDS.

Critics, including the American Civil Liberties Union, assailed name reporting as an invasion of privacy that carries social and economic risks. They claimed that any benefit that would result from reporting names could not override the negative consequences (such as ostracism and the potential loss of jobs and health insurance) of being classified as infected. They added that name reporting discourages those at risk for HIV from coming forward to seek testing and timely treatment.

Name-based reporting became the norm in 2013 because the Ryan White HIV/AIDS Treatment Extension Act of 2009 required grantees to convert to name-based reporting by fiscal year (FY) 2013 or risk the loss of funding. The name-reporting debate subsided in 2013, with the states acquiescing to federal requirements.

Previous HIV Testing among Adults and Adolescents Newly Diagnosed with HIV Infection

In 2006 the Centers for Disease Control and Prevention (CDC) recommended HIV testing for adults, adolescents, and pregnant women in health care settings and HIV testing at least annually for people who were at high risk for HIV infection. The three populations at highest risk for HIV in the United States are men who have sex with men (MSM), injection drug users (IDUs), and high-risk heterosexuals. The CDC collects information from all these groups.

The most recent data that have been analyzed are from 18 jurisdictions participating in the CDC National HIV Surveillance System. In "Previous HIV Testing among Adults and Adolescents Newly Diagnosed with HIV Infection—National HIV Surveillance System, 18 Jurisdictions, United States, 2006–2009" (*Morbidity and Mortality Weekly Report*, vol. 61, no. 24, June 22, 2012), the CDC observes that many people diagnosed with HIV infection have never been tested previously. Between 2006 and 2009, 40.8% were diagnosed with HIV infection at their first HIV test, and 59.2% had a negative test at some point before HIV diagnosis. (See Table 8.1.) The highest percentage of people testing HIV negative less than 12 months before HIV diagnosis were those aged 13 to 29 years (33%), males with HIV transmission attributed to MSM (29%), and whites (28%).

Contact Tracing/Partner Notification

A by-product of testing is contact tracing, or partner notification. When individuals test positive for HIV, health officials ask them to provide, with the promise of anonymity, the names of those with whom they have had sexual contact or shared needles. The CDC asks counselors to inform contacts if the patient is reluctant to do so and strongly endorses contact-tracing programs, but results vary. States struggling under the strain of many HIV/AIDS cases continue to support programs that

TABLE 8.1

Percentage of people diagnosed with HIV infection with a negative HIV test before HIV diagnosis, 2006–09

Characteristic	No.	No.	(%)	No.	(%)[a]	No.	(%)[a]
		\<\<Diagnosis of HIV infection\>\>					
		\<\<HIV diagnoses with testing history information\>\>					
				Previous negative HIV test		**No previous test**	
Total[b]	125,104	57,476	(45.9)	34,049	(59.2)	23,427	(40.8)
Age group at diagnosis (yrs)							
13–29	38,521	21,734	(56.4)	14,220	(65.4)	7,513	(34.6)
30–39	32,339	14,816	(45.8)	9,386	(63.4)	5,430	(36.7)
40–49	33,179	13,244	(39.9)	7,252	(54.8)	5,992	(45.2)
≥50	21,065	7,683	(36.5)	3,191	(41.5)	4,492	(58.5)
Race/Ethnicity							
Black/African American	62,824	29,945	(47.7)	16,756	(56.0)	13,188	(44.0)
Hispanic/Latino[c]	25,234	11,135	(44.1)	6,490	(58.3)	4,644	(41.7)
White	33,377	14,781	(44.3)	9,846	(66.6)	4,935	(33.4)
Other	3,669	1,616	(44.0)	957	(59.2)	659	(40.8)
Transmission category (males)							
Male-to-male sexual contact	65,908	31,493	(47.8)	20,317	(64.5)	11,176	(35.5)
Injection drug use	8,889	3,104	(34.9)	1,431	(46.1)	1,674	(53.9)
Male-to-male sexual contact and injection drug use	3,696	1,781	(48.2)	1,151	(64.6)	630	(35.4)
Heterosexual contact[d]	14,167	6,186	(43.7)	2,710	(43.8)	3,476	(56.2)
Other[e]	188	48	(25.7)	17	(35.8)	31	(64.2)
Subtotal	92,849	42,613	(45.9)	25,627	(60.1)	16,986	(39.9)
Transmission category (females)							
Injection drug use	5,330	2,306	(43.3)	1,356	(58.8)	950	(41.2)
Heterosexual contact[d]	26,776	12,499	(46.7)	7,048	(56.4)	5,451	(43.6)
Other[e]	149	58	(39.1)	18	(31.2)	40	(68.9)
Subtotal	32,255	14,863	(46.1)	8,422	(56.7)	6,441	(43.3)

HIV = Human Immunodeficiency Virus.

[a]Percentage among those for whom testing history information was available.

[b]Because column totals for estimated numbers were calculated independently of the values for the subpopulations, the values in each column might not sum to the column total.

[c]Hispanics/Latinos might be of any race.

[d]Heterosexual contact with a person known to have, or to be at high risk for, HIV infection.

[e]Includes hemophilia, blood transfusion, perinatal exposure, and any risk factor not reported or not identified.

Notes: Estimated numbers resulted from statistical adjustment that accounted for reporting delays and missing risk factor information, but not for incomplete reporting. Data used to determine whether a person had a negative HIV test result before HIV diagnosis. Those with a negative HIV test at any point before the first positive HIV test. The 18 jurisdictions contributing data for the 2006—2009 national HIV incidence estimate were the states of Alabama, Arizona, Colorado, Connecticut, Florida, Indiana, Louisiana, Michigan, Mississippi, New Jersey, New York, North Carolina, South Carolina, Texas, Virginia, and Washington, and the cities of Chicago, Illinois, and Philadelphia, Pennsylvania.

SOURCE: "Table 1. Estimated Number and Percentage of Adults and Adolescents Diagnosed with HIV Infection, with HIV Testing History Information, Having a Negative HIV Test before HIV Diagnosis, by Selected Characteristics—National HIV Surveillance System, 18 Jurisdictions, 2006–2009," in "Previous HIV Testing among Adults and Adolescents Newly Diagnosed with HIV Infection—National HIV Surveillance System, 18 Jurisdictions, United States, 2006–2009," *MMWR*, vol. 61, no. 24, June 22, 2012, http://www.cdc.gov/mmwr/pdf/wk/mm6124.pdf (accessed July 30, 2013) encourage the infected people to notify partners on their own. Contact-tracing programs in states with fewer HIV/AIDS cases are more likely to contact partners. Many patients who are HIV infected or have AIDS fear that promises of confidentiality will be broken; others fear retribution from those they may have infected.

Binwei Song et al. explain in "Partner Referral by HIV-Infected Persons to Partner Counseling and Referral Services (PCRS)—Results from a Demonstration Project" (*Open AIDS Journal*, vol. 6, 2012) that "the success of partner notification depends on whether [patients] are willing to provide information about their partners, the content of the information that they provide (i.e., whether they provide names and locating information of their partners), and how they choose to inform their partners that they have been exposed to HIV." The researchers report on their research to determine factors associated with refusal and agreement to provide partner information. They find that clients who were aged 25 years and older, male, or reported MSM or injection drug use in the past 12 months were more likely to refuse to provide partner information. Song et al. posit that MSM and IDUs may be more reluctant to share personal information because of social stigma or more negative feelings about being HIV positive. The proportion of partners that were located, notified, and counseled differed by approach used, ranging from 38% when patients agreed to notify their partners within a certain time frame or else a health care professional would notify them to 98% when patients notified their partners with a health professional present.

ETHICAL, LEGAL, AND MORAL DILEMMAS OF PARTNER NOTIFICATION. Worldwide, there is increasing emphasis on partner notification as a strategy with the potential not only to prevent HIV transmission to partners at risk but also to promote early diagnosis and prompt treatment for those found to be infected. Barnabas N. Njozing et al. of Umeå University assert in "'If the Patients Decide Not to Tell What Can We Do?'—TB/HIV Counsellors' Dilemma on Partner Notification for HIV" (*BMC International Health and Human Rights*, vol. 11, June 3, 2011) that counselors are often frustrated by HIV-positive patients' reluctance to voluntarily notify their sexual partners. The researchers interviewed counselors to identify the issues surrounding confidentiality and partner notification.

Njozing et al. find that all counselors encouraged voluntary notification but that counselors responded differently to people who refused to voluntarily notify their partners of their HIV status. One group believed in absolute respect of patients' autonomy and that it is not the counselors' responsibility to inform partners at risk without the patients' consent. The researchers note that legal counsel endorsed this position. A second group of counselors acknowledged the importance of respecting patients'

autonomy, but also felt a responsibility for their partners' safety. They used strategies such as couples counseling and continuous reminders of the benefits of disclosure to encourage reluctant patients.

A third group of counselors wanted solutions that inform sexual partners who are at risk of HIV infection and legal protection for counselors. Njozing et al. state that this group believed "upholding confidentiality in absolute terms was morally wrong, and patients who refused to inform their partners about their status were selfish by not considering the health and wellbeing of their partners." Some of these counselors admitted that as a last resort they occasionally threatened patients to pressure them to inform partners. These counselors were very conflicted about their roles in terms of respecting patient confidentiality and informing sexual partners. They explained that this conflict was exacerbated when they were acquainted with the patients' sexual partners.

A fourth group of counselors felt that HIV/AIDS should be treated as any other chronic disease and advocated routine HIV testing and partner notification. Their goal is to destigmatize and normalize the diagnosis of HIV so that it is a medical condition like any other, for which diagnosis and disclosure are conducted based on medical necessity rather than on legal or ethical bases.

INTERNET-BASED PARTNER NOTIFICATION. Because research indicates that a substantial number of new HIV cases and sexually transmitted infections (STIs) are acquired by MSM who meet new sexual partners on the Internet, health professionals wondered if the same medium could be used to convey information to men, such as in e-mails or e-cards informing them that they had sex with someone with an STI and providing links about the STI and where to get tested for it. In "Evaluation of inSPOTLA.org: An Internet Partner Notification Service" (*Sexually Transmitted Diseases*, vol. 39, no. 5, May 2012), Aaron Plant et al. evaluated inSPOTLA.org, an STI partner notification website that primarily targets MSM. Between December 2005 and 2009 the site received more than 400,000 visitors and resulted in nearly 50,000 e-mail postcards sent. Users of inSPOTLA choose from six different e-cards, which vary in tone from serious to humorous. They select their STI from a pull-down menu of 10 different diseases. E-cards may be sent anonymously to as many as six partners at once or can include a personal note from the sender. E-card recipients receive an e-mail from getchecked@inspotla.org. Although the site had many visitors, Plant et al. find that community awareness and utilization of the site were low. Nonetheless, the researchers believe that sites such as inSPOTLA have the potential to enhance traditional partner notification efforts.

Rapid Testing

One way to increase access to HIV testing is through rapid testing, which may be readily performed in a variety of settings, such as correctional facilities, military battlefield operations, and worksites where occupational exposures may occur. Several rapid HIV antibody tests have been approved by the U.S. Food and Drug Administration (FDA) for use in the United States. Table 2.5 in Chapter 2 lists the FDA-approved rapid HIV screening tests and provides their features. The tests contain test strips with HIV antigens. If the blood or sputum they come in contact with contains HIV antibodies, then the antibodies bind to the antigens and a reagent in the test kit creates a color change. The tests are interpreted visually and, like conventional HIV enzyme immunoassays, require additional testing by a Western blot or immunofluorescent assay to confirm a positive response.

Because rapid HIV testing informs clients with reactive test results that it is highly likely that they are HIV positive, compared with receiving no test result information at the conclusion of a visit where a conventional HIV test specimen is drawn, it is vitally important for health care workers to explain the meaning of preliminary positive results. Counseling for patients who receive rapid HIV testing is somewhat different from conventional testing and involves determining how prepared clients are to receive test results in the same session.

In July 2012 the FDA approved the first rapid response test for home use. The OraQuick In-Home HIV Test does not require sending a sample to a laboratory for analysis. It provides a test result in 20 to 40 minutes. As with other rapid tests, positive test results must be confirmed by follow-up laboratory-based testing.

Home Testing

Home HIV tests were developed during the mid-1980s but were opposed by the FDA and some HIV/AIDS organizations and health care agencies. The FDA was concerned about telephone counseling for those who tested positive, the accuracy of the tests, and confidentiality. In 1996 the FDA reversed its position, deciding that despite the limitations of home testing, the benefits outweigh the risks.

Public health officials explain that many people are afraid of obtaining testing at a physician's office or public clinic because of the associated stigma. They assert that home testing may be the only way some of these people will learn their HIV status and argue that more people will then enter treatment and take precautions to prevent spreading the infection.

Some home tests use saliva, which does not require a needle stick, and others use blood samples. When blood is tested, the patient draws a few drops of blood from a fingertip, places it on filter paper, and mails the paper to a company laboratory, which performs the standard HIV assay. If the results are positive, a confirmation test is performed. An HIV test kit called the Home Access Express HIV-1 Test System, manufactured by Home Access Health Corporation and approved by the FDA in 1996, was the only HIV home test kit approved by the agency as of 2013. Seven days (or sooner if express service is requested) after Home Access Health receives the test kit, results and counseling are available by calling a 24-hour toll-free number and giving an identification code. Home Access claims an accuracy rate of 99.9%.

Critics of home testing suggest that news of HIV infection is not as easy to accept as the results of other in-home tests, such as those for pregnancy and cholesterol. They claim that most people cannot properly prepare themselves for the news that they have a life-threatening disease. They advocate the expansion of current testing sites to include mobile vans, sports clubs, and other places that are not exclusively associated with HIV testing, but where in-person counseling can be provided.

Military Practices

The U.S. Department of Defense (DOD) regularly screens all members of the armed services as well as those seeking to join for HIV. The DOD states in "Department of Defense: Instruction" (June 7, 2013, http://www.dtic.mil/whs/directives/corres/pdf/648501p.pdf) that its policy is to "deny eligibility for military service to persons with laboratory evidence of HIV infection for appointment, enlistment, pre-appointment, or initial entry training for military service." Biannual HIV testing is required of all personnel on active duty, as well as of all members of the reserves and National Guard. In 1995, after two months of debate in Congress, federal legislators scrapped a discharge provision that would have forced the DOD to dismiss members of the military within six months of testing positive for HIV. Along with HIV infection, a number of chronic conditions, including asthma, cancer, diabetes, heart disease, or complications of pregnancy, place troops on limited assignment, precluding them from overseas service or combat.

In "Epidemiology of Sexually Transmitted Infections among Human Immunodeficiency Virus Positive United States Military Personnel" (*Journal of Sexually Transmitted Diseases*, March 2013), Jeff S. Tzeng et al. look at the incidence and prevalence of STIs in HIV-positive military personnel between 2000 and 2010. The researchers find higher rates of STIs in the period following the HIV diagnosis and conclude that despite intensive counseling, "high-risk sexual behavior continues to occur in the HIV-positive military population."

Pregnant Women and Newborns

The issue of testing newborns has placed the rights of mothers at odds with those of their newborns. States have kept HIV test results anonymous to preserve a mother's right to privacy. Civil libertarians (those that actively support the strengthening and protecting of individual rights and freedoms) and some groups that represent women, gays, and lesbians support anonymous testing, claiming that attaching names to test results would start local, state, and federal governments down the "slippery slope" of mandatory testing of adults. They also raise further privacy concerns, contending that once names are known, there is no guarantee they will not fall into the hands of employers, insurance companies, and others who might discriminate on the basis of HIV status.

The CDC recommends HIV testing of all pregnant women as a standard part of prenatal care to identify and treat HIV and to prevent transmission of HIV to infants. Testing is also advised for any newborn whose mother's HIV status is unknown. When treatment begins early in pregnancy, the risk of mother-to-child HIV transmission is reduced to 2% or less.

In May 1996 the U.S. House of Representatives and the U.S. Senate passed bills that would cut off federal money for HIV/AIDS treatment to states that failed to comply with the new disclosure requirements. In June 1996 New York became the first state to mandate that health officials tell parents the results of HIV tests that the state routinely performs on all newborns. Before June 1996 parents in New York did not receive results unless they requested them, as was still the case in many states in 2013.

NEW JERSEY LEGISLATION MANDATES TESTING OF PREGNANT WOMEN AND SOME NEWBORNS. In June 2007 New Jersey legislators approved a bill requiring pregnant women and some newborns—infants born to mothers who have tested positive or those whose HIV status is unknown at the time of birth—to be tested for HIV. The law requires that pregnant women be tested twice for HIV, once early and once late during the pregnancy, unless the mother specifically requests not to be tested.

Supporters of this legislation contend that the requirement for testing will save children's lives. Detractors argue that all infants of HIV-infected mothers test positive for HIV antibodies because they inherit their mother's antibodies. This initial positive result does not necessarily mean the infant is infected. Because it takes several months for the mother's antibodies to clear from the infant, it may be more prudent to test infants when they are between three and six months old to determine their HIV status. According to the Kaiser Family Foundation, in "New Jersey Legislature Approves Bill Requiring Pregnant Women, Some Infants to Receive HIV Tests" (June 25, 2007, http://www.kaiserhealthnews .org/daily-reports/2007/june/25/dr00045784.aspx?referrer =search), the American Civil Liberties Union and women's health advocacy groups assert that the legislation "deprives women of authority to make medical decisions."

Although the CDC recommends routine opt-out HIV screening of all pregnant women and newborn testing if the mother's HIV status is unknown, state policies vary. The National HIV/AIDS Clinicians' Consultation Center at the University of California, San Francisco, reports in *Compendium of State HIV Testing Laws—Perinatal Quick Reference Guide: Guide to States' Perinatal HIV Testing Laws for Clinicians* (http://www.nccc.ucsf.edu/ docs/Perinatal_QRG.pdf) that as of April 2011, 20 states, the District of Columbia, and Puerto Rico had no specific provisions regarding prenatal testing. The balance of the states had provisions for prenatal testing. Ten states had opt-out HIV testing—it is part of routine prenatal care and pregnant women are tested unless they refuse or "opt-out." The remaining 40 states had opt-in HIV testing of pregnant women—an HIV test is not part of routine prenatal care and pregnant women must specifically request or "opt-in" to receive an HIV test.

Health Care Workers

There has been a continuing debate over whether health care workers should be required to obtain HIV tests. As of 2013, there was no law requiring health care workers to submit to HIV testing, although many employers require it as a condition of employment. They cannot, however, discriminate against health care workers on the basis of their HIV status because like other employees, they are covered by the Americans with Disabilities Act of 1990, the federal law that prohibits discrimination against individuals with disabilities.

According to the CDC, in "HIV Transmission" (June 3, 2013, http://www.cdc.gov/hiv/basics/transmission.html), the risk of health care workers becoming infected with HIV on the job is very low, especially if they follow prudent safety measures known as universal precautions—gloves, goggles, and masks to prevent HIV and other bloodborne infections. The largest risk is posed by accidental needle-stick injuries, but even this risk is less than 1%.

Testing Policies in U.S. Prisons

Guidelines for the testing of inmates for HIV exist in all 50 states, in the District of Columbia, and in the regulations of the Federal Bureau of Prisons. However, the timing of testing varies. In "HIV in Correctional Settings" (July 24, 2012, http://www.cdc.gov/hiv/topics/ correctional/), the CDC recommends that HIV screening be provided on entry into prison and before release and that voluntary HIV testing be offered periodically during incarceration.

The CDC acknowledges that some correctional systems face logistical, security, and financial constraints that hamper testing. Using rapid HIV tests within the first 24 hours after incarceration may overcome issues such as quick turnover of jail inmates. The laboratory costs associated with HIV testing may be obstacles for some correctional systems. Another obstacle may be that health care providers in correctional settings lack familiarity with confidentiality and reporting requirements; knowledge of local and state public health confidentiality laws may increase HIV testing.

PREVENTION
Critics Fault Programs' Focus and Funding

The objective of HIV prevention programs is to reduce the number of new cases to as close to zero as possible. All prevention efforts are based on the belief that individuals can be educated in a way that will lead to changes in behavior, which will help bring an end to the spread of HIV/AIDS. However, many AIDS advocacy groups have long been critical of the ways the CDC has communicated this message. In 1987 CDC officials chose to emphasize the universality of AIDS, instead of focusing efforts on those most at risk: MSM and IDUs. According to AIDS advocates, this strategy misdirected the spending of available prevention dollars during the first decade of the epidemic. In 2013, although the number of infected people outside of these two groups was growing, HIV/AIDS was still largely a threat to MSM, IDUs, their partners, and their children. Most women with HIV/AIDS were IDUs or were sex partners of IDUs.

CDC Prevention Activities

The CDC's HIV prevention strategy, as described in "About the Division of HIV/AIDS Prevention (DHAP)" (October 29, 2013, http://www.cdc.gov/hiv/dhap/about .html), aims to reduce the incidence and prevalence of HIV infection as well as the morbidity (illnesses) and mortality (deaths) that result from HIV infection by working with communities and other partners. The agency's efforts focus on four areas:

- Capacity building—strengthening and supporting the HIV prevention workforce

- Program evaluation—assessing the effectiveness, costs, and impact of HIV prevention strategies, policies, and programs

- Communication—developing and disseminating scientific and informative communications on HIV/ AIDS for providers, people at risk, and the public

- Research—conducting research to design and test interventions to prevent HIV transmission

The prevention strategy capitalizes on rapid test technologies, interventions that bring people unaware of their HIV status to HIV testing, and behavioral interventions that provide prevention skills to people living with HIV/AIDS. To carry out its strategy, the CDC works in conjunction with governmental and nongovernmental partners to implement, evaluate, and further develop and strengthen effective HIV prevention efforts nationwide. Along with direct programs and service, the CDC provides financial and technical support for:

- Disease surveillance

- HIV antibody counseling, testing, and referral services

- Street and community outreach

- Risk-reduction counseling

- Prevention case management

- Prevention and treatment of other STIs

- Public information and education

- School-based AIDS education

- International research studies

- Technology transfer systems

- Organizational capacity building

- Program-relevant epidemiological, sociobehavioral, and evaluation research

CDC health education and disease prevention efforts continue to emphasize that the most reliable ways to avoid HIV infection or virus transmission are by abstaining from sexual intercourse; maintaining a mutually monogamous, long-term relationship with a partner who is uninfected; and/or refraining from sharing needles and syringes in drug use. Although seemingly logical, critics contend that the CDC's emphasis on abstinence burdens people with an unrealistic expectation. Critics also point to the insistence on abstinence policies as a condition of U.S. government assistance for other countries' health programs to be an ill-advised foreign policy intrusion.

According to the Kaiser Family Foundation, in the fact sheet "U.S. Federal Funding for HIV/AIDS: The President's FY 2014 Budget Request" (May 23, 2013, http://kff.org/hivaids/fact-sheet/u-s-federal-funding-for-hivaids-the-presidents-fy-2014-budget-request/), for FY 2014 the CDC was allocated $836 million for domestic HIV/AIDS prevention activities conducted by the National Center for HIV/AIDS, Viral Hepatitis, STD, and TB Prevention, a 1.6% increase from FY 2012.

High-Impact Prevention

In the fact sheet "HIV Prevention in the United States—High-Impact Prevention: Saving Lives and Money" (August 2011, http://www.cdc.gov/hiv/strategy/hihp/pdf/dhap _policy_maker.pdf), the CDC explains that HIV prevention saves money by avoiding the high lifetime health care costs of infection—an estimated $360,000 per person living with HIV/AIDS. Prevention efforts saved more than $125 billion in direct medical costs between 1991 and 2006. Figure 8.1 shows how effective prevention efforts avert thousands of new infections and save billions of dollars.

FIGURE 8.1

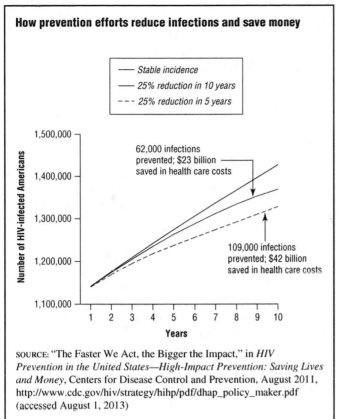

How prevention efforts reduce infections and save money

— Stable incidence
— 25% reduction in 10 years
--- 25% reduction in 5 years

62,000 infections prevented; $23 billion saved in health care costs

109,000 infections prevented; $42 billion saved in health care costs

Years

SOURCE: "The Faster We Act, the Bigger the Impact," in *HIV Prevention in the United States—High-Impact Prevention: Saving Lives and Money*, Centers for Disease Control and Prevention, August 2011, http://www.cdc.gov/hiv/strategy/hihp/pdf/dhap_policy_maker.pdf (accessed August 1, 2013)

CDC high-impact prevention programs consider not only program effectiveness but also the overall impact of these prevention efforts on the course of the epidemic. They combine scientifically proven, cost-effective, and scalable interventions targeted to the right populations in the right geographic areas. Proven tools include expanding HIV testing, increasing access to condoms and sterile syringes, and providing antiretroviral therapy for HIV-infected people to reduce the risk of transmission and screening and treatment for other STIs.

High-impact prevention also involves accurately funding prevention efforts so that they reach their target populations. Figure 8.2 shows how FY 2016 funding will be allocated to provide HIV testing and treatment in the geographic areas with the greatest burden of HIV.

EDUCATING YOUTH

The CDC estimates in "Basic Statistics" (April 23, 2013, http://www.cdc.gov/hiv/topics/surveillance/basic.htm) that in 2011, 15,538 new cases of HIV infection and 5,858 new cases of AIDS were reported for people aged 20 to 29 years. With an average incubation period of 10 years, it is likely that most of these young people were infected while they were teenagers. Because some people begin having sexual relationships and using injection drugs at earlier ages, many health officials fear the number of HIV-positive young people will grow.

Most states offer prevention programs for students in public schools. However, youths who are not in school may not have ready access to such programs. Many homeless shelters and local health departments employ roving counselors who seek out these young people to offer prevention information and direct them to health and social service agencies.

Sexual Health Education

Many education programs offer students sufficient information about STIs and HIV/AIDS, but only high-quality education affects behavior. In "The Effectiveness of Group-Based Comprehensive Risk-Reduction and Abstinence Education Interventions to Prevent or Reduce the Risk of Adolescent Pregnancy, Human Immunodeficiency Virus, and Sexually Transmitted Infections: Two Systematic Reviews for the Guide to Community Preventive Services" (*American Journal of Preventive Medicine*, vol. 42, no. 3, March 2012), Helen B. Chin et al. examine group-based interventions that address the sexual behavior of adolescents such as use of condoms by sexually active teenagers and aim to reduce the incidence of pregnancy, HIV, and other STIs in this group. They also look at group-based abstinence education, which has as its exclusive purpose teaching the social, psychological, and health gains to be realized by abstaining from sexual activity.

Chin et al. find that group-based comprehensive risk reduction programs significantly improved one or more sexual behaviors. The programs acted by delaying or decreasing sexual behaviors or by increasing condom and contraceptive use. Although the abstinence education interventions showed a potentially meaningful effect on sexual activity, the researchers find that these interventions did not have a significant effect on the frequency of sexual activity. Therefore, Chin et al. are unable to draw clear conclusions about their effects on the rates of STIs.

The provision of comprehensive sex education remained controversial in 2013. Some people do not agree that information about sexual health or decisions should be offered in public schools, preferring that parents instill their own values in their children. However, others point out that some parents never talk to their children about sex and drugs and that school may be the only place a child can get reliable information. According to the Guttmacher Institute, in "State Policies in Brief: Sex and STI/HIV Education" (November 1, 2013, http://www.guttmacher.org/statecenter/spibs/spib_SE.pdf), 33 states and the District of Columbia required HIV/AIDS prevention education in 2013. Twenty states and the District of Columbia required HIV education and sex education, and 13 only required HIV education. Twenty-two states and the District of Columbia required schools to notify parents that HIV education or sex education will be

FIGURE 8.2

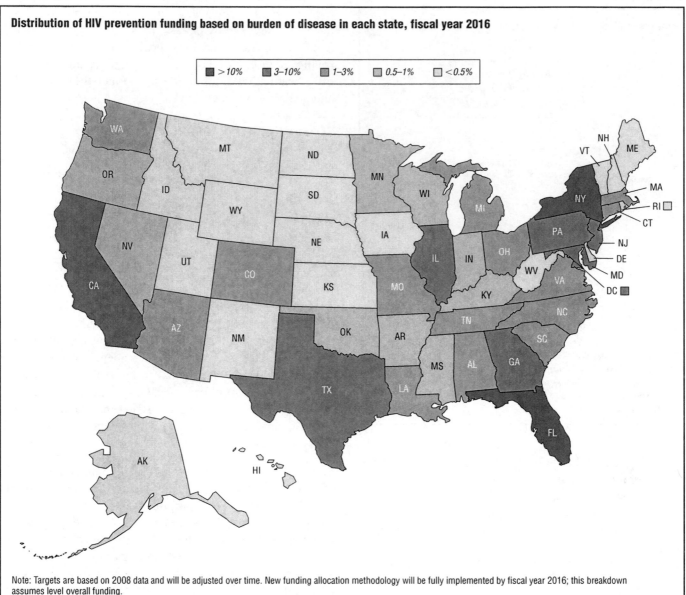

Distribution of HIV prevention funding based on burden of disease in each state, fiscal year 2016

■ >10%   ■ 3–10%   ■ 1–3%   □ 0.5–1%   □ <0.5%

Note: Targets are based on 2008 data and will be adjusted over time. New funding allocation methodology will be fully implemented by fiscal year 2016; this breakdown assumes level overall funding.

SOURCE: "Targeted Distribution of CDC Core HIV Prevention Funding—FY2016, Based on Proportion of All Americans Diagnosed with HIV Who Live in Each State," in *The Future of HIV Prevention*, Centers for Disease Control and Prevention, February 2013, http://www.cdc.gov/nchhstp/newsroom/docs/ HIVFactSheets/Future-508.pdf (accessed August 1, 2013).

provided to students. Although laws vary from state to state, and some allow local school districts to decide on curricula, many of these states have one or more mandates determining the material that may be taught in the programs. The mandates range from requiring age-appropriate materials, to teaching comprehensive sex education programs (advocating contraceptive and condom use), to providing programs in which abstinence from premarital sex is presented as the only 100% effective means of preventing HIV/AIDS. The Guttmacher Institute notes that in 2013 only 12 states required the information that is taught be medically accurate.

Federal funding for abstinence-only educational programs was initiated in 1998. Proponents of these

programs claim they change attitudes about casual sex by reducing both teen pregnancies and rates of STIs. They also maintain that teaching students about contraceptive and condom use condones, or even encourages, unsafe sexual behavior. Critics of these programs argue that there is no reliable evidence that abstinence-only programs are effective. In addition, they contend that for the five out of 10 teens aged 15 to 19 years who do choose to have sex, lack of knowledge about contraception and condom use will only result in continued teen pregnancies, STIs, and HIV infections.

The U.S. Department of Health and Human Services concludes in *Review of Comprehensive Sex Education Curricula* (May 2007) that abstinence-only education is ineffective. The review finds that students given abstinence-only education were no more likely to abstain from sex, that those who had sex did so with a similar number of partners as those who had not received abstinence-only education, and that students first had sex at the same age, independent of the type of education they had received.

In *Cuts, Consolidations, and Savings* (April 2013, http://www.whitehouse.gov/sites/default/files/omb/budget/fy2014/assets/ccs.pdf), the White House notes that between FYs 2012 and 2014 federal funding for abstinence-only education decreased by $5 million. The Sexuality Information and Education Council of the United States explains in "The President's FY 2014 Budget" (2013, http://www.siecus.org/index.cfm?fuseaction=Feature.showFeature&featureid=2269&parentid=478) that the $5 million is a discretionary abstinence-only-until-marriage grant program and that abstinence-only funding is estimated to total $37 million in FY 2014 based on state funding requests. Critics of abstinence-only education are disheartened by continued funding of such programs in view of the dearth of evidence of their efficacy (the ability of an intervention to produce the intended diagnostic or therapeutic effect in optimal circumstances).

CONDOM USE

In the fact sheet "Condoms and STDs: Fact Sheet for Public Health Personnel" (March 25, 2013, http://www.cdc.gov/condomeffectiveness/latex.htm), the CDC indicates that studies provide compelling evidence that latex condoms are highly effective in protecting against HIV infection when used properly for every act of intercourse. However, the agency warns that "the most reliable ways to avoid transmission of sexually transmitted diseases (STDs), including human immunodeficiency virus (HIV), are to abstain from sexual activity or to be in a long-term mutually monogamous relationship with an uninfected partner."

The CDC's analysis of data from the Youth Risk Behavior Surveys conducted between 1991 and 2011 finds that U.S. high school students are engaging in fewer HIV-related risk behaviors—decreasing percentages of students reported being sexually active and having had sexual intercourse with four or more people during their life. Condom use increased between 1991 and 2003, but since then has leveled off. Condom use among sexually active students rose from 46.2% in 1991 to 60.2% in 2011. (See Table 5.5 in Chapter 5.)

Other Forms of Protection

In 1993 the FDA approved Reality, a female condom that serves as a mechanical barrier to viruses. The condom is designed for women to protect themselves from STIs, including HIV. It is made of polyurethane (a resin made of two different compounds used in elastic fibers, cushions, and various molded products) and is unlikely to rip or tear. The condom is prelubricated and is intended for use during only one sex act.

The use of female condoms is low. Margaret R. Weeks et al. cite in "Initial and Sustained Female Condom Use among Low-Income Urban U.S. Women" (*Journal of Women's Health*, vol. 22, no. 1, January 2013) the findings of a Hartford, Connecticut, study—that 29% of women had ever used female condoms before the study but after a demonstration of their use and given free samples, nearly three-quarters (73%) of never users reported sustained use. Weeks et al. assert that women will use female condoms when they are educated about them and given free trial samples and call for inclusion of this approach in standard clinical practice and public health education.

CIRCUMCISION MAY SLOW THE SPREAD OF HIV

According to the press release "WHO and UNAIDS Announce Recommendations from Expert Consultation on Male Circumcision for HIV Prevention" (March 28, 2007, http://www.who.int/hiv/mediacentre/news68/en/index.html), in 2007 the World Health Organization (WHO) and the Joint United Nations Programme on HIV/AIDS recommended circumcision as a strategy to prevent heterosexually acquired HIV infection in men. Circumcision (the surgical removal of the foreskin from the penis) has long been thought to reduce men's susceptibility to HIV infection because the skin cells in the foreskin are especially vulnerable to the virus. Kevin De Cock, the director of the WHO HIV/AIDS Department, asserted that "countries with high rates of heterosexual HIV infection and low rates of male circumcision now have an additional intervention which can reduce the risk of HIV infection in heterosexual men. Scaling up male circumcision in such countries will result in immediate benefit to individuals. However, it will be a number of years before we can expect to see an impact on the epidemic from such investment."

Charles Shey Wiysonge et al. conclude in "Male Circumcision for Prevention of Homosexual Acquisition of HIV in Men" (*Cochrane Database of Systematic Reviews*, no. 6, June 15, 2011), an exhaustive review of the relevant medical literature that included 21 studies of 71,693 subjects, that "current evidence suggests that male circumcision may be protective among MSM who practice primarily insertive anal sex, but the role of male circumcision overall in the prevention of HIV and other sexually transmitted infections among MSM remains to be determined. Therefore, there is not enough evidence to recommend male circumcision for HIV prevention among MSM at present." The researchers call for completion of a randomized controlled trial, the most rigorous type of clinical research, to definitively determine whether male circumcision protects against HIV transmission.

Three randomized clinical trials conducted in sub-Saharan Africa demonstrate that circumcision reduces HIV incidence. In "The Long Term Efficacy of Medical Male Circumcision against HIV Acquisition" (*AIDS*, July 3, 2013), Supriya D. Mehta et al. look at 2,784 men aged 18 to 24 years who were randomly assigned to immediate circumcision in December 2006 or to a control group, which was not circumcised. The men were followed through September 2010 and circumcision was found to reduce HIV infection by 60%.

SYRINGE EXCHANGE PROGRAMS

IDUs often share the syringes they use to inject drugs into their body. When an HIV-positive IDU uses a syringe, he or she may contaminate it with HIV-positive blood that can then spread the disease to other IDUs who use that syringe. Syringe exchange programs (SEPs) attempt to prevent the spread of HIV in this manner by encouraging IDUs to bring in their used, unsafe syringes and exchange them for new, safe syringes. The reasoning behind these programs is that if people are going to use drugs, at least an effort can be made to make sure they do not contract HIV because of it. Proponents of these programs point out that the spread of HIV among IDUs threatens everyone, as people who contract HIV through drug use can then pass it on to their sexual partners and children.

Despite these arguments, SEPs are highly controversial due to their connection to drug use. Some opponents see them as helping IDUs avoid the consequences of their actions, or even providing them with the means to continue their illegal activities. In April 1998, after much debate, the Clinton administration decided not to lift a nine-year-old ban on federal financing for programs to distribute clean needles to drug addicts. This meant that state and local governments that received federal block grants for HIV/AIDS prevention were not permitted to use this money for SEPs. Public health experts and advocates for people with HIV/AIDS criticized the decision. The ban was lifted in 2009 and state and local health authorities sought and obtained federal funds for SEPs. However, the ban was reinstated in late 2011 and was still in full force as of October 2013.

The Foundation for AIDS Research (amfAR) details in "Syringe Exchange Program Coverage in the United States 2012" (April 2012, http://www.amfar.org/uploadedFiles/_amfarorg/On_the_Hill/3_29_12_SEP_Map_FINAL.pdf) the location of SEPs by state. In 2012 there were 203 SEPs in 34 states, the District of Columbia, Puerto Rico, and the Native American nations. Overall, 186 cities had SEPs, and 31 cities operated 10 or more SEPs.

In "2011 National Survey of Syringe Exchange Programs: Summary of Results" (2011, http://www.nasen.org/news/categories/survey/), a survey of SEPs funded by amfAR, the Elton John AIDS Foundation, and the Irene Diamond Foundation, Don C. Des Jarlais et al. find that 36.9 million syringes were exchanged in 2011. Besides exchanged syringes, most of the SEPs provided other public health and social services. Of the 144 SEPs responding to the survey, 75 provided on-site medical services. Nearly seven out of 10 (69%) held 501-C3 status, meaning they operated as tax-exempt nonprofit organizations, and just 10% received federal funding before the ban was reinstated.

According to Des Jarlais et al., the majority (68%) of SEP participants injected heroin, 18% each injected cocaine by itself or in combination with heroin, 17% injected methamphetamine, and 16% injected other opiates. Three-quarters of SEPs reported the lack of funding and resources as a problem encountered in 2011 and 56% suffered staff shortages. Thirty percent said they lacked political support, 28% suffered from staff burnout, and 24% were unable to conduct enough outreach.

Helping IDUs Saves Lives

In "Spatial Access to Syringe Exchange Programs and Pharmacies Selling Over-the-Counter Syringes as Predictors of Drug Injectors' Use of Sterile Syringes" (*American Journal of Public Health*, vol. 101, no. 6, June 2011), Hannah L. Cooper et al. look at relationships between access to SEPs and pharmacies selling over-the-counter syringes and the behaviors of 4,003 IDUs in New York City between 1995 and 2006. The researchers find that greater access to SEPs and pharmacies that sell syringes over-the-counter improved IDUs' abilities to engage in risk-reduction practices that reduce the likelihood and frequency of both HIV and hepatitis C virus transmission.

In "Demographic, Risk, and Spatial Factors Associated with Over-the-Counter Syringe Purchase among Injection Drug Users" (*American Journal of Epidemiology*, vol. 176, no. 1, July 1, 2012), Thomas J. Stopka et al. look at the experience in California, where since 2005 over-the-counter (OTC) syringe sales are permitted in many jurisdictions. The researchers used a combination of geographic information system and statistical analyses to determine the factors associated with OTC syringe purchase by IDUs. Stopka et al. find that the distance from the IDU's residence to the nearest OTC syringe-selling pharmacy was not significantly associated with OTC purchase but that the prevalence of OTC syringe purchase among African American IDUs was significantly lower compared with that among white IDUs. The latter finding was thought to relate to the fact that several predominantly African American neighborhoods had few or no OTC syringe-selling pharmacies, meaning more extensive travel was required for IDUs wishing to purchase syringes.

Alexandra Lutnick, Patricia Case, and Alex H. Kral opine in "Injection Drug Users' Perspectives on Placing HIV Prevention and Other Clinical Services in Pharmacy Settings" (*Journal of Urban Health*, vol. 89, no. 2, April 2012) that expanding pharmacy services to IDUs may help address the low utilization of health care services in this population. The researchers interviewed 11 IDUs in San Francisco to find out their feelings about accessing health services in pharmacies. They find that while those surveyed would like to see additional services offered in pharmacies, respondents were concerned about being judged or treated poorly by pharmacists and other pharmacy personnel. Lutnick, Case, and Kral observe that "pharmacy-based interventions will only be of use to IDUs if the interventions are delivered in a professional manner."

PHYSICIANS SUPPORT ACCESS TO STERILE SYRINGES FOR IDUS. In many states syringe prescription laws effectively block access to sterile syringes for IDUs. Pharmacists may be reluctant to sell syringes to suspected IDUs, and police may take possession of syringes or arrest IDUs who cannot demonstrate a medical need, other than injection drug use of illegal drugs, for the syringes they possess. These barriers could be eliminated by physician prescription of syringes.

Grace E. Macalino et al. conducted the first national survey of physicians to determine their willingness to prescribe syringes for IDUs and reported the results in "A National Physician Survey on Prescribing Syringes as an HIV Prevention Measure" (*Substance Abuse Treatment, Prevention, and Policy*, vol. 4, June 8, 2009). The researchers find that despite the fact that physicians have, in general, never actually prescribed syringes to IDUs, most would consider doing so. Macalino et al. conclude, "The physicians in our study were generally amenable to participating in syringe prescription programs, but physician willingness to act can be supported by better communication of what constitutes evidence-based practice, alleviation of legal concerns, and explicit validation by peers and professional organizations. Requiring substance abuse as a subject in medical training and continuing medical education would also promote better care for IDUs."

Legal Barriers to Federal Funding of SEPs

Despite the preponderance of evidence from myriad sources that SEPs are effective strategies for the prevention of HIV transmission, the federal government, as well as most local and state governments, have not made them legal. They argue that taxpayers should not finance illicit drug use. Since 1988 Congress has passed at least six laws that contain provisions that specifically prohibit or restrict the use of federal funds for SEPs and activities. The Comprehensive Alcohol Abuse, Drug Abuse, and Mental Health Amendments Act of 1988 requires states, as a condition for receiving block grant funds, to agree that funds will not be used "to carry out any program of distributing sterile needles for the hypodermic injection of any illegal drug or bleach for the purpose of cleansing needles for such hypodermic injection."

SEP advocates were heartened by a February 2011 determination by Regina Benjamin (1956–), the U.S. surgeon general. In "Determination That a Demonstration Needle Exchange Program Would Be Effective in Reducing Drug Abuse and the Risk of Acquired Immune Deficiency Syndrome Infection among Intravenous Drug Users" (*Federal Register*, vol. 76, no. 36, February 23, 2011), Benjamin opined that SEPs "would be effective in reducing drug abuse and the risk of infection with the etiologic agent for acquired immune deficiency syndrome" and that the scientific evidence supporting the health benefits of SEPs fulfills "the statutory requirement permitting the expenditure of Substance Abuse Prevention and Treatment (SAPT) Block Grant funds."

In February 2011 the Obama administration designated needle exchanges as a drug treatment program, allowing federal money allocated to treat addictions to be used to distribute syringes and needles to IDUs. According to Scott McCabe, in "White House Moves to Fund Needle Exchanges as Drug Treatment" (WashingtonExaminer.com, March 19, 2012), Benjamin indicated "that needle exchange programs can serve as a gateway to treatment for drug addiction, HIV and other diseases" and endorsed the use of federal funds. However, later that year Congress reinstated the ban.

William Martin observes in "Marijuana Prohibition: Going up in Smoke? and Sterile Syringes for Injecting Drug Users" (Rice University James A. Baker III Institute for Public Policy, *2013 Policy Recommendations for the Obama Administration*, 2013) that U.S. medical and public health workers and professional societies—including the National Academy of Science, the CDC, the American Medical Association, the Institute of Medicine, the National Institutes of Health, the American Public Health Association, and the American Bar Association—"overwhelmingly support making sterile syringes available to injecting drug users." He reports that 49 states and the District of Columbia permit syringe exchange, but notes that "resistance to funding at federal, state, and local levels has hampered the success of SEPs in some areas."

Martin explains that research conclusively demonstrates that access to sterile needles does not encourage people to start injecting drugs nor does it increase drug use by IDUs. He also observes that the cost-savings are substantial, pointing out that a clean needle costs "less than a dime." Martin recommends that the federal government "remove the ban on the use of federal funds to programs and projects that provide sterile syringes to injecting drug users as a proven means of reducing the spread of blood-borne diseases such as HIV/AIDS and hepatitis C" and "authorize federal funding and encourage other forms of governmental and nongovernmental funding for programs that increase the availability of sterile syringes to injecting drug users." He also advises the Obama administration to "allow funds from the President's Emergency Plan for AIDS Relief (PEPFAR) to be used to provide sterile syringes to injecting drug users."

CHAPTER 9
HIV AND AIDS WORLDWIDE

Even as the global economic recovery remains uncertain, our vision of getting to zero new HIV infections, zero discrimination and zero AIDS-related deaths remains high on the international agenda.

—Michel Sidibé, Joint United Nations Programme on HIV/AIDS Executive Director and Under Secretary-General of the United Nations, *Global Report: UNAIDS Report on the Global AIDS Epidemic, 2012* (2012)

SCOPE OF THE PROBLEM

Few factors have changed global demographics as inalterably as the HIV/AIDS pandemic (worldwide epidemic). According to the Joint United Nations Programme on HIV/ AIDS (UNAIDS), in *Global Report: UNAIDS Report on the Global AIDS Epidemic, 2012* (2012, http://www.unaids.org/ en/media/unaids/contentassets/documents/epidemiology/ 2012/gr2012/20121120_UNAIDS_Global_Report_2012 _with_annexes_en.pdf), an estimated 34 million people were living with HIV/AIDS at the end of 2011.

The number of new HIV infections reported each year continues to decline from a peak of 3.2 million in 1997 to approximately 2.5 million in 2011. The decline in HIV incidence is attributable not only to the efficacy (the ability of an intervention to produce the intended diagnostic or therapeutic effect in optimal circumstances) of HIV prevention activities but also to the natural course of HIV epidemics. The prevalence of HIV in a population does not increase indefinitely, because at some point the population is saturated. Generally, after the initial spread of HIV there is likely to be a decrease in the incidence of infection, which results in a decrease in prevalence.

The HIV/AIDS pandemic is actually many separate epidemics, each with its own distinctive origin and shaped by specific geography and populations. Each epidemic involves different risk behaviors and practices, such as unprotected sex with multiple partners or sharing injection drug equipment. According to UNAIDS, some

countries have made tremendous strides in expanding and ensuring access to treatment. It also notes that there has been progress in advancing HIV prevention programs— new HIV infections are declining in many countries that have been hardest hit by the epidemic and some of the big epidemics in sub-Saharan Africa have stabilized or are beginning to decline.

However, the epidemics are not subsiding everywhere. In countries in eastern Europe and Central Asia—Bangladesh, Georgia, Guinea-Bissau, Indonesia, Kazakhstan, Kyrgyzstan, the Philippines, the Republic of Moldova, and Sri Lanka—the incidence of HIV rose by more than 25% between 2001 and 2011.

UNAIDS indicates that women continue to account for more than half of all people living with HIV infection. Outside of sub-Saharan Africa, HIV disproportionately affects injection drug users (IDUs), men who have sex with men (MSM), and sex workers. More women (68%) than men (47%) receive antiretroviral therapy (ART) in low- and middle-income countries and more adults (58%) than children (28%) receive treatment. Nonetheless, the Kaiser Family Foundation (KFF) reports in "The Global HIV/ AIDS Epidemic" (October 10, 2013, http://kff.org/global- health-policy/fact-sheet/the-global-hivaids-epidemic/) that most people living with HIV/AIDS or at risk for HIV do not have access to prevention, care, and treatment.

Global Trends

UNAIDS explains in *Global Report: UNAIDS Report on the Global AIDS Epidemic, 2012* that although fewer people are becoming HIV infected and fewer are dying from AIDS, HIV/AIDS remains a global health problem of unprecedented dimensions.

According to the KFF, in "The Global HIV/AIDS Epidemic," the global prevalence rate (the percentage of people aged 15 to 49 years who are infected) has leveled since 2001 and was 0.8% in 2011. The KFF explains that

HIV disproportionately affects people during their most productive years—about 40% of all new infections occur in people under the age of 25 years. In the early 21st century the pandemic is beginning to stabilize. The number of people newly HIV infected and the number of AIDS-related deaths have declined. Rafael Lozano et al. report in "Global and Regional Mortality from 235 Causes of Death for 20 Age Groups in 1990 and 2010: A Systematic Analysis for the Global Burden of Disease Study 2010" (*Lancet*, vol. 380, no. 9859, December 15, 2012) that deaths from HIV/AIDS peaked at 1.7 million in 2006. Also heartening is the fact that even in countries with few resources, more people with HIV are being treated—in 2003 just over 400,000 people were receiving treatment; by 2011 this number increased to 8 million.

In "A New Infectious Disease Model for Estimating and Projecting HIV/AIDS Epidemics" (*Sexually Transmitted Infections*, vol. 8, suppl. 2, December 2012), Le Bao of Pennsylvania State University observes that as the global HIV pandemic enters its fourth decade, countries have collected more surveillance data, and the AIDS-related mortality has been substantially reduced by the increasing availability and use of ART. Bao presents a model that enables the HIV infection rate to change over the years in response to past prevalence and the past infection rate as the epidemic in a country stabilizes. This model also considers the impact of prevention programs and helps policy makers and planners grade their epidemics as generalized, concentrated, or low level. In generalized epidemics HIV prevalence is more than 1% in pregnant women in urban areas. By contrast, in low-level and concentrated epidemics HIV infection is not at a significant level in the general population, although in concentrated epidemics it is high in at-risk populations such as IDUs and MSM.

PATTERNS OF INFECTION

Globally, HIV/AIDS is primarily a sexually transmitted infection (STI) that is transmitted through unprotected sexual intercourse between men and women or MSM. Like some other STIs, HIV infection can also be spread through blood, blood products, donated organs, semen, or vaginal fluids and perinatally from a pregnant mother to her unborn child. The majority of worldwide cumulative (over the entire time that statistics have been kept) HIV infections in adults are estimated to have been transmitted through heterosexual intercourse, although the relative proportion of infections resulting from heterosexual contact as opposed to MSM varies greatly in different parts of the world.

More than 90% of children with HIV acquired the virus perinatally, during birth, or through breastfeeding. The balance were infected by contaminated injections,

transfusion with infected blood, sexual abuse, or sexual intercourse.

HIV-1 and HIV-2

Kevin Peterson et al. explain in "Antiretroviral Therapy for HIV-2 Infection: Recommendations for Management in Low-Resource Settings" (*AIDS Research and Treatment*, February 9, 2011) that two types of HIV have been recognized and identified: HIV-1, the predominant worldwide virus, and HIV-2. HIV-2 has much lower rates of progression and infectivity than does HIV-1, and the majority of people that become infected are likely to be long-term nonprogressors (people who become infected but do not develop AIDS). HIV-2 also responds differently to antiretroviral drugs and is frequently resistant to two of the major classes of antiretroviral drugs—the fusion inhibitors and the nonnucleoside reverse transcriptase inhibitors—that are the standard treatment for HIV-1.

HIV-1 and HIV-2 also show an extraordinary difference in global distribution. In North and South America HIV-1 has reached pandemic proportions among certain risk groups, primarily through MSM and IDUs. Some African and Asian countries have also experienced extensive heterosexual transmission of HIV-1. HIV-2 is largely restricted to West Africa, where it is mostly attributable to heterosexual transmission and accounts for one-third of the HIV prevalence cases. Other countries with sizable populations infected with HIV-2 are European countries with colonial links to West Africa, such as France, Portugal, and the United Kingdom, as well as other countries with previous Portuguese ties, such as Angola, Brazil, India, and Mozambique.

In "Characteristics of HIV-2 and HIV-1/HIV-2 Dually Seropositive Adults in West Africa Presenting for Care and Antiretroviral Therapy: The IeDEA-West Africa HIV-2 Cohort Study" (*PLoS One*, vol. 8, no. 6, June 18, 2013), Didier K. Ekouevi et al. observe that HIV-2 is widespread in West Africa and many people are infected with both HIV-1 and HIV-2. The researchers also note that HIV-2 may be underreported because antibody cross-reactivity between HIV-1 and HIV-2 is common and often results in misdiagnosis of HIV-2 as HIV-1 or dual infection. Ekouevi et al. assert that clinical trials to determine optimal treatment for people with dual infection are needed.

DIFFERENCES IN EPIDEMIOLOGY, INCIDENCE, AND TRANSMISSION. The epidemiological characteristics (factors such as distribution, incidence, and prevalence that determine the presence, extent, or absence of a disease) of HIV-2 are different from those of HIV-1. Perhaps reflecting these differences, the international spread of HIV-2 is quite limited. During the early course of infection, people with HIV-2 are less infectious than those with HIV-1. This is due to the low levels of the virus isolated from the blood of immunodeficient people with HIV-2. Over time, as an individual's immunodeficiency progresses, HIV-2 probably becomes more infectious, but this more infectious period is relatively shorter than for HIV-1 and tends to occur in older individuals.

According to Elizabeth Pádua et al., in "Assessment of Mother-to-Child HIV-1 and HIV-2 Transmission: An AIDS Reference Laboratory Collaborative Study" (*HIV Medicine*, vol. 10, no. 3, March 2009), multiple studies demonstrate evidence that HIV-2 is not frequently transmitted from mother to child. Although the mechanics of perinatal transmission are not completely understood, advanced immunodeficiency of the mother is certainly a risk factor. Low levels of the virus are not sufficient to transmit to the baby, and higher levels of virus infection in women past childbearing years may explain why perinatal transmission is less frequent. This is the most likely explanation for the observation that HIV-2 infection is so rare in children.

Interactions and HIV Transmission

One of the major concerns of public health officials worldwide is the possible interaction between HIV and other infections. The same risky behaviors that expose individuals to potential HIV infection also expose them to other STIs, such as gonorrhea, syphilis, and chancroid (a genital ulcer). Considerable data suggest that STIs, particularly herpes simplex, chancroid, and syphilis (which all cause ulcerative lesions), promote the transmission of HIV.

In "Herpes Simplex Virus Type 2: Epidemiology and Management Options in Developing Countries" (*Postgraduate Medical Journal*, vol. 84, no. 992, 2008), Gabriela Paz-Bailey et al. observe that genital herpes simplex virus type 2 is highly prevalent worldwide and is an increasingly important cause of genital ulcer disease, which in turn increases the risk of HIV transmission and acquisition. The researchers call for actions "to improve recognition of genital herpes, to prevent its spread and also to prevent its potential to promote HIV transmission in developing countries."

TUBERCULOSIS. HIV infection is recognized as the strongest known risk factor for the development of active tuberculosis (TB), because people with a latent TB infection are more apt to develop the disease once their immune system has been compromised by HIV. According to the World Health Organization (WHO), in *Guidelines for Intensified Tuberculosis Case-Finding and Isoniazid Preventive Therapy for People Living with HIV in Resource-Constrained Settings* (2011, http://whqlibdoc.who.int/publications/2011/9789241500708_eng.pdf), people with HIV have 20 to 37 times the risk of developing TB as people without HIV infection. More than one-quarter of all deaths of people with HIV are attributable to TB.

UNAIDS confirms in *Global Report: UNAIDS Report on the Global AIDS Epidemic, 2012* that although TB was still a leading cause of death among people with HIV between 2004 and 2011, TB-related deaths among people living with HIV/AIDS fell 25% worldwide, which translates into an estimated 1.3 million lives saved. Nearly 80% of all people living with HIV/AIDS and TB are in sub-Saharan Africa.

People infected with HIV who test tuberculin-positive are not only more likely to develop TB but also are more likely to develop TB more rapidly than people without HIV infection. An even more disastrous consequence is that half of all people infected with both will develop contagious TB, which they could then spread to susceptible people, even those not infected with HIV.

The WHO 2011 guidelines offer recommendations that are intended to reduce TB in people living with HIV/AIDS, their families, and their communities via a combination of screening for TB and preventive therapy. The guidelines advise screening all people with HIV for TB and treating those with positive test results prophylactically (to prevent the disease). Furthermore, they advise starting all HIV-infected people who also have active TB on ART regardless of their CD4 cell counts.

ART reduces the risk of TB among HIV-infected people by 65%. However, UNAIDS reports that fewer than half (48%) of the people living with both HIV and TB received ART in 2011. In sub-Saharan Africa only 46% of the people living with both HIV and TB began HIV treatment. Although there are high rates of infection with HIV and TB in 41 countries, there are only six countries (Angola, Brazil, Cambodia, Burma [Myanmar], Rwanda, and Sudan) in which more than 75% of such patients are receiving ART.

Highly Drug-Resistant Tuberculosis

In *HIV and Tuberculosis: Ensuring Universal Access and Protection of Human Rights* (March 2010, http://data.unaids.org/pub/ExternalDocument/2010/20100324_unaidsrghrtsissuepapertbhrts_en.pdf), UNAIDS observes that people living with HIV/AIDS are more likely to have multidrug-resistant tuberculosis (MDR-TB; this type of TB does not respond to two first-line anti-TB drugs—rifampicin and isoniazid) than people who are not HIV infected. Extensively drug-resistant tuberculosis (XDR-TB; this type of TB does not respond to first- and second-line anti-TB drug treatment) is associated with extremely high mortality rates in people with HIV/AIDS.

To a large extent, drug-resistant TB occurs in response to inadequate TB control, poor patient or clinician adherence to TB treatment regimens, poor-quality drugs, or a lack of drug supplies. People living with HIV/AIDS are particularly vulnerable to developing drug-resistant TB because of their compromised immune system, which makes them more susceptible to infection and more likely to progress to active TB.

Disparities in access to health care and the quality of health care exacerbate the problem of drug-resistant TB in developing countries. MDR- and XDR-TB arose largely in response to inadequate care of poor and neglected populations. Inappropriate drug choices, drug doses, and duration of treatment, as well as an irregular supply of drugs, poorly trained personnel, and poor adherence to treatment, all act to increase the development and transmission of drug-resistant TB.

Promising Research

New anti-TB drugs are urgently needed to overcome drug resistance and to eliminate TB as a public health threat. Keith D. Green and Sylvie Garneau-Tsodikova explain in "Resistance in Tuberculosis: What Do We Know and Where Can We Go?" (*Frontiers in Microbiology*, vol. 4, July 23, 2013) that current strategies focus on generating compounds that will avoid or overcome the defenses of Mycobacterium tuberculosis (Mtb). Research is being carried out to find new compounds that will disrupt deoxyribonucleic acid, cell membrane biosynthesis, and general cellular metabolism. Other studies combine drugs to achieve effects greater than those achieved by either alone.

In "Antituberculosis Thiophenes Define a Requirement for Pks13 in Mycolic Acid Biosynthesis" (*Nature Chemical Biology*, vol. 9, no. 8, August 2013), Regina Wilson et al. report on a new class of compounds that kill Mtb by dissolving its protective fatty coating. The compounds, known as thiophenes, killed Mtb in the laboratory by disabling an enzyme that connects the fatty acids that coat the bacterium. More important, it appears that TB does not develop resistance to this class of compounds. Researchers hope that these compounds may be used to develop more effective TB treatment.

UNAIDS Calls for TB Testing of Every Person Living with HIV/AIDS

In the press release "UNAIDS Calls for Zero Parallel Systems for HIV and TB" (March 24, 2013, http://www.unaids.org/en/resources/presscentre/pressreleaseandstatementarchive/2013/march/20130324psworldtbday/), Michel Sidibé (1952–), the executive director of UNAIDS, calls for zero parallel systems for HIV and TB. This means "every person living with HIV/AIDS is tested for TB and that every person with TB is offered an HIV test, and people with TB who are HIV-positive are started on antiretroviral treatment immediately."

Geographic Differences

In North America and Europe during the 1980s and early 1990s, HIV was transmitted predominantly through unprotected sexual intercourse among MSM and through IDUs with contaminated needles. During the late 1990s heterosexual intercourse and injection drug use became the prevailing modes of HIV transmission in North America and Europe.

In sub-Saharan Africa the overwhelming mode of transmission has been heterosexual intercourse. In this part of the world, transmission through MSM contact or through injection drug use is slight. Because many women have been infected, preventing perinatal transmission is increasingly important. UNAIDS notes in *Global Report: UNAIDS Report on the Global AIDS Epidemic, 2012* that the increasing numbers and percentages of HIV-infected pregnant women receiving antiretroviral drugs (57%) to prevent mother-to-child transmission of HIV has effectively reduced transmission. Nonetheless, in 32 countries, including 12 with high prevalence of HIV infection, some pregnant women were not receiving the optimal regimen of ART to prevent transmission in 2011.

The rates of MSM transmission in Latin America are similar to those of Europe and the United States, injection drug use transmission is less frequent, and heterosexual transmission is considerably higher. Furthermore, there are high rates of transmission among IDUs and sex workers and their clients. In South and Southeast Asia the rapid increase of HIV can be traced to shared contaminated injection equipment and heterosexual intercourse. According to UNAIDS, in *2012 China AIDS Response Progress Report* (March 31, 2012, http://www.unaids.org/en/dataanalysis/knowyourresponse/countryprogressreports/2012countries/ce_CN_Narrative_Report[1].pdf), in 2011 almost half of HIV-infected people living in China were infected via sexual transmission. Infections resulting from sexual transmission increased from 33.1% in 2006 to 76.3% in 2011. Of these, 13.7% were attributable to homosexual transmission in 2011, up from 2.5% in 2006. More than one-quarter (28.4%) of infections resulted from IDUs.

Similarly, Aditi Tandon reports in "Punjab Has Highest HIV Rate among Injecting Drug Users" (TribuneIndia.com, December 1, 2012) that Indian government data show that contaminated injection drug equipment is also a significant risk factor for HIV infection in India, with an overall prevalence rate of 7.1%. The highest reported rates were in Punjab (21.1%), Delhi (18.3%), Maharashtra (14.2%), Manipur (12.9%), Mizoram (12%), Chandigarh (7.2%), Odisha (7.2%), and Meghalaya (6.4%).

The highest national HIV infection levels in Asia continue to be found in Southeast Asia, where combinations of unsafe practices with sex workers and MSM, along with IDUs, continue to fuel and maintain the epidemics. Although the HIV infection rate has peaked and leveled off in other parts of the world, it is escalating in Bangladesh, China, Indonesia, Pakistan, and Vietnam, largely from heterosexual intercourse and through sex workers.

Unless otherwise noted, the following data and statistics, which describe the epidemics in various regions and countries, are drawn from UNAIDS reports. UNAIDS and the WHO provide the most recent and reliable estimates of HIV incidence and prevalence, generally from 2009 to 2011.

AFRICA
North Africa and the Middle East

Unreliable and often inadequate HIV surveillance systems complicate an accurate assessment of the patterns and trends of the epidemics in many countries in North Africa and the Middle East, especially among high-risk populations—IDUs, MSM, and sex workers and their clients. UNAIDS (November 2012, http://www.unaids.org/en/media/unaids/contentassets/documents/epidemiology/2012/gr2012/2012_FS_regional_mena_en.pdf) reports that the number of new HIV infections in the region increased more than 35%, from 27,000 in 2001 to 37,000 in 2011. In 2011 approximately 300,000 people in the region were living with HIV/AIDS.

The Middle East and North Africa is the only region where there has not yet been a reduction in the number of children newly infected with HIV. This is likely due to the fact that there has been little progress made in the provision of ART to prevent mother-to-child transmission—only 7% of HIV-positive pregnant women were estimated to have received treatment in 2011. Similarly, the percentage of people eligible for ART that received it was also low—just 15%. Access and continuity of HIV treatment is a critical issue in the epidemic in the Middle East and North Africa and as a result the region experienced an increase of 17% in AIDS-related deaths, from 20,000 in 2005 to 23,000 in 2011.

Improved data collection and surveillance in some countries such as Algeria, Iran, Libya, and Morocco show that HIV epidemics do exist across the region and that an epidemic continues in Sudan. In Algeria and Morocco the majority of reported HIV infections are attributable to unprotected sex, and women make up a growing proportion of people living with HIV/AIDS.

The largest epidemic in the region is in Sudan. The HIV epidemic in Sudan is attributable to heterosexual transmission of the virus. Here, as in other countries, an increasing number of women are acquiring the virus from husbands or boyfriends who became infected from injection drug use or paid sex. UNAIDS indicates in *Global AIDS Response Progress Reporting 2010–2011: Sudan* (March 2012, http://www.unaids.org/en/data analysis/knowyourresponse/countryprogressreports/2012 countries/ce_SD_Narrative_Report[1].pdf) that in 2012 rates of HIV testing among MSM were low, ranging from 3.3% to 15.4%, and that between 8% and 25.8% of men reported the use of a condom the last time they had anal sex with a male

partner. Fewer than 10% of eligible adults and children received ART and just 6.7% of young people aged 15 to 24 years had comprehensive knowledge of HIV transmission.

Unparalleled Infection Rates

UNAIDS reports in *Global Report: UNAIDS Report on the Global AIDS Epidemic, 2012* that in 2011, 69% (23.5 million) of the people living with HIV/AIDS worldwide were in sub-Saharan Africa. Although it remains the most severely affected region, the number of new HIV infections in the region decreased 25% between 2001 and 2011, from an estimated 2.4 million to 1.8 million. In 13 countries new infections decreased by 50% or more. The region is home to 92% of pregnant women living with HIV/AIDS, but in 2011 more than half (59%) received ART.

Despite these decreases, 71% of the adults and children newly infected in 2011 were in sub-Saharan Africa. Although AIDS deaths decreased 32% between 2005 and 2011, the region still accounted for 70% of all AIDS-related deaths in 2011.

The national prevalence rates (the number of cases of the disease present in a specified population at a given time) of HIV infection among adults vary widely, even within a given country. For example, Swaziland has the highest HIV prevalence in the region. In *Swaziland Country Report on Monitoring the Political Declaration on HIV and AIDS* (March 2012, http://www.unaids.org/en/dataanalysis/knowyourresponse/countryprogressreports/2012countries/ce_SZ_Narrative_Report[1].pdf), UNAIDS reports that 173,619 adults and 21,780 children were living with HIV/AIDS in 2010, and 41.1% of pregnant women were HIV positive. The highest prevalence rates were among women aged 25 to 29 years (49.2%) and men aged 35 to 39 years (44.9%). However, 40.8% of people aged 20 to 24 years and 20.4% of people aged 15 to 19 years were living with HIV/AIDS. Regardless, treatment rates are improving—80% of eligible people were receiving ART by the close of 2011.

SEVERAL MODES OF TRANSMISSION. Because heterosexual transmission is the predominant mode of transmission in Africa, men and women have been almost equally infected. However, UNAIDS finds that nearly six out of 10 (58%) people living with HIV/AIDS in sub-Saharan Africa were women and that social and economic inequality limit women's access to care and their ability to take measures to prevent infection, such as by insisting on condom use.

Sex workers and their customers play a significant role in the spread of HIV in many countries. For example, in 2011, 70% of sex workers in Swaziland were HIV infected. Besides migrant workers and prisoners, sex workers are considered to be the most at-risk population.

Mother-to-child transmission also contributes to the pandemic in eastern and southern Africa. UNAIDS (November 2012, http://www.unaids.org/en/media/unaids/contentassets/documents/epidemiology/2012/gr2012/2012_FS_regional_ssa_en.pdf) indicates that although the numbers of children newly infected with HIV in Burundi, Kenya, Namibia, South Africa, Togo, and Zambia declined between 40% and 59% from 2009 to 2011 and 14 other countries reported more modest declines, the numbers of new HIV infections in children increased in Angola, Congo, Equatorial Guinea, and Guinea-Bissau.

PAYING THE PRICE FOR YEARS OF EVASION. Although Kenya had experienced the ravages of AIDS for about a decade, the Kenyan parliament and cabinet did not debate the issue publicly until 1993. Physicians diagnosed the first AIDS cases in 1984, but the government did not issue national statistics until 1986, when it announced one AIDS-related death. The nation's president and vice president regularly warned the public in speeches to avoid infection, and national officials instructed district administrators, including local tribal chiefs, to encourage their people to practice safe sex and limit their partners, but there had been no official statement.

Since then, Kenya has instituted programs to address its epidemic. The National AIDS Control Council and the National AIDS and STI Control Programme report in *The Kenya AIDS Epidemic: Update 2011* (2012, http://www.unaids.org/en/dataanalysis/knowyourresponse/countryprogressreports/2012countries/ce_KE_Narrative_Report.pdf) that as of December 2011, 1.6 million people in Kenya were living with HIV/AIDS. The prevalence of HIV infection among adults was 6.2%, about 40% lower than the prevalence at the peak of the epidemic in 1993. The number of new infections in 2010 was about 33% lower than the number at the epidemic's peak, and the number of AIDS-related deaths in 2011 was approximately one-third the number of deaths reported each year between 2002 and 2004.

Some of this decline may be attributable to changing behaviors. Kenyans are less than half as likely to have multiple sex partners than they were during the late 1990s and condom use has increased dramatically. However, it is also believed that the lower prevalence of HIV infection may reflect the saturation of the infection in the at-risk population, meaning that the peak of the epidemic has passed and/or that deaths from AIDS have served to reduce HIV prevalence.

Gender inequality, sexual violence, and HIV stigma increase HIV risk and vulnerability, while long-standing social and cultural practices promote HIV transmission. For example, "wife inheritance," which was once a socially useful tradition, continues to contribute to the spread of HIV/AIDS. In western Kenya, when a woman is widowed, her former husband's family takes care of her and her children. For generations, a brother-in-law or male cousin took her in with his family. Initially, tradition frowned on his having sexual relations with the inherited wife. Eventually, the inheritors began to ignore this restriction and had sex with the widow. If the widow's former husband had died of AIDS, she was likely to be infected and could pass the virus on to her inheritor, who would pass it on to his wife, causing the disease to spread.

UGANDA'S EFFORTS TO REDUCE HIV INFECTION. Scientists think that during the early 1980s truck drivers first spread HIV in Uganda's Rakai District, which lies along a Lake Victoria trade route to the capital city of Kampala. Because commercial sex is widely available along the trade route, HIV quickly spread throughout Uganda and all of Africa. At one time, Uganda had the world's highest HIV infection rates. At the turn of the 21st century, it was one of only two developing nations (Thailand is the other) where there was nationwide evidence of declining HIV rates in response to strong prevention programs.

Uganda was the first African country to respond powerfully to its HIV/AIDS epidemic. The government began by gathering religious and traditional leaders, along with representatives of other sectors of society, in an effort to reach agreement that the problem had to be confronted. Prevention efforts targeted specific populations or communities. For example, prevention programs that focused on safe sex practices and/or delaying sex were presented in schools. Community groups were formed to counsel and support those living with the virus. Condom use was heavily promoted.

Unlike Kenya, Uganda began an aggressive campaign against the spread of HIV/AIDS during the mid-1980s, when it had the highest number of recorded HIV cases in Africa. With virtually every family touched by HIV/AIDS, much of the cultural, religious, and psychological stigma disappeared in Uganda, where HIV infection rates declined from a high of 18.5% in 1992 to 6.7% in 2011. Although education did prompt behavior changes that in turn resulted in lower HIV prevalence among pregnant women in Kampala and other cities from the early 1990s through the first decade of the 21st century, the decline was also due in part to increased AIDS mortality.

According to UNAIDS, a rise in multiple concurrent partnerships and a shift in the epidemic from people in casual relationships to those in long-term relationships has prevented the prevalence rate from declining further. UNAIDS reports in *Country Progress Report: Uganda* (April 2012, http://www.unaids.org/en/dataanalysis/knowyourresponse/countryprogressreports/2012countries/ce_UG_Narrative_Report[1].pdf) that the peak prevalence of the epidemic in 2011 was among people aged 35 to

39 years (10.3%). Comprehensive knowledge about how to prevent sexual transmission of HIV remained low in 2011—just 36.7% of women aged 15 to 24 years and 37.8% of men the same age.

The populations at greatest risk of HIV infection are female sex workers and their clients, MSM, people living in fishing communities, and plantation workers. The lowest HIV prevalence is among university students, presumably in large part because they have knowledge of how to prevent infection.

The number of new infections per year increased 11.4% between 2007–08 and 2009–10 and the number of new infections (128,980) was the fourth highest of the 53 countries in Africa. New infections in children under the age of 15 years fell 6.2% in part because ART coverage of expectant mothers increased. The percentage of HIV-infected pregnant women who received ART to reduce the risk of transmission rose from 73.1% in 2010 to 86.2% in 2011.

In "The Effects of an HIV Project on HIV and Non-HIV Services at Local Government Clinics in Urban Kampala" (*BMC International Health and Human Rights*, vol. 11, suppl. 1, March 9, 2011), Toru Matsubayashi et al. observe that there is "widespread consensus that weak health systems hamper the effective provision of HIV/AIDS services." The researchers examine the effects of an HIV/AIDS program that was funded by the President's Emergency Plan for AIDS Relief. Specifically, the program provided health care delivery to six government-run general clinics in Kampala. Besides analyzing the volume of services provided, the researchers interviewed patients to compare perceptions of the experiences of patients receiving HIV care and those receiving non-HIV care. More than 90% of all patients reported high levels of satisfaction with care. Matsubayashi et al. conclude that "when a collaboration is established to strengthen existing health systems, in addition to providing HIV/AIDS services in a setting in which other primary health care is being delivered, there are positive effects not only on HIV/AIDS services, but also on many other essential services," such as treatment for malaria and TB as well as for pediatric care and immunization. They also note that "there was no evidence that the HIV program had any deleterious effects on health services offered at the clinics studied."

EUROPE
Western and Central Europe
HIV in western and central Europe is spread primarily through MSM. However, according to UNAIDS (November 2012, http://www.unaids.org/en/media/unaids/contentassets/documents/epidemiology/2012/gr2012/2012_FS_regional_nawce_en.pdf), in 2011 less than one out of three MSM were tested for HIV in the past 12 months. In 2011,

900,000 people were living with HIV/AIDS, up from 640,000 in 2001. The number of new infections rose slightly, from 29,000 in 2001 to 30,000 in 2011. The number of AIDS-related deaths decreased from 7,800 in 2005 to 7,000 in 2011.

THE UNITED KINGDOM. According to UNAIDS, in *UNGASS Country Progress Report: United Kingdom* (July 2010, http://www.unaids.org/en/dataanalysis/knowyourresponse/countryprogressreports/2010countries/unitedkingdom_2010_country_progress_report_en.pdf), at the close of 2008 an estimated 83,000 people were living with HIV/AIDS in the United Kingdom. Of this total, more than one-quarter (27%) of these were unaware of their infection status. Fifty percent of the 7,382 new HIV infections diagnosed in 2008 were attributable to heterosexual transmission and 42% were in MSM. Just 185 (2.5% of cases) were diagnosed as IDUs. The low prevalence of HIV in IDUs is attributable to the institution of needle exchange programs during the 1980s. UNAIDS reports in *Global Report: UNAIDS Report on the Global AIDS Epidemic, 2012* that just 1% of IDUs were living with HIV/AIDS in 2011. Furthermore, 81% of IDUs said they had used sterile injecting equipment the last time they injected drugs in 2009.

Since the mid-1990s AIDS diagnoses have declined significantly, from a peak of 1,882 in 1994 to 700 in 2008; likewise, AIDS-related deaths decreased during this same period, from 1,726 to 571. In 2011 less than 500 deaths were attributable to AIDS. Rates of diagnosis of HIV in pregnant women have increased, from 70% in 1999 to 90% in 2008, and 95% of pregnant women received HIV testing.

THE NETHERLANDS. UNAIDS (2013, http://www.unaids.org/en/regionscountries/countries/netherlands/) reports that in the Netherlands an estimated 25,000 people were living with HIV/AIDS in 2011, up from 19,000 in 2001. Less than 200 deaths were attributable to AIDS and there were less than 500 orphans aged 0 to 17 years.

In *Global Report: UNAIDS Report on the Global AIDS Epidemic, 2012*, UNAIDS indicates that HIV prevalence was 0.2% in 2011. An estimated 15% of MSM and less than 10% of IDUs were living with HIV/AIDS. About three-quarters (74%) of IDUs received an HIV test in the preceding 12 months and knew their test results. An even higher percentage (82%) of sex workers had been tested in the past 12 months and knew their results. However, safe sex practice was not as high; in 2011 just 42% of men said they had used a condom the last time they had anal sex with a male partner and only 58% of MSM said they had an HIV test in the past 12 months and knew their results.

SPAIN. Historically, Spain had the highest number of HIV/AIDS cases per capita in the European Union. The

Institute of Health Carlos III (2013, http://www.isciii.es/) indicates that the first case of HIV was reported in Spain in 1981; by the end of 2001, 110,000 to 150,000 people were living with HIV/AIDS. UNAIDS estimates in *Global Report: UNAIDS Report on the Global AIDS Epidemic, 2012* that 150,000 people were living with HIV/AIDS in 2011. The number of deaths attributable to AIDS decreased dramatically, from 2,100 in 2001 to fewer than 100 in 2011.

In 2011 just 2% of sex workers were living with HIV/AIDS, a decrease of one percentage point from 2009. During the same period the percentage of IDUs living with HIV/AIDS fell from 20% to 16%. However, the percentage of MSM who had an HIV test in the past 12 months and knew the results fell from 87% in 2009 to 44% in 2011. Likewise, the percentage of men who reported using a condom the last time they had anal sex with a man fell from 66% in 2009 to 59% in 2011.

The article "Spain's War on AIDS Visits the Prado" (NYTimes.com, August 27, 1997) explains that drug use in Spain began to increase during the 1970s and 1980s, after the long Francisco Franco (1892–1975) dictatorship ended. Isabel Noguer of the Ministry of Health describes this period as a time of heavy heroin use, with addicts sharing infected needles. In 1997 IDUs still made up the highest risk group, whereas unprotected heterosexual relations was the next most common form of transmission. By 2003 HIV prevalence among IDUs declined in cities that had instituted effective long-standing harm reduction programs. In *Global Report: UNAIDS Report on the Global AIDS Epidemic, 2010* (2010, http://www.unaids.org/globalreport/documents/20101123_GlobalReport_full_en.pdf), UNAIDS notes that in 2006 Spain was one of just eight countries that provided comprehensive harm reduction programs, which included needle and syringe exchange and treatment programs for IDUs in prisons.

Marta Torrens et al. observe in "Methadone Maintenance Treatment in Spain: The Success of a Harm Reduction Approach" (*Bulletin of the World Health Organization*, vol. 91, no. 2, February 2013) that during the 1980s and 1990s Spain was the European country with the highest number of AIDS cases attributable to injection drug use. The researchers describe the HIV epidemic in Spanish prisons and how the implementation of comprehensive harm reduction, including needle and syringe exchange programs, significantly reduced both the incidence and prevalence of HIV/AIDS.

Eastern Europe and Central Asia

The HIV pandemic did not reach eastern Europe until the mid-1990s. According to UNAIDS, in *Global Report: UNAIDS Report on the Global AIDS Epidemic, 2012*, after sub-Saharan Africa, eastern Europe and Central Asia is one of the regions hardest hit by the epidemic, with 1% of

adults living with HIV/AIDS in 2011. Changes in HIV prevalence in eastern Europe and Central Asia varied by country. For example, between 2001 and 2011 it was unchanged in Armenia and Ukraine but increased in Azerbaijan, Belarus, Georgia, Kazakhstan, and Kyrgyzstan. The numbers of people living with HIV/AIDS increased throughout the region. Between 2001 and 2011 the most dramatic increases were in Belarus, where the number rose from 4,900 to 20,000, and in Kazakhstan, where the number rose from 9,200 to 19,000.

Between 2001 and 2011 the numbers of new infections decreased in Belarus but increased in Georgia, Kazakhstan, Kyrgyzstan, the Republic of Moldova, and Tajikistan. The sharpest increase in new infections was reported in Kyrgyzstan, which had less than 500 in 2001 and an estimated 3,000 in 2011.

Just one-quarter of people eligible to receive ART were receiving it in 2011. The percentage of women receiving ART to prevent mother-to-child transmission varied by country, from lows of 15% in Armenia and Tajikistan to more than 95% in the Russian Federation and Ukraine. The number of newly infected children decreased 13% from 2009 to 2011. Between 2001 and 2011 AIDS-related deaths increased 21% throughout the region, more than doubling in Ukraine from 9,000 in 2001 to 22,000 in 2011.

UNAIDS indicates that although injection drug use is the "main mode of HIV transmission" in the region, there are few harm reduction programs in place, and there is very limited access to drug rehabilitation services. Furthermore, because possession of even small amounts of narcotics is harshly punished in many countries in eastern Europe and Central Asia, IDUs are understandably reluctant to participate in needle exchange programs.

ASIA

Asia could eventually overtake Africa as the continent most affected by HIV. The HIV/AIDS pandemic arrived in Asia much later than in the rest of the world. Until the mid-1990s HIV/AIDS was uncommon, but because the average incubation period is approximately 10 years, more people are now beginning to die from the disease. UNAIDS estimates in *Global Report: UNAIDS Report on the Global AIDS Epidemic, 2012* that in South and Southeast Asia 4 million adults and 280,000 children were infected with HIV in 2011. The number of children acquiring HIV infection also declined 12% between 2009 and 2011. In 2011 an estimated 780,000 people in China, 15,000 in South Korea, 7,900 in Japan, and less than 1,000 in Mongolia were living with HIV/AIDS.

Thailand

The spread of HIV in Thailand is unprecedented. Thailand's commercial sex industry is notorious, and travel packages based on the availability of sex workers in Thailand are common in Asia (as they are in other countries, including the United States). In the capital city of Bangkok, brothels are found in virtually every neighborhood. Cheewanan Lertpiriyasuwat, Tanarak Plipat, and Richard Jenkins find in "A Survey of Sexual Risk Behavior for HIV Infection in Nakhonsawan, Thailand, 2001" (*AIDS*, vol. 17, no. 13, September 5, 2003) that in 1990, 20% of all Thai men reported having paid for sex in the previous year. After a military coup in 1991, the transitional government instituted a comprehensive HIV/AIDS education program, which included a media campaign and condom distribution to brothels and massage parlors. Brothels that refused to use condoms were closed down. Although the anti-HIV program came too late for those infected during the mid- to late 1980s, Thailand recorded a drop in new HIV infections until the late 1990s.

In *Thailand AIDS Response Progress Report 2012 Reporting Period: 2010–2011* (2012, http://www.unaids.org/en/dataanalysis/knowyourresponse/countryprogressreports/2012countries/ce_TH_Narrative_Report[1].pdf), UNAIDS notes that HIV continued to spread during the first decade of the 21st century in the general population, with no decreases in new infections or prevalence in key at-risk populations—female sex workers, MSM, and IDUs. In 2010 HIV prevalence among IDUs was 21.9% and some drug treatment centers report rates as high as 50%. At the close of 2011, 225,272 people living with HIV/AIDS were receiving ART—82% of women and 54% of men received treatment.

Deaths attributable to HIV were higher in adults than in children (8.9% versus 4.2%) and higher in men than in women (10.3% versus 7%). Late diagnosis and/or delayed entry into care and treatment are responsible for many of these deaths.

Some efforts to combat the epidemic have proven effective, whereas others have not been as successful as hoped. For example, HIV prevalence among female sex workers has steadily decreased from 2.8% in 2008 to 1.8% in 2011. More than 95% of female sex workers said they used condoms with their customers, and in 2008–10, 81% had been tested for HIV and knew the results of the test, up from 57% in 2004–07. In contrast, there have been declines in HIV knowledge and understanding and increases in high-risk behaviors—multiple sex partners and low rates of condom use—among youth.

Other Southeast Asian Countries

In other parts of Southeast Asia data about the epidemics reveal different patterns.

Cambodia has been the hardest hit country in the region. However, there is evidence that the epidemic is subsiding. In *Global Report: UNAIDS Report on the Global AIDS Epidemic, 2012*, UNAIDS finds that in 2011 there were an estimated 64,000 adults and children living with HIV/AIDS and 1,400 deaths attributable to AIDS. HIV prevalence in Cambodia is declining. UNAIDS indicates in *Cambodia Country Progress Report* (March 2012, http://www.unaids.org/en/dataanalysis/knowyourresponse/countryprogressreports/2012countries/ce_KH_Narrative_Report[1].pdf) that in 2011 HIV prevalence among adults was 0.6%, down from 0.9% in 2006. Although heterosexual transmission and injection drug use remain the primary modes of transmission, the epidemic disproportionately affects at-risk populations—sex workers, MSM, transgender people, and IDUs. In 2010, 24% of IDUs, 13.9% of sex workers, and 2.1% of MSM were HIV infected.

An estimated 53,100 people aged 15 years and older were living with HIV/AIDS in 2011, and there were 2,400 AIDS-related deaths. The number of people living with HIV/AIDS is steadily declining in response to fewer new infections, increased ART coverage, and effective HIV prevention programs. Increased ART coverage has also served to reduce the mortality rate of HIV-infected people.

Although Cambodia aims to reduce HIV transmission by half by 2015, young people's knowledge of how to prevent transmission did not improve between 2005 and 2010 and in some instances even decreased. The percentages of people reporting multiple partners decreased, but there was only a slight increase in condom use at last intercourse, from 39.9% in 2005 to 40.6% in 2010. However, condom use was high among teens, with 100% of males and females aged 15 to 19 years reporting their use; HIV prevalence in this age group fell from 0.4% in 2006 to 0.2% in 2010. There has also been a steady increase in the percentage of pregnant women receiving ART, from just 1.2% in 2003 to 63.5% in 2011.

India

At the International AIDS Conference held in Vancouver, Canada, in July 1996, a United Nations official reported that India had emerged as the country with the most people infected with HIV. This news came as a surprise to many of the conferees because HIV was not detected in India until 1986. According to UNAIDS, in *Global Report: UNAIDS Report on the Global AIDS Epidemic, 2010*, in 2009, the most recent year for which data were available as of October 2013, approximately 2.4 million people in India were HIV positive, down from 2.5 million in 2001. Of this total, an estimated 880,000 were women. In 2009, 170,000 deaths were attributable to AIDS.

In *UNGASS Country Progress Report: India* (March 31, 2010, http://www.unaids.org/en/dataanalysis/knowyourresponse/countryprogressreports/2010countries/india_2010_country_progress_report_en.pdf), UNAIDS notes that the epidemic is declining in most states in India. Most HIV infections are attributable to unprotected heterosexual relationships, and there is also overlap of IDUs and sex workers. Researchers speculate that more than 90% of women with HIV acquired the virus from their regular partners, who were infected during paid sex.

Sex trafficking and female sex workers contribute to the epidemic in many states. Jhumka Gupta et al. examine in "History of Sex Trafficking, Recent Experiences of Violence, and HIV Vulnerability among Female Sex Workers in Coastal Andhra Pradesh, India" (*International Journal of Gynecology and Obstetrics*, vol. 142, no. 2, August 2011) associations between sex trafficking and recent violence experiences and HIV vulnerability among female sex workers in Andhra Pradesh. The researchers find that one out of five female sex workers met the United Nations definition of sex trafficking (exploitation and abuse of people for revenue through sex) and that these sex workers were at increased risk for both violence and HIV.

According to Puspen Ghosh et al., in "Factors Associated with HIV Infection among Indian Women" (*International Journal of STD and AIDS*, vol. 22, no. 3, March 2011), the most common risk factor for HIV transmission for women is an exclusive sexual relationship with their husband. The researchers analyzed data from the National Family Health Survey 2005–06 to identify other risk factors. They find that women at highest risk were those aged 26 to 35 years, were impoverished, and had more than one sexual partner during their lifetime. Women with a history of a genital sore (a marker for other STIs) were also at increased risk. Because most HIV transmission in women takes place within marriage, Ghosh et al. advocate targeting risk-reduction programs to this population, especially in view of their finding of a low percentage of condom use by married men with their wife and other sexual partners.

China

The first HIV case in China was identified in 1985, but the disease did not begin to spread until the early 1990s, when changes in the structure of the economy produced an increase in drug use and prostitution. The U.S. embassy in China indicates in *Flying Blind on a Growing Epidemic: AIDS in China* (2002) that the government of China estimated in 1997 that between 100,000 and 300,000 people were living with HIV/AIDS. By the beginning of 1998 this estimate had doubled. According to UNAIDS, in *2012 China AIDS Response Progress Report*, in 2011 an estimated 780,000 people were living with HIV/AIDS in China. Of these, 46.5% were infected through heterosexual transmission, 28.4% through injection drug use, 17.4% through MSM, 6.6% were former blood donors or transfusion recipients, and 1.1% were infected via mother-to-child transmission. That same year

an estimated 39,183 new cases were diagnosed and 21,234 deaths were attributed to AIDS.

As in other countries, HIV transmission and infection in China have migrated from the traditional high-risk populations—sex workers, IDUs, and the overlap of these populations—to the general population, and as a result the number of HIV infections in women is growing. Although the HIV epidemic remains one of low prevalence overall, infections resulting from heterosexual transmission increased from 33.1% in 2006 to 76.3% in 2011. Likewise, the proportion arising from homosexual transmission increased from 2.5% in 2006 to 13.7% in 2011.

In 2011 HIV prevalence among sex workers was 0.3%. The percentage of sex workers that was tested for HIV in the past 12 months and knew their test results increased from 36.9% in 2009 to 38.2% in 2011. During the same period the percentage of sex workers using a condom during the last sex act increased from 85.1% to 87.5%.

In 2011 HIV prevalence among MSM was 6.3%. The percentage of MSM that was tested for HIV in the past 12 months and knew their test results increased from 44.9% in 2009 to 50.4% in 2011. During the same period the percentage of MSM using a condom during the last sex act was unchanged—74.1%.

The percentage of IDUs infected with HIV fell from 9.3% in 2009 to 6.4% in 2011. Over 900 needle and syringe exchange sites have been established in 19 provinces, and they distribute more than 12 million clean needles and syringes each year.

The total number of people ever receiving and currently receiving ART rose from 81,739 and 65,481, respectively, in 2009 to 155,530 and 126,448, respectively, in 2011. About three-quarters (74.1%) of HIV-positive pregnant women received ART in 2011. Because of this preventive measure, HIV prevalence in children born to women living with HIV/AIDS decreased from 8.1% in 2009 to 7.4% in 2011. The majority (85.2%) of HIV-positive children received ART.

Although AIDS deaths have declined in China, some observers, such as Jane Qiu, in "Stigma of HIV Imperils Hard-Won Strides in Saving Lives" (*Science*, vol. 332, no. 6035, June 10, 2011), Talha Khan Burki, in "Discrimination against People with HIV Persists in China" (*Lancet*, vol. 377, no. 9762, January 2011), and Laurie Abler et al., in "Affected by HIV Stigma: Interpreting Results from a Population Survey of an Urban Center in Guangxi, China" (*AIDS and Behavior*, July 27, 2013), are concerned that stigma about homosexuality and discrimination against people living with HIV/AIDS may hamper China's efforts to further reduce the size of its epidemic. People with HIV are often barred from education and employment opportunities and may be demoted or forced to resign. Hospitals and universities frequently disclose workers' HIV test results to employers and policies regarding confidentiality and consent vary from one province to the next.

CENTRAL AND SOUTH AMERICA

UNAIDS (November 2012, http://www.unaids.org/en/media/unaids/contentassets/documents/epidemiology/2012/gr2012/2012_FS_regional_la_caribbean_en.pdf) indicates that the number of new HIV infections in Central and South America is on the decline. In 2011 there were an estimated 83,000 new cases of HIV, down from 93,000 in 2001, and the number of newly infected children dropped 24% between 2009 and 2011. Approximately 1.4 million adults and children in Central and South America were living with HIV/AIDS in 2011. There were 54,000 AIDS-related deaths in 2011, down from 60,000 in 2005.

About two-thirds (68%) of eligible people received ART in the region in 2011, but there was considerable variation by country. More than 80% of eligible people received ART in Cuba, the Dominican Republic, Mexico, and Guyana, and over 60% were treated in Argentina, Brazil, Chile, Ecuador, El Salvador, Jamaica, Nicaragua, Paraguay, Peru, and Venezuela. By contrast, less than 20% of eligible people received ART in Bolivia.

The majority of HIV/AIDS cases in Central and South America can be traced to MSM and men who have sex with both men and women. There were high rates of HIV prevalence among MSM in 2011—23% in Panama, 20% in Chile, and greater than 15% in Argentina and Mexico. Social stigma continues to challenge efforts to identify, educate, and prevent infection among MSM. Only Belize and Guatemala reported high levels (greater than 75%) of condom use by MSM; in other countries the rates varied between 50% and 74%.

Sex workers continue to contribute to the epidemics in many countries. In the Dominican Republic, HIV prevalence among sex workers was 4.7% in 2011, compared with a national prevalence of 0.7%. Similarly, HIV prevalence among sex workers in Brazil was 4.9%, compared with a national prevalence of 0.3%.

THE CARIBBEAN

The first suspected AIDS cases in the Caribbean appeared in Jamaica in 1982. UNAIDS indicates in *Global Report: UNAIDS Report on the Global AIDS Epidemic, 2012* that after sub-Saharan Africa, the Caribbean is the region most affected by HIV, with 1% of adults affected in 2011. However, it also had the sharpest drop in new infections—a 42% decrease between 2001 and 2011. The number of newly infected children also fell 32%, largely in response to more pregnant women receiving ART—79% of HIV-positive pregnant women received ART in 2011, up more than 30% from 2010. The Caribbean also had a significant decrease in AIDS-related deaths—48% between 2005 and 2011.

HIV prevalence varies by country, from a low of 0.2 in Cuba, 0.7 in the Dominican Republic, and 1 in Barbados to highs of 1.8 in both Haiti and Jamaica and 2.8 in the Bahamas.

Since its inception, the HIV/AIDS epidemic has changed from a mostly homosexual phenomenon to a largely heterosexual one, attributable to unprotected sex between partners and sex workers. In Jamaica HIV prevalence among MSM was 38% in 2011, but condom use among MSM was 77%. The Bahamas, Jamaica, and Saint Kitts and Nevis also reported high rates of condom use among MSM.

About two-thirds (67%) of those eligible to receive ART were receiving it in 2011. In Cuba more than 80% of those in need of ART received it.

UNAIDS (November 2012, http://www.unaids.org/en/media/unaids/contentassets/documents/epidemiology/2012/gr2012/2012_FS_regional_la_caribbean_en.pdf) notes that an estimated 230,000 people in the Caribbean were living with HIV/AIDS in 2011, and approximately 13,000 had contracted the infection during that year. Although these numbers reflect a decline in the region's epidemic that is at least in part attributable to behavior changes and improved access to antiretroviral drugs, AIDS remains a leading cause of death among people aged 15 to 44 years in the Caribbean and was responsible for an estimated 10,000 deaths in 2011.

CHALLENGES

Although great strides have been made in the treatment of HIV infection and AIDS and in raising public awareness about the nature of the disease and preventing its spread, several issues, challenges, and controversies continue to hamper the unity of purpose that is required to effectively combat HIV/AIDS worldwide.

In June 2013 UNAIDS and the Lancet Commission met for the first time in Lilongwe, Malawi. The commission will develop strategies to advance the global AIDS movement with the goal of achieving zero new HIV infections, zero discrimination, and zero AIDS-related deaths in the coming decades. In "Defeating AIDS— Advancing Global Health" (2013, http://www.unaids.org/en/resources/campaigns/post2015/defeatingaidsadvancingglobalhealth/), UNAIDS explains that the commission will consider three questions:

- What will it take to end AIDS?

- How can lessons from the AIDS response inform global health?

- How must the global health and AIDS architecture be modernised to achieve sustainable global health?

Among its goals, UNAIDS states in *UNAIDS 2011–2015 Strategy: Getting to Zero* (2010, http://www.unaids.org/en/media/unaids/contentassets/documents/unaidspublication/2010/JC2034_UNAIDS_Strategy_en.pdf) that by 2015 it hopes to reduce sexual transmission of HIV by half, eliminate mother-to-child transmission of HIV, and prevent new infections among IDUs. It also aims to provide "universal access to antiretroviral therapy for people living with HIV/AIDS who are eligible for treatment," reduce TB deaths by half, and end discrimination against people affected by HIV by 2015.

Cost of Drugs

The high price of HIV/AIDS drugs has been and continues to be a contentious issue. In "International Consultation Focuses on Access to HIV Medicines for Middle-Income Countries" (June 13, 2013, http://www.unaids.org/en/resources/presscentre/featurestories/2013/june/20130613brazil/), UNAIDS observes that the high price of medication places the WHO-recommended first-line treatment—the one-pill-a-day, three-drug, fixed-dose combination—out of reach of some countries such as Brazil, China, and the Russian Federation. The high cost of drugs threatens even middle-income countries' ability to provide optimal treatment for people affected by HIV. Although much attention has been paid to improving access to treatment in lower-income countries, middle-income countries do not benefit from international initiatives that are aimed at improving access to drugs. Most middle-income countries rely on government funding or out-of-pocket expenditure for drugs, and UNAIDS is uncertain as to whether it is feasible for these countries to provide long-term treatment for the growing numbers of people who will need it.

Increasing Access to HIV/AIDS Drugs in Developing Countries

The Clinton Health Access Initiative (CHAI; http://www.clintonhealthaccess.org/) was founded by the former U.S. president Bill Clinton (1946–) to assist countries to implement large-scale prevention and treatment programs. CHAI works with the governments of countries in Africa, the Caribbean, and Asia and provides technical assistance and human and financial resources to ensure the delivery of quality care and treatment. The initiative also provides access to reduced prices for HIV/AIDS drugs and diagnostics to countries. In total, CHAI represents over 90% of people living with HIV/AIDS in developing countries.

In "About CHAI" (2013, http://www.clintonhealthaccess.org/about), CHAI reports that as of 2013 it had successfully negotiated price reductions for antiretroviral drugs that have benefitted 3.9 million people in 70 countries. CHAI's efforts resulted in price reductions of 60% to 90% and have saved countries more than $1 billion. CHAI works in concert with governments to support and strengthen their capacities to care for their citizens. For example, in South Africa CHAI is assisting the government to extend ART to more than 2.3 million people and to offer HIV testing to more than 15 million.

UNITAID is an international drug purchase facility that was established in 2006 by Brazil, Chile, France, Norway, and the United Kingdom. UNITAID is an innovative funding mechanism that focuses on speeding access to quality drugs and diagnostics for HIV/AIDS, malaria, and TB in countries where these diseases pose serious threats to the health of their residents. UNITAID works with CHAI, the WHO, and the United Nations Children's Fund. UNITAID indicates in "Role in Global Health Landscape" (2013, http://www.unitaid.eu/en/who/role-in-global-health-landscape) that at the close of 2011 approximately 84% of its funds were directed to low-income countries, 13% to low-middle-income countries, and 3% to upper-middle-income countries.

According to UNITAID, in "HIV Diagnostics—Point-of-Care and Decentralized Testing and Monitoring" (2013, http://www.unitaid.eu/en/what/hiv/16-home/994-hiv-diagnostics-point-of-care-and-decentralized-testing-and-monitoring), in 2012 it committed more than $140 million to point-of-care testing, which enables patients to receive their HIV test results quickly and conveniently. In "Adult Second-Line HIV/AIDS Project" (2013, http://www.unitaid.eu/en/secondline), UNITAID notes that besides expanding access to, availability, and affordability of antiretroviral drugs, its accomplishments include price reductions of up to 60% for the more-potent ART drugs many patients need when first-line drugs no longer keep the virus in check and enabling more than 100,000 patients per year to obtain these lifesaving drugs.

President's Emergency Plan for AIDS Relief

The President's Emergency Plan for AIDS Relief (PEPFAR) is a U.S. government initiative to help people suffering from HIV/AIDS worldwide. Launched by President George W. Bush (1946–) in 2003, PEPFAR is responsible for saving millions of lives. In "Bush Signs Bill to Triple AIDS Funding" (Associated Press, July 30, 2008), Katharine Euphrat describes the program as "one of the major achievements of the Bush presidency." In 2008 the program was renewed for five years and the controversial requirement that 33% of prevention funds be used for abstinence-until-marriage programs was eliminated.

Abstaining from sexual intercourse does prevent the sexual transmission of HIV, although most experts, who agree that it is not realistic to expect sexual abstinence from many segments of the population, stress that condom use is essential to stop the spread of the disease. Abstinence education remains a key component of PEPFAR, although in 2007 the program's prevention strategy was broadened to include "ABC—Abstain, Be faithful, and correct and consistent Condom use," the prevention of mother-to-child transmission, activities that focus on blood safety, and interventions aimed at IDUs.

PEPFAR was reauthorized by the Tom Lantos and Henry J. Hyde United States Global Leadership against HIV/AIDS, Tuberculosis, and Malaria Reauthorization Act in July 2008. The reauthorization act stipulates that "in countries with generalized HIV epidemics, at least half of all money directed towards preventing sexual HIV transmission should be for activities promoting abstinence, delay of sexual debut, monogamy, fidelity, and partner reduction," but it does not mandate abstinence-only education and prevention programs as a requirement for receiving funds.

The number of people served by PEPFAR was 5.1 million in fiscal year (FY) 2012. (See Table 9.1.) The launch of PEPFAR significantly increased U.S. spending to support the fight against the global HIV/AIDS pandemic—it increased from $2.3 billion in FY 2004 to $6.9 billion in FY 2010. (See Table 9.2.) For FY 2014 President Barack Obama (1961–) requested $6.7 billion, including nearly $4.9 billion for bilateral HIV/AIDS programs and $1.7 billion for the Global Fund.

On June 18, 2013, in an address marking the 10th anniversary of PEPFAR, John Kerry (1943–; http://www.pepfar.gov/press/releases/2013/210773.htm), the U.S. secretary of state, announced that the one-millionth baby was born HIV-free in June 2013 as a result of the success of PEPFAR-supported prevention of mother-to-child transmission programs. Kerry also observed that there are 13 countries "at the programmatic tipping point in their AIDS epidemic—the point where the annual increase in adults on treatment is greater than the number of annual new adult HIV infections." Table 9.3 shows the countries where annual increases in treatment are outpacing new infections.

TABLE 9.1

Number of people receiving antiretroviral treatment supported by U.S. government as of September 30, 2012

Treatment: Direct fiscal year 2012 antiretroviral treatment results[a]

Countries	Number of individuals
Angola[b]	NA
Botswana	5,300
Burundi	NA
Cambodia	13,100
Cameroon	NA
China	2,300
Côte d'Ivoire	81,400
Democratic Republic of the Congo	6,800
Dominican Republic	4,600
Ethiopia	275,000
Ghana[b]	NA
Guyana	2,600
Haiti	41,000
India[b]	NA
Indonesia[b]	NA
Kenya	579,000
Lesotho	93,800
Malawi	119,200
Mozambique	242,700
Namibia	113,100
Nigeria	488,800
Russia[b]	NA
Rwanda	68,000
South Africa	1,651,800
Sudan[b]	NA
Swaziland	60,100
Tanzania	364,300
Thailand[b]	NA
Uganda	364,200
Ukraine[b]	NA
Vietnam	40,800
Zambia	445,200
Zimbabwe	80,000
Regions	
Caribbean region[b]	NA
Central America[b]	NA
Central Asia[b]	NA
Total[c]	**5,143,100**

Notes: All numbers greater than 100 have been rounded off to the nearest 100.
[a]The number of individuals is as of September 30, 2012.
[b]"NA" refers to countries where the U.S. government did not directly support treatment programs.
[c]Due to several country updates, the total results are slightly higher than the reported results in the PEPFAR Blueprint and the 2012 World AIDS Day FACT Sheet. All results still reflect accomplishments through September 20, 2012.

SOURCE: "Treatment: Direct FY2012 Antiretroviral Treatment Results," in *Annual Report to Congress on the President's Emergency Plan for AIDS Relief, Ninth Annual Report to Congress on PEPFAR (2013)*, 2013, http://www.pepfar.gov/press/207534.htm (accessed August 9, 2013)

TABLE 9.2

President's Emergency Plan for AIDS Relief funding, fiscal years 2004–14

[$ in millions]

Programs	Fiscal year 2004 enacted	Fiscal year 2005 enacted	Fiscal year 2006 enacted	Fiscal year 2007 enacted	Fiscal year 2008 enacted	Fiscal year 2009 enacted	Fiscal year 2010 enacted	Fiscal year 2011 enacted[b]	Fiscal year 2012 enacted	Total enacted[c]	Fiscal year 2013 requested	Fiscal year 2014 enacted
Bilateral HIV/AIDS programs[a]	1,643	2,263	2,654	3,699	5,028	5,503	5,574	5,440	5,083	36,887	4,537	4,881
Global fund	547	347	545	724	840	1,000	1,050	1,046	1,300	7,399	1,650	1,650
Bilateral TB program	87	94	91	95	163	177	243	239	256	1,445	232	199
Total PEPFAR (w/o malaria)	**2,277**	**2,704**	**3,290**	**4,518**	**6,031**	**6,680**	**6,867**	**6,725**	**6,639**	**45,731**	**6,419**	**6,730**

[a]Bilateral HIV/AIDS programs includes funding for bilateral country/regional programs, UNAIDS, IAVI, Microbicides and NIH HIV/AIDS research.
[b]Fiscal year 2011 enacted level includes across-the board and HHS agency-wide rescissions.
[c]Includes enacted funding for fiscal years 2004–2012.
PEPFAR = President's Emergency Plan for AIDS Relief.
HIV = Human Immunodeficiency Virus.
AIDS = Acquired Immunodeficiency Syndrome.
TB = Tuberculosis.
UNAIDS = United Nations Programme on HIV/AIDS.
IAVI = International AIDS Vaccine Initiative.
NIH = National Institutes of Health.
Note: All funding amounts have been rounded to the nearest million, so the numbers shown in the table may not sum to the totals. Information as of April 2013.

SOURCE: "FY 2004–FY 2014 PEPFAR Funding ($ in Millions)," in *Working toward an AIDS Free Generation: Latest PEPFAR Funding*, The United States President's Emergency Plan for AIDS Relief, April 2013, http://www.pepfar.gov/documents/organization/189671.pdf (accessed August 9, 2013)

TABLE 9.3

Countries where annual increases in treatment are outpacing new infections, 2012

Country	2011 adult HIV infections	2011 increase in adult patients on treatment	Ratio of new HIV infections to increase in patients on treatment
Botswana	8,500	17,811	0.5
Burundi	1,900	3,566	0.5
Ethiopia	11,000	40,507	0.3
Ghana	10,000	14,176	0.7
Guyana	199	349	0.6
Haiti	5,400	5,344	1.0
Kenya	91,000	93,912	1.0
Malawi	31,000	96,614	0.3
Namibia	8,000	14,539	0.6
Rwanda	9,000	11,456	0.8
Swaziland	12,000	11,751	1.0
Zambia	42,000	66,479	0.6
Zimbabwe	60,000	142,155	0.4

SOURCE: "Thirteen Countries at Programmatic Tipping Point," in "Secretary of State John Kerry Marks Tenth Anniversary of PEPFAR," The United States President's Emergency Plan for AIDS, June 18, 2013, Relief http://www.pepfar.gov/press/releases/2013/210773.htm (accessed August 9, 2013)

CHAPTER 10

KNOWLEDGE, AWARENESS, BEHAVIOR, AND OPINION

CONCERN ABOUT HIV/AIDS

During the first decade of the 21st century the U.S. public appeared less concerned about HIV/AIDS and its impact on health care than ever before. According to the Gallup Organization, the number of Americans who named AIDS as the most urgent health problem facing the country has declined steadily when compared with 68% of Americans in 1988. It declined to 41% in 1992 and to 29% in 1997. By late 2012 just 1% of Americans considered AIDS the most urgent health problem. (See Table 10.1.)

Access to health care and health care costs overshadowed diseases as the most pressing health problems facing the country. (See Table 10.1.) Interestingly, obesity was the most frequently named health problem, outpacing cancer, heart disease, diabetes, AIDS, and flu.

Americans' Understanding of the HIV/AIDS Epidemic

The publication *Washington Post/Kaiser Family Foundation 2012 Survey of Americans on HIV/AIDS* (July 2012, http://kaiserfamilyfoundation.files.wordpress.com/2013/01/8334-f.pdf) describes trends in public opinions, attitudes, knowledge, and awareness of HIV/AIDS and related issues. The 2012 survey was one of several that have been conducted by the Kaiser Family Foundation (KFF) since 1995, so it reveals how Americans' attitudes toward HIV/AIDS have changed over time.

The 2012 survey finds that the percentage of Americans identifying HIV/AIDS as the "most urgent health problem facing the nation" plummeted from 44% in 1995 to 10% in 2012. A slightly higher percentage considered HIV/AIDS to be the world's most pressing health problem, but this percentage decreased over time as well, from 34% in 2006 to 16% in 2012. The vast majority (89%) of Americans believed it is possible for people with HIV to lead healthy productive lives, but they were evenly divided about whether to characterize HIV as a manageable chronic disease comparable to diabetes or high blood pressure.

Perhaps concern has diminished because media attention has waned or because other health messages predominate. The survey participants reported seeing and hearing less about HIV/AIDS in the United States than they did in the past. The proportion claiming to have seen or heard "a lot" or "some" about the problem fell from 70% in 2004 to 43% in 2012. Even the global HIV/AIDS pandemic appears to have receded from Americans' awareness. Seventy-one percent recalled hearing about the magnitude of the problem in Africa in 2004, the first year that the President's Emergency Plan for AIDS Relief (PEPFAR) was funded, but by 2012, 51% said they had heard or read "a lot" or "some" about the problem in Africa and just 24% had heard about HIV/AIDS elsewhere in the world.

More than half (54%) of Americans and nearly two-thirds (63%) of African Americans indicated that the epidemic has disproportionately affected African Americans. Furthermore, the majority (87%) recognized that access to medication is a problem in developing countries.

Three-quarters of Americans acknowledged that there is prejudice and discrimination against people living with HIV/AIDS. Forty percent said there is a lot and 35% said there is some prejudice and discrimination.

Concern about Becoming Infected with HIV

According to the 2012 survey, 52% of respondents were not at all concerned about becoming infected with HIV and an additional 23% were not too concerned. Just 13% of Americans were very concerned about the possibility of becoming HIV infected and 11% were somewhat concerned. Less than one out of five (18%) was concerned about a family member becoming infected with HIV, down from 24% in 2011.

TABLE 10.1

Percent of people naming AIDS as the most urgent health problem, November 2012

WHAT IS THE MOST URGENT HEALTH PROBLEM FACING THIS COUNTRY AT THE PRESENT TIME?

[Open-ended]

	NOV 15–18, 2012
Access	23
Cost	19
Obesity	16
Cancer	13
Gov't interference	2
Heart disease	2
Diabetes	2
AIDS	1
Flu	0
Finding cures for diseases	1
Drug/alcohol abuse	*
Smoking	*
Bioterrorism	*
Other	6
No opinion	15

*Less than 0.5%.

SOURCE: Elizabeth Mendes, "What Is the Most Urgent Health Problem Facing This Country at the Present Time?" in "In U.S., More Cite Obesity as Most Urgent Health Problem," The Gallup Organization, December 5, 2012, http://www.gallup.com/poll/159083/cite-obesity-urgent-health-problem.aspx (accessed August 9, 2013) Copyright © 2013 Gallup, Inc. All rights reserved. The content is used with permission; however, Gallup retains all rights of republication.

More than four out of 10 (41%) of those surveyed had talked with a doctor or health care provider about HIV/AIDS and just 46% had discussed it with a partner or spouse. Nearly three-quarters (72%) felt that home HIV tests, which are sold over the counter, are a good idea because they encourage people to learn their HIV status. Interestingly, when it comes to their own testing, more survey respondents expressed a preference for having the test performed in a physician's office or clinic (59%) than at home (30%).

KNOWLEDGE AND TOLERANCE GROW, BUT MISCONCEPTIONS PERSIST

In the three decades since HIV/AIDS was first identified, aggressive community health education and awareness programs have sought to increase the public's knowledge about the prevention, transmission, and treatment of HIV/AIDS. Based on the findings of the 2012 survey, although public understanding and awareness have improved in many areas, misconceptions and stigmatizing attitudes about HIV/AIDS persist.

For example, 27% of Americans mistakenly believed that HIV can be transmitted by sharing a drinking glass. Another 17% believed that HIV can be transmitted via shared toilet seats and 11% thought swimming in a pool with a person who is infected may transmit HIV. The KFF finds that one out of three (34%) survey respondents

gave an incorrect answer when queried about these three ways that HIV cannot be transmitted.

In contrast, some knowledge about HIV treatment had increased by 2012. For example, 49% of respondents knew of the relatively recent finding that treatment can effectively prevent transmission of HIV.

There is, however, an understanding that the U.S. HIV epidemic has had a profound effect on U.S. culture and society as well as on personal behaviors. Historically, the KFF surveys and other polling organizations have found that about half of Americans feel there has been considerable discrimination against people with AIDS. However, the results of the 2012 survey indicate that some, but not all, of the stigmas and discrimination that are associated with HIV/AIDS may be diminishing. Some of the observed changes in attitudes and declining stigmas may be attributable to how widespread HIV/AIDS has become. In 2012, 45% of Americans, up from 41% in 2011, said they had personal contact with HIV/AIDS—either they knew someone who is infected with HIV, someone who has AIDS, or someone who has died from an AIDS-related illness.

Spending for HIV/AIDS in the United States

Since 1995, when the KFF began surveying Americans about HIV/AIDS, the majority of survey respondents have felt that too little money is being devoted to combating HIV/AIDS domestically. The 2012 survey indicates that, despite continuing economic uncertainty and instability that remained following the recession (which lasted from late 2007 to mid-2009), support for spending on HIV/AIDS was strong in 2012—56% of Americans concurred with experts that increasing funding will advance progress to counter the epidemic. Half of the survey respondents said the federal government is spending too little to combat the domestic epidemic. When asked to compare HIV/AIDS funding and spending with expenditures for other diseases such as cancer and heart disease, 43% felt that spending is too low and 35% felt that the current level of spending is about right.

Although the 2012 survey finds continued support for spending on HIV/AIDS prevention and treatment, Americans were divided about the outcomes of such spending. Fifty-four percent felt spending will produce significant progress and slow the epidemic, whereas 39% felt HIV/AIDS prevention programs will make no difference and 34% felt the same way about HIV/AIDS treatment.

Is Enough Being Done?

According to the 2012 survey, Americans felt that most of the stakeholders were not doing enough to help solve the problem of HIV/AIDS in the United States. Nearly half (47%) believed that President Barack Obama

(1961–) and his administration are not doing enough and 61% felt the same way about Congress.

Approximately half of Americans wanted to see greater involvement in HIV/AIDS initiatives and efforts from pharmaceutical companies (51%), public schools (51%), and religious leaders and institutions (50%).

Nevertheless, 51% of Americans said the United States is making progress in terms of the problem of HIV/AIDS, and an even higher percentage (58%) said the world is making progress. Nearly four out of 10 (41%) expected a cure for AIDS in the next 10 years, 41% anticipated a cure during their lifetime, and 55% felt it is possible to achieve the goal of an AIDS-free generation worldwide by 2050.

DIFFERING OPINIONS: AIDS DISSIDENTS AND DENIALISTS

In 1987 Peter Duesberg of the University of California, Berkeley, published "Retroviruses as Carcinogens and Pathogens: Expectations and Reality" (*Cancer Research*, vol. 47, no. 5, March 1, 1987), in which he asserts that HIV does not cause AIDS. Duesberg believes that HIV is a harmless virus and one of many of the organisms that may reside in humans but will not harm them. One of his arguments is that most viruses make people ill very quickly, before they can mount an immune response. People infected with HIV may not become ill for more than a decade. Duesberg posits that it is the use of illicit drugs that compromises the immune system, not infection with HIV. He feels that maintaining a healthy diet and abstaining from harmful drug use is sufficient to prevent and even cure AIDS. Duesberg is considered by many to be at the forefront of a small but vocal minority of people who do not accept the direct connection between HIV infection and AIDS.

Besides rejecting HIV as the cause of AIDS, others argue that the risks of antiretroviral drugs far outweigh the benefits. Some even assert that antiretroviral therapy (ART) is poison and is promoted to generate profits for pharmaceutical companies. Other dissidents aver that there is no AIDS epidemic in sub-Saharan Africa. They feel that the deaths attributed to AIDS resulted from malnutrition and the lack of clean, safe water supplies—circumstances that most observers believe have hindered efforts to stem the epidemic but did not cause it.

Critics of Duesberg and other AIDS denialists contend that the adoption of their beliefs has led to the premature death of hundreds of thousands of people affected by HIV. In "Death by Denial: The Campaigners Who Continue to Deny HIV Causes AIDS" (TheGuardian.com, February 12, 2012), Brian Deer reports that the denialist beliefs of Thabo Mbeki (1942–), who as president of South Africa from June 1999 to September 2008

delayed widespread use of ART, resulted in more than 300,000 deaths and 35,000 preventable infections.

Other denialists seek to promote alternative treatment to ART. For example, Matthias Rath (1955–), a German physician, urges people living with HIV/AIDS to abandon prescribed treatment in favor of high doses of vitamins and other nutrients. Rath claims that his vitamin regimens will prevent or even cure AIDS as well as other chronic diseases. Michael Specter notes in "The Denialists" (NewYorker.com, March 12, 2007) that Rath has been criticized by many organizations, including the Joint United Nations Programme on HIV/AIDS and the South African Medical Association, and that the U.S. Food and Drug Administration deems material on Rath's website to be misleading.

AIDS denialism persists in the 21st century. In "'There Is No Proof That HIV Causes AIDS': AIDS Denialism Beliefs among People Living with HIV/AIDS" (*Journal of Behavioral Medicine*, vol. 33, no. 6, December 2010), Seth C. Kalichman, Lisa Eaton, and Chauncey Cherry report the results of their study of the prevalence of AIDS denialism beliefs and their association to health-related outcomes among people living with HIV/AIDS. The researchers surveyed African American men and women living with HIV/AIDS. One out of five survey participants expressed the belief that there is no proof that HIV causes AIDS and that treatment does more harm than good. The respondents who held these beliefs were less likely to be on ART and as a result were in poorer health. Kalichman, Eaton, and Cherry conclude, "Openly discussing the baseless views of AIDS denialists and exposing the pseudo-science behind AIDS denialism is key to diluting its impact.... Ignoring AIDS denialism undermines our best efforts to test, engage, and care for people living with HIV/AIDS."

HIV/AIDS AWARENESS EFFORTS

Many national and global initiatives and observances are conducted in an effort to inform the public, heighten awareness, and improve understanding of the HIV/AIDS pandemic. This section describes some of the activities, individuals, and groups that are involved in the ongoing effort to educate, motivate, and mobilize people to prevent the spread of HIV and to assist those who are living with HIV/AIDS.

The U.S. Department of Health and Human Services (2013, http://www.aids.gov/news-and-events/awareness-days/) designates the annual observation of HIV/AIDS Awareness Days. These include:

- February 7, National Black HIV/AIDS Awareness Day—this annual awareness day was created by a community-based coalition to raise awareness among

African Americans about HIV/AIDS and its disproportionate and devastating impact on African American communities.

- March 10, National Women and Girls HIV/AIDS Awareness Day—this day aims to raise awareness of the increasing impact of HIV/AIDS on the lives of women and girls.

- March 20, National Native HIV/AIDS Awareness Day—this day was created to increase awareness of the impact of HIV/AIDS on Native Americans, Alaskan natives, and native Hawaiians.

- May 18, HIV Vaccine Awareness Day—this day recognizes and acknowledges the people who are working to help find an HIV preventive vaccine, such as the clinical trial volunteers, the nurses, the community educators/recruiters, and the researchers.

- May 19, National Asian and Pacific Islander HIV/AIDS Awareness Day—this awareness day intends to increase awareness among Asians and Pacific Islanders in the United States about the ruinous impact of HIV/AIDS.

- June 8, Caribbean American HIV/AIDS Awareness Day—this day is a national mobilization effort that is designed to encourage Caribbean American and Caribbean-born individuals across the United States and its territories to become better informed and educated, obtain testing, and seek treatment.

- June 27, National HIV Testing Day—this day aims to provide opportunities for testing, especially for those who have never been tested or who have engaged in high-risk behavior since their last test, and to help dispel the myths and stigmas that are associated with HIV.

- September 18, National HIV/AIDS and Aging Awareness Day—this day aims to heighten awareness of the impact of HIV/AIDS on older adults. It intends to focus on HIV prevention, care, and treatment of people aged 50 years and older.

- September 27, National Gay Men's HIV/AIDS Awareness Day—this day aims to regain and refocus the attention of a community that has been disproportionately affected by the HIV/AIDS epidemic at a time when the United States confronts the simultaneous challenges of a resurgence of new HIV infections among gay men and growing complacency about HIV/AIDS among gay men.

- October 15, National Latino AIDS Awareness Day—this awareness day marks an opportunity to communicate the devastating and disproportionate effects AIDS is having on the Hispanic community.

- December 1, World AIDS Day—started by the World Health Organization in 1988, this day serves to focus global attention on the HIV/AIDS pandemic. Observance of this day provides an opportunity for governments, national AIDS programs, churches, community organizations, and individuals to demonstrate the importance of the fight against HIV/AIDS.

The AIDS Memorial Quilt

The AIDS Memorial Quilt is not only an ongoing community art project that pays tribute to and commemorates the lives claimed by AIDS but also serves as a powerful visual way to inform, educate, and heighten awareness of the lives lost in this epidemic. The AIDS Memorial Quilt notes in "History of the Quilt" (2013, http://www.aidsquilt.org/about/the-aids-memorial-quilt) that the quilt consists of cloth panels that have been designed and made by friends and families of people who died from AIDS-related illnesses. Cleve Jones, a San Francisco, California, gay rights activist, had the idea for the quilt in November 1985 and the quilt was "born" in June 1987, when Jones and a group of his friends in San Francisco decided to memorialize people who had died from AIDS-related illnesses.

The first public display of the quilt was at the National Mall in Washington, D.C., in October 1987. It contained 1,920 panels and was larger than a football field. The quilt, and enthusiasm for it, grew quickly. One year later the quilt had grown to 8,288 panels. Each time the quilt was displayed the names of those honored by it were read aloud by celebrities, politicians, family members, and friends.

The AIDS Memorial Quilt states that over 18 million people have seen the 1.3-million-square-foot (121,000-square-m) quilt and that it contains over 94,000 names. The quilt has traveled around the world, raising awareness and money (more than $4 million) for AIDS-related research and programs. It has been the subject of stories, papers, articles, and books and was nominated for a Nobel Peace Prize in 1989. That same year a feature-length documentary about it, *Common Threads: Stories from the Quilt*, won an Academy Award.

In "The AIDS Quilt, and Hoping for 'The Last One'" (CNN.com, July 24, 2012), Julie Rhoad of the NAMES Project Foundation, an international nonprofit organization that is the caretaker of the AIDS Memorial Quilt, states: "Throughout its 25-year history, [it] has been used to fight prejudice, and to raise awareness and funding for direct service and advocacy groups. The Quilt is a catalyst and conduit, a tool for healing and grief therapy, a springboard for frank dialogue.... It gives voice to far too many lives lost, telling us that never again should we ever leave a community in need and dying, ignored and uncared for. It is a stark reminder that we can never forget that we are all inextricably linked in life."

AIDS Activists

AIDS activists have been credited with raising awareness and attracting money and media attention to the pandemic. Many groups, individuals, and celebrities have taken on the cause and become champions of HIV/AIDS research, prevention, and treatment. Others have agitated to change the course of national and government policy and to improve access to and availability of quality care, especially affordable drug treatment. Still others have defended the rights of people living with HIV/AIDS in an effort to counter stigmatization and discrimination. Using a variety of approaches—from fund-raising campaigns and political lobbying to protests and guerrilla theater (dramatization of a social issue, often performed outdoors in a park or on the street)—AIDS activists have raised their voices and the consciousness of people around the world.

Although there are many groups and organizations engaged in AIDS activism, the most effective and vibrant organization is probably the AIDS Coalition to Unleash Power (ACT UP). ACT UP (2013, http://www.actupny.org/) describes itself as "a diverse, non-partisan group of individuals united in anger and committed to direct action to end the AIDS crisis." It states, "We advise and inform. We demonstrate. We are not silent. Silence = Death." ACT UP has thousands of members in more than 70 chapters in the United States and worldwide. The organization advocates nonviolent direct action through vocal demonstrations and acts of civil disobedience that are intended to make the public aware of the crucial issues of the AIDS crisis. During a span of more than 25 years, ACT UP members have staged scores of protests and demonstrations and have often been arrested, usually for civil disobedience.

AIDS United (2013, http://www.aidsunited.org/about/), another national organization, has as its slogan "Every Person, Every Community," which conveys the group's commitment to "end the AIDS epidemic within the United States. We seek to fulfill our mission through strategic grantmaking, capacity building, and advocacy." AIDS United has played a key role in the development and implementation of public health policies to improve the quality of life for Americans who are HIV positive. It also works with the public health community to enhance HIV prevention programs and care and treatment services.

The AIDS Treatment Activists Coalition is also a national coalition of AIDS activists who work together to end the AIDS epidemic by advancing research on HIV/AIDS. The coalition's mission statement (2013, http://www.thebody.com/content/art53683.html) describes its goals as:

- To encourage greater and more effective involvement of people with HIV/AIDS in the decisions that affect their lives by identifying, mentoring and empowering treatment activists in all communities affected by the epidemic

- To develop within all communities affected by HIV/AIDS and related coinfections the leadership to provide the knowledge and skills needed to advocate for improved research, treatment and access to care

- To enable treatment activists to speak with a united, powerful voice to provide meaningful input into issues concerning HIV disease and related complications and coinfections

- To facilitate communications and set agenda items ... between HIV/AIDS treatment activists and government, industry and academia in matters affecting research, treatment and access [and] among HIV/AIDS treatment activists and the larger HIV community in keeping up to date with the latest developments in research, treatment and access

CELEBRITIES SHINE A SPOTLIGHT ON HIV/AIDS. When celebrities endorse or lend their name to charitable causes, the causes often benefit from increased media attention and visibility. When celebrities actively work to promote their chosen causes, the results can be even more dramatic. For example, Martyn Wraight of HepC and HIV Haven, a nonprofit organization that focuses on HIV drug development, research, and campaigns, lists in "Celebrities Who Support HIV" (HIVHaven.com, 2013) over 30 celebrities—from President Clinton and Microsoft chairman Bill Gates (1955–); to the actors George Clooney (1961–), Matt Damon (1970–), Richard Gere (1949–), Whoopi Goldberg (1955–), and Sharon Stone (1958–); and to the musicians Bono (1960–), Miley Cyrus (1992–), Lady Gaga (1986–), Elton John (1947–), and Alicia Keys (1981–)—who are active in contributing their time, energy, and money to combat the HIV/AIDS pandemic.

Many young celebrities have also taken up the cause. The article "Celebrities Changing the World for HIV-Positive People" (HIVPlusMag.com, July 21, 2013) indicates that Snoop Lion (formerly Snoop Dog; 1971–), Khloe Kardashian (1984–), and Vinny Guadagnino (1988–) have promoted HIV prevention. The music industry has also taken up the cause. Educational material about HIV and free condoms were offered at Tour Outreach (2013, http://lifebeat.org/programs/outreach/) concerts by Madonna (1958–), Kendrick Lamar (1987–), Wiz Khalifa (1987–) and Mac Miller (1992–), and Lil' Kim (1975–) in 105 cities. A program called Hearts & Voices (2013, http://lifebeat.org/programs/hearts-voices/) brings concerts to hospitals, residential facilities, and day-treatment programs. Among the musicians and groups that have participated are Destiny's Child, LL Cool J (1968–), Jewel (1974–), Jon Secada (1962–), Maroon 5, and Kanye West (1977–).

Bono uses his celebrity to champion the fight against HIV/AIDS. In 2002 he formed the organization Debt AIDS Trade Africa (DATA), an advocacy organization that was dedicated to eradicating extreme poverty and AIDS in Africa. In 2005 Bono was named *Time*'s Person of the Year along with Bill Gates and Melinda Gates (1964–). The following year he was nominated for a Nobel Peace Prize.

In January 2008 DATA merged with ONE (http://www.one.org/us/), a global antipoverty organization that pursues high-level global advocacy in concert with grassroots mobilization efforts. Like DATA, ONE's (2013, http://www.one.org/international/about/faqs/what-is-ones-mission/) mission is to "fight extreme poverty and preventable disease in the poorest places on the planet, particularly in Africa." ONE partners with other global relief and HIV/AIDS initiatives, including the Bill and Melinda Gates Foundation, Bread for Life, CARE, Islamic Relief, Malaria No More, Oxfam America, Physicians for Peace, (RED), Save the Children, and the White Ribbon Alliance for Safe Motherhood.

(RED) (2013, http://www.red.org) involves the private and public sectors in a joint fund-raising initiative. Companies whose products carry the (RED) insignia pledge to contribute a significant percentage of their sales or a portion of their profits from those products to the Global Fund to finance AIDS programs in Africa, with an emphasis on the health of women and children. The Global Fund (2013, http://www.red.org/en/learn/the-global-fund), which is supported by the funds that (RED) generates, is the world's leading financer of programs to fight AIDS, tuberculosis, and malaria. Since its launch in 2002, the Global Fund has earmarked $23 billion for programs in 151 countries. Since 2003 PEPFAR and the Global Fund have provided funding for free antiretroviral drugs to countries where they are urgently needed.

In 2013 Apple, Beats by Dr. Dre, Belvedere, Coca-Cola, Live Nation Entertainment, SAP, Starbucks, and Telcel and Claro were partners in (RED). MySpace.com was the program's first media sponsor in the United Kingdom. In "Learn" (2013, http://www.red.org/en/learn), (RED) indicates that 14 million people have been reached through programs supported by Global Fund–financed grants that (RED) supports. Since its inception in 2006, (RED) has raised over $215 million for the Global Fund. (RED) provides funding for programs in Ghana, Kenya, Lesotho, Rwanda, South Africa, Swaziland, Tanzania, and Zambia that promote HIV/AIDS prevention, administer antiretroviral therapy for people with HIV infection, educate children who have been orphaned by AIDS, and supply antiretroviral therapy to prevent mother-to-child transmission.

IMPORTANT NAMES
AND ADDRESSES

ACT UP/New York
332 Bleecker St., Ste. G5
New York, NY 10014
URL: http://www.actupny.org/

AIDS United
1424 K St. NW, Ste. 200
Washington, DC 20005
(202) 408-4848
FAX: (202) 408-1818
URL: http://www.aidsunited.org/

**American Foundation for
AIDS Research**
120 Wall St., 13th Floor
New York, NY 10005-3908
(212) 806-1600
FAX: (212) 806-1601
URL: http://www.amfar.org/

America's Essential Hospitals
1301 Pennsylvania Ave. NW, Ste. 950
Washington, DC 20004
(202) 585-0100
FAX: (202) 585-0101
E-mail: info@essentialhospitals.org
URL: http://essentialhospitals.org/

Center for Women Policy Studies
1776 Massachusetts Ave. NW, Ste. 450
Washington, DC 20036
(202) 872-1770
FAX: (202) 296-8962
E-mail: cwps@centerwomenpolicy.org
URL: http://www.centerwomenpolicy.org/

**Centers for Disease Control
and Prevention**
1600 Clifton Rd.
Atlanta, GA 30333
1-800-232-4636
URL: http://www.cdc.gov/

Human Rights Campaign
1640 Rhode Island Ave. NW
Washington, DC 20036-3278

(202) 628-4160
1-800-777-4723
FAX: (202) 347-5323
URL: http://www.hrc.org/

**Joint United Nations Programme on
HIV/AIDS**
20 Ave. Appia
CH-1211 Geneva 27 Switzerland
(011-41-22) 791-3666
FAX: (011-41-22) 791-4187
URL: http://www.unaids.org/

Kaiser Family Foundation
2400 Sand Hill Rd.
Menlo Park, CA 94025
(650) 854-9400
FAX: (650) 854-4800
URL: http://www.kff.org/

**National Hemophilia
Foundation**
116 W. 32nd St., 11th Floor
New York, NY 10001
(212) 328-3700
1-800-424-2634
FAX: (212) 328-3777
E-mail: handi@hemophilia.org
URL: http://www.hemophilia.org/

**National Institute of Allergy and
Infectious Diseases**
6610 Rockledge Dr., MSC 6612
Bethesda, MD 20892-6612
(301) 496-5717
1-866-284-4107
FAX: (301) 402-3573
URL: http://www.niaid.nih.gov/

National Minority AIDS Council
1931 13th St. NW
Washington, DC 20009-4432
(202) 483-6622
FAX: (202) 483-1135

E-mail: communications@nmac.org
URL: http://www.nmac.org/

**National Prevention Information
Network**
PO Box 6003
Rockville, MD 20849-6003
(404) 679-3860
1-800-458-5231
FAX: 1-888-282-7681
E-mail: info@cdcnpin.org
URL: http://www.cdcnpin.org/scripts/
index.asp

**National Women's Health
Network**
1413 K St. NW, Fourth Floor
Washington, DC 20005
(202) 682-2640
FAX: (202) 682-2648
E-mail: nwhn@nwhn.org
URL: http://www.nwhn.org/

ONE
1400 Eye St. NW, Ste. 600
Washington, DC 20005
(202) 495-2700
URL: http://www.one.org/us/

**U.S. Department of Health and Human
Services
AIDSinfo**
PO Box 4780
Rockville, MD 20849-6303
1-800-448-0440
FAX: (301) 315-2818
E-mail: contactus@aidsinfo.nih.gov
URL: http://aidsinfo.nih.gov/

**U.S. Food and Drug
Administration**
10903 New Hampshire Ave.
Silver Spring, MD 20993
1-888-463-6332
URL: http://www.fda.gov/cder

RESOURCES

The Centers for Disease Control and Prevention (CDC) provides the most current accounting of the HIV/AIDS epidemic in the United States. Publications cited in this text include "1993 Revised Classification System for HIV Infection and Expanded Surveillance Case Definition for AIDS among Adolescents and Adults" (Kenneth G. Castro et al., December 1992), "About the Division of HIV/AIDS Prevention (DHAP)" (October 2013), "Basic Statistics" (April 2013), "Current Trends Update: Acquired Immunodeficiency Syndrome—United States, 1981–1990" (June 1991), "Current Trends Update: Impact of the Expanded AIDS Surveillance Case Definition for Adolescents and Adults on Case Reporting—United States, 1993" (March 1994), *Epidemiology of HIV Infection through 2011* (June 2013), "HIV among African Americans" (May 2013), "HIV in Correctional Settings" (June 2012), "HIV Prevention in the United States—High-Impact Prevention: Saving Lives and Money" (August 2011), "HIV Transmitted from a Living Organ Donor—New York City, 2009" (March 2011), "Impact of an Innovative Approach to Prevent Mother-to-Child Transmission of HIV—Malawi, July 2011–September 2012" (Frank Chimbwandira et al., March 2013), "Integrated Prevention Services for HIV Infection, Viral Hepatitis, Sexually Transmitted Diseases, and Tuberculosis for Persons Who Use Drugs Illicitly: Summary Guidance from CDC and the U.S. Department of Health and Human Services" (Hrishikesh Belani et al., November 2012), "Pregnant Women, Infants, and Children" (May 2013), "Revised Surveillance Case Definitions for HIV Infection among Adults, Adolescents, and Children Aged <18 Months and for HIV Infection and AIDS among Children Aged 18 Months to <13 Years—United States, 2008" (Eileen Schneider et al., December 2008), "The Role of STD Detection and Treatment in HIV Prevention—CDC Fact Sheet" (September 2010), "STDs in Adolescents and Young Adults" (December 2012), "STD Trends in the United States: 2011 National Data for Chlamydia, Gonorrhea, and Syphilis" (March 2013), and *Weekly Surveillance Report, 1985* (December 1985).

HIV Surveillance Reports are prepared by the CDC and describe and quantify transmission categories, risk factor combinations, demographics, and people living with HIV/AIDS. Other CDC publications that were used to prepare this publication include *HIV Surveillance in Men Who Have Sex with Men (MSM)* (May 2012), *HIV Surveillance Report: Diagnoses of HIV Infection in the United States and Dependent Areas, 2011* (February 2013), *HIV Surveillance in Women* (June 2013), *Pediatric HIV Surveillance* (June 2013), and "Surveillance of Occupationally Acquired HIV/AIDS in Healthcare Personnel, as of December 2010" (May 2011).

The CDC National Center for Health Statistics publishes findings from the Youth Risk Behavior Surveys, the National HIV Behavioral Surveillance System, the *National Vital Statistics Reports*, and *Health, United States, 2012* (May 2013).

The U.S. Department of Justice's *HIV in Prisons, 2001–2010* (Laura M. Maruschak, September 2012) provides information on HIV/AIDS in U.S. prisons and jails, inmate deaths from HIV/AIDS, and testing policies for the virus antibody by states.

Information about the worldwide effects of HIV/AIDS, as well as global projections, were provided by reports including the Joint United Nations Programme on HIV/AIDS's *Global Report: UNAIDS Report on the Global Aids Epidemic, 2010* (2010), *Global Report: UNAIDS Report on the Global AIDS Epidemic, 2012* (2012), "UNAIDS 2011–2015 Strategy: Getting to Zero" (2010), and *UNAIDS World AIDS Day Report, 2012* (2012); the World Health Organization's *Guidelines on HIV and Infant Feeding 2010: Principles and Recommendations for Infant Feeding in the Context of HIV and a Summary of Evidence* (2010), *Guidelines for Intensified Tuberculosis Case-Finding and Isoniazid Preventive Therapy for People Living with HIV in Resource-Constrained Settings* (2011), and "WHO Issues New

HIV Recommendations Calling for Earlier Treatment" (June 13, 2013); the United Nations Children's Fund's "Orphan Estimates" (April 2013); and the Kaiser Family Foundation's "The Global HIV/AIDS Epidemic" (October 2013).

Medical and scientific journals provide a wealth of information about the HIV/AIDS pandemic. Articles cited in this publication were published in *AIDS and Behavior*, *AIDS Research and Treatment*, *American Journal of Epidemiology*, *American Journal of Preventive Medicine*, *American Journal of Public Health*, *Annals of Internal Medicine*, *Antiviral Chemistry and Chemotherapy*, *Archives of Oral Biology*, *Archives of Surgery*, *BMC International Health and Human Rights*, *BMC Public Health*, *Brain, Behavior, and Immunity*, *British Medical Journal*, *Bulletin of the World Health Organization*, *Clinical Infectious Diseases*, *Clinics in Perinatology*, *Cochrane Database of Systematic Reviews*, *Emerging Infectious Diseases*, *Frontiers in Microbiology*, *Hematology*, *HIV Clinician*, *HIV Medicine*, *Indian Journal of Experimental Biology*, *International Journal of Gynecology and Obstetrics*, *International Journal of STD and AIDS*, *Issues in Mental Health Nursing*, *Journal of Acquired Immune Deficiency Syndrome*, *Journal of Experimental Medicine*, *Journal of the International AIDS Society*, *Journal of Managed Care Pharmacy*, *Journal of the National Cancer Institute*, *Journal of Sexually Transmitted Diseases*, *Journal of Telemedicine and Telecare*, *Journal of Urban Health*, *Journal of Virology*, *Lancet*, *Lancet Infectious Diseases*, *Maternal and Child Health Journal*, *Nature*, *Nature Chemical Biology*, *Nature Medicine*, *New England Journal of Medicine*, *Obstetrics and Gynecology*, *Open AIDS Journal*, *Pediatric Research*, *PLoS Medicine*, *PLoS ONE*, *PLoS Pathogens*, *Postgraduate Medical Journal*, *Proceedings of the American Thoracic Society*, *Psychosomatics*, *Science*, *Science Translational Medicine*, *Sexually Transmitted Diseases*, *Sexually Transmitted Infections*, and *Substance Abuse Treatment, Prevention, and Policy*.

Timely information about many facets of HIV/AIDS may be found at the website TheBody.com. The National Coalition for the Homeless, the National AIDS Housing Coalition, and the U.S. Department of Housing and Urban Development provided information on housing opportunities for people with HIV/AIDS.

The Kaiser Family Foundation publications *Washington Post/Kaiser Family Foundation 2012 Survey of Americans on HIV/AIDS* (July 2012) and "U.S. Federal Funding for HIV/AIDS: The President's FY 2014 Budget Request" (May 2013) were used to prepare this publication. The Kaiser Family Foundation also provides daily updates about a variety of issues that are related to HIV/AIDS on its website (http://www.kff.org/).

We are grateful to the Gallup Organization for permitting us to present the results of its renowned opinion polls and graphics depicting Americans' feelings about HIV/AIDS.

INDEX

HIV-infected pregnant women, 63, 67, 69

international issues, 126

life expectancy, 17

middle stage HIV, 18, 20

mother-infant treatment timing, 69*t*

pneumocystis carinii pneumonia, 9–10

postexposure prophylaxis, 83, 90

President's Emergency Plan for AIDS Relief, 126–127, 127*t*, 128(*t*9.2)

risks *vs.* benefits, 131

tuberculosis, 117

World Health Organization testing and treatment guidelines, 27–28

ART. *See* Antiretroviral therapy

Ashe, Arthur, 95

Asia, 122–125

Asian and Pacific Islanders, 132

Asimov, Isaac, 97

Atlanta, GA, 80

At-risk populations

hemophiliacs, 55, 57–59

injection drug users, 47–49

men who have sex with men, 51

older adults, 51–52

prisoners, 52–53, 55

sex workers, 55

women, 49–50

Autonomy, 105

AVERT, 55

Azidothymidine, 65–66

B

Barré-Sinoussi, Françoise, 1, 93

Benjamin, Regina, 113

Berenson, Berry, 96

Birth defects, 61

Blood supply safety, 22–23

Blood tests, 24–25

Blood transfusions

AIDS cases due to, decline in, 39

hemophiliacs, 55, 57–59

HIV transmission modes, 21

Bodily fluids, 21, 25

Bone marrow cells, 8

Bone marrow transplantation, 13

Bono, 133–134

Breastfeeding, 64–65

Brown, Timothy Rae, 91, 93

Bush, George W., 126

C

Calypte Biomedical Corporation, 25

Cambodia, 123

Canada

blood supply safety, 23

hemophiliacs, HIV-infected, 57–58

Cancer

HIV and antiretroviral therapy relationship to, 20–21

retroviruses, 3

susceptibility to, 11–12

Caribbean Americans, 132

Caribbean countries, 125

Casual contact, 21

Caucasians, 89

CCR2 gene, 89

CCR5 gene, 67, 69–70, 89

CD4+ T cells

AIDS definition, 15–16

early antiretroviral therapy, 12

elite suppressors, 90

final stage HIV, 20

HIV classification in children, 63, 63*t*

HIV to AIDS progression, 9, 17–18

molecular structure of HIV, 6

Option B+ treatment, 66

progression of HIV, 8, 8*f*

CDC. *See* Centers for Disease Control and Prevention

Celebrities, 95–97, 133–134

Centers for Disease Control and Prevention (CDC)

AIDS definition, 15–16

AIDS mortality trends, 1–2

blood supply safety, 22

condom use, 111

contact tracing and partner notification, 104–105

health care worker to patient transmission, 83

high-impact prevention program, 108–109

HIV case definitions in children, 62

HIV prevalence statistics, 29

HIV stages, 17*t*

HIV testing recommendations, 26–27, 27*f*

HIV transmission modes, 47

HIV-infected health care workers, guidelines for, 81–82

HIV-infected pregnant women, treatment recommendations for, 69

occupational exposure among health care workers, 82

older people with HIV/AIDS, 97

pregnant women, testing of, 107

prevention strategies, 108, 109*f*

prisoners, testing of, 107–108

testing recommendations, 103–104

women with HIV/AIDS, 49–50

Centers of Excellence program, 79

Central Africa, 4

Central America, 125

Central Asia, 122

Central nervous system, 20

Cesarean sections, 50

CHAI (Clinton Health Access Initiative), 126

Children

AIDS prevalence and incidence, 29, 36*f*, 66–67, 67*t*

drug resistance, 66

global HIV infection among, 70–71

HIV prevalence, 29, 31*f*, 40

HIV progression, 61, 69–70

HIV/AIDS definitions, 62, 62*t*, 63*t*

orphans, 71

Romania, 23

treatments, 65–66

China, 124–125

Chlamydia, 73, 74(*f*5.4)

Circumcision, 111–112

Class-action lawsuits, 58

Classifications of HIV infection in children, 62, 63, 63*t*

Clinical trials. *See* Research

Clinton, Bill, 126, 133

Clinton Health Access Initiative (CHAI), 126

Clooney, George, 133

Community-based health care, 27, 80

Compensation for HIV-infected hemophiliacs, 57–59

Comprehensive Alcohol Abuse, Drug Abuse, and Mental Health Amendments Act, 113

Comprehensive sex education, 109–110

Concentrated clotting factor, 57

Condom use, 72(*t*5.5), 111

Contact tracing, 100, 104–105

Costs

health care, 83–85

home testing kits, 25

housing programs, cost-effectiveness of, 100

international considerations, 126

lifetime costs of care for HIV-infected people, 77

Office of AIDS Research budget, 86*t*

postexposure treatment, 90

prevention, cost-effectiveness of, 79–80

syringe exchange programs, 113–114

treatment research, 86–87

Counseling and counselors

contact tracing and partner notification, 104–105

rapid testing, 106

Cuba, 125

Cultural issues, 120

Cyrus, Miley, 133

Cytokines, 8–9

D

Dale and Betty Bumpers Vaccine Research Center, 93

Damon, Matt, 133

De Cock, Kevin, 111

Death benefits, 85

CPSIA information can be obtained
at www.ICGtesting.com
Printed in the USA
FFOW01n0111180315
11949FF